Principles and Practice
of
Critical Care

Principles and Practice of Critical Care

P.K. Verma, MD
Senior Specialist, Anaesthesiology and Intensive Care,
In Charge, Intensive Care Unit,
Deptt. of Anaesthesia & Intensive Care,
Safdarjang Hospital, New Delhi
Reader in Anaesthesia,
Vardhman Mahavir Medical College,
New Delhi

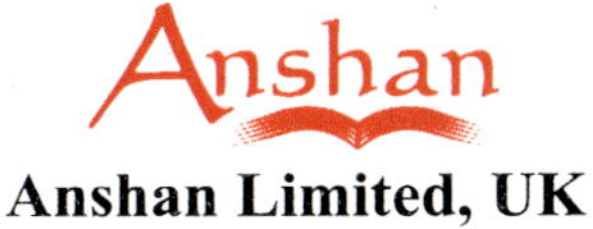

Anshan Limited, UK

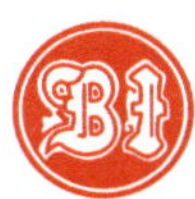

Anshan Limited
6 Newlands Road
Tunbridge Wells
Kent TN4 9AT, UK

Tel/Fax: +44 (0) 1892 557767
e-mail: info@anshan.co.uk
Web site: www.anshan.co.uk

Notice - Every effort has been made that the drug dosage schedules in this book are accurate and in accord with the standards accepted at the time of publication. However, the reader is urged to consult drug manufacturer's printed instructions, particularly regarding the recommended dose, indications and contraindications for administration and adverse reactions, before administering any of the drugs.

Published 2006

British Library Cataloguing in Publication Data
A catalogue record for this book is available from the British Library

Not for sale in India, Pakistan, Nepal, Sri Lanka and Bangladesh

ISBN-10   1-904798-90-X
ISBN-13   978-1-904798-90-3

This edition is co-published by B.I. Publications Pvt Ltd, New Delhi, India, and Anshan Limited, Kent, UK.
Printed at Saurabh Printers Pvt Ltd, Noida, India.

To my parents :
Thank you for the education and the values

To my wife, Poonam and children, Prateek and Parichay :
Thank you for the love, support, and encouragement

Foreword

> " पुस्तकस्था तु या विद्या परहस्तगतंधनम् ,
> कार्य कालेसमुत्पन्ने न सा विद्या न तद्धनम् "

(old Sanskrit proverb)

"All the knowledge stored in the books and all your wealth deposited with some-one else are totally useless if they cannot be produced at the moment of need"

Intensive care medicine is one of the fastest developing branches of medical science. As a result, any book written on this subject may become outdated even before it is published. Shelves of major medical libraries are bursting with books on intensive care medicine ranging from slim, pocket size versions to superfat volumes. Unfortunately, many of these books in trying to draw knowledge from other specialities have simply summarized their conventional wisdom, resulting in dull, insipid and scattered collection of techniques and procedures.

When Dr Pardeep Kumar Verma requested me to go through his second book on intensive care medicine, I must confess, I opened the pages with a bit of scepticism. But soon, I was sitting up and enjoying the precise arrangement of information in each chapter and the lucid language. Dr Verma has commendably explained the logic behind each step which will answer most of the queries that arise in the mind of a reader while following a particular protocol.

This book will not only fulfil the requirements of a beginner admirably, but will be an excellent companion of the seasoned intensivist as well. The reader will easily be able to translate the knowledge imbibed from this book into practice.

I am especially overjoyed that the author of this book is incharge of the intensive care unit of Safdarjang Hospital where the concept of critical care took shape in the early sixties and where the first intensive care facility in India was established under the supervision of the legendary Prof BL Bhattacharjee.

In fact, my only regret is that such a book was not available to us, when as the first generation of young graduates, we were learning intensive care medicine in this country.

A Bhattacharya
Ex-Professor and Head
Department of Anaesthesiology,
Critical Care and Pain Medicine.
University College of Medical Sciences
and GTB Hospital, Delhi
Senior Consultant, Anaesthesiology,
Critical Care & Pain Medicine,
Sir Ganga Ram Hospital, New Delhi

Preface

In the past few years texts and manuals on critical care have proliferated. Nonetheless, I believe that my user-friendly book meets a need not met before – the need to provide specific information required by a patient care team faced with making decisions.

Knowledge of the principles is essential in making correct decisions, but principles can be hard to remember in the heat of battle – or in the management of an acutely ill patient. This book serves not only as a quick reference and a guide but also a means of confirming the accuracy of one's decisions at these times.

The text includes commonly performed procedures, management approaches and frequently encountered diseases in a multidisciplinary intensive care unit. The topics have been presented in a uniform pattern consisting of introductory comments relating to the understanding and practical management of the topic concerned, followed by a step-wise approach towards the management. Each step carries an explanation, so that the reader can understand the rationale for its existence. An extra effort has been put to answer the questions asked frequently by residents on daily rounds in the ICU. Although the material presented here is based on the latest available literature, yet with the ever-changing concepts in critical care medicine, these guidelines should not be taken as rigid rules but only as a guide to patient care. Moreover, these guidelines may evolve over time, as the clinical and institutional experience with them grows. The approach, the style, and the content of this book are the result of many years of clinical experience at the bedside, both in managing the patients and in teaching the management of critically ill patients. I am confident that these guidelines will be of immense help to the readers in understanding critical care.

The information presented here has been taken from various sources. All that I have done is to arrange it with a specific aim in mind. My task has been that of the weaver and the dyer and I take no credit at all for the cotton and the thread.

How to read this book: Read one or two guidelines at a time. Reflect on them in silence. Try to correlate with the patient's symptoms/signs or the practical clinical situation, you are presented with. Decide whether these guidelines can be applied as such or need to be modified. Let these guidelines be in your mind, let them make you restless or stimulate you to look for more details from various sources, and let yourself be transformed. Even if you read this book only for curiosity, there is no guarantee that an occasional guideline will not slip through your defenses and explode when you least expect it to.

I am grateful to the patients from whom I got the impetus for writing this book. I must also thank Drs Sita Lakshmi, Harish Sachdeva, Vandana Talwar, Suniti Kale, Charu Bamba, Krishan Kumar, Monica, and Aikta, and Mr YR Chadha, Publishing Director, B.I. Publications, for their help in giving this book its final shape.

It is impossible to express my indebtedness to those authors of monographs and articles, from which I have gained so much information. I can only hope that some measure of my gratitude is expressed by the references I have given to their works.

PK Verma

Contents

Tracheal Suctioning

1

Introduction

- Presence of endotracheal or tracheostomy tube prevents effective coughing, swallowing, and secretion removal. It also promotes the development of a viscous biofilm, which promotes bacterial growth and adherence.
- Suctioning is done to remove secretions, maintain patency of the tubes, decrease airway resistance, improve gas exchange and to reduce the risk of infection. It is also done to obtain samples of tracheal secretions for laboratory analysis.
- Suctioning should be performed only for a clinical indication and not as a routine, fixed scheduled treatment. The indications include one or more of the following: clinically apparent increased work of breathing, visible secretions in the airway, patient's inability to generate an effective spontaneous cough, presence of coarse breath sounds, increased peak inspiratory pressures during volume-controlled mechanical ventilation or increased respiratory rate/ decreased tidal volume during pressure-controlled ventilation, changes in monitored flow and pressure graphics, deterioration in arterial blood gases, suspected aspiration of gastric contents or upper airway secretions, and radiological changes consistent with retention of pulmonary secretions, e.g. pulmonary atelectasis.
- A closed tracheal suction system (Fig. 1.1) permits mechanical ventilation and PEEP (positive end-expiratory pressure) to continue during suctioning. The need to use a closed tracheal suction system could arise in any of the following situations:
    - (a) High ventilatory requirements
        - (i)   PEEP $\geq$ 10 cm H_2O
        - (ii) Mean airway pressure $\geq$ 20 cm H_2O
        - (iii) Inspiratory time $\geq$ 1.5 seconds and
        - (iv) $FiO_2 \geq 0.6$.
    - (b) Mechanically ventilated patients receiving frequent suctioning ($\geq$ 6/24hr).
    - (c) Haemodynamic instability associated with ventilator disconnection.
    - (d) Mechanically ventilated patients with active tuberculosis, and
    - (e) Patients receiving inhalational agents that cannot be interrupted by ventilator disconnection (e.g. nitric oxide, heliox).
- The use of chest-wall percussion in critical care is waning, due to critiques on its efficacy in acute care. However, percussion may have value in suppurative, chronic lung diseases such as bronchiectasis and cystic fibrosis.

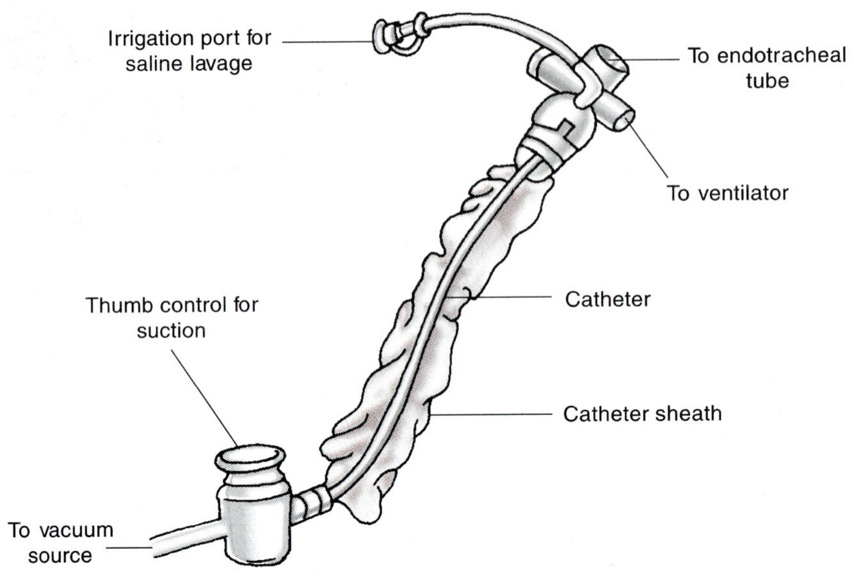

Fig. 1.1: Closed tracheal suction system

GUIDELINES FOR TRACHEAL SUCTIONING

A. Open Tracheal Suction Technique

1. **Explain the procedure to the patient.**
   Reassures the patient.

2. **Wash hands and wear sterile gloves.**
   Reduces the risk of transmission of micro-organisms. Standard precautions.

3. **Make the patient supine and monitor the patient.**
   - Tracheal suction causes vagal stimulation, hypoxia and may stimulate bronchospasm.
   - Monitor the patient before, during and after the procedure. The parameters to be monitored include: breath sounds, cyanosis, arterial oxygen saturation, respiratory rate and pattern, pulse rate, blood pressure, ECG, sputum characteristics (colour, volume, consistency), cough effort, ventilatory parameters (peak inspiratory pressure, plateau pressure, tidal volume) and ventilator waveform graphics, if available.

4. **Turn on suction apparatus and set vacuum regulator to appropriate pressure (Fig. 1.2 a,b).**
   The higher the level of vacuum pressure applied to a suction catheter, the greater will be the degree of mucosal damage. Greater suction pressure does not mean increased secretion removal. Recommended suction pressure for different age groups are: infants 80-100 mmHg, children 100-125 mmHg, and adults 120-150 mmHg.

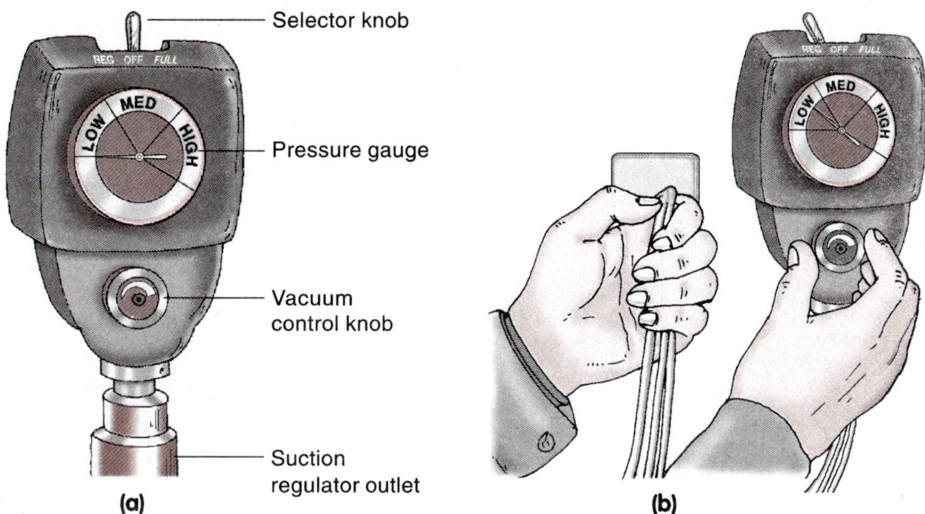

Fig. 1.2a,b: (a) Ohmeda Medical continuous vacuum regulator with a three-position selector knob. **(b)** Appropriate level of negative pressure can be set by pinching the vacuum tubing and adjusting the vacuum control knob.

5. Secure one end of the connecting tube to the suction machine and hold the other end with left hand.

6. Take a sterile suction catheter of appropriate size in the right hand and hold it in such a way that it does not touch any unsterile surface. Secure the catheter to the connecting tube.

   The diameter of the suction catheter should be less than half the inner diameter of the endotracheal tube (ETT) or tracheostomy tube, to prevent hypoxia. A simple formula to find out the appropriate size of the suction catheter is as follows:

$$\frac{\text{Size of ETT (mm)} \times 3}{2}$$

7. Take 100-200 ml of sterile normal saline solution or water in a sterile container. Used as flush solution.

8. Check suction by suctioning a small amount of sterile solution from the container.
   - Ensures proper functioning of the equipment.
   - This act also wets the outer surface of suction catheter and allows it to pass easily into the endotracheal tube or tracheostomy tube.

9. Hyperoxygenate the patient for at least 30 seconds either by increasing the baseline inspired fraction of oxygen on the ventilator to 1.0 or by pressing the button meant for suction hyperoxygenation.

   This is done to prevent suction related hypoxemia. The aim should be to maintain oxygen saturation above 90-92%.

10. Perform hyperinflation of the lungs.
    - Lessens hypoxemia, presumably by reinflating collapsed lung segments. Hyperinflation, generally involves delivering several breaths before suctioning, and after each pass of the suction catheter, using either a manual resuscitation bag or the ventilator circuit. Each of these breaths is set to approximately 1.5 times the patient's visual tidal volume, or peak inspiratory pressure (PIP) is increased approximately 10 cm H_2O above the settings.
    - Hyperinflation may be harmful in patients prone to air trapping and in those with elevated intracranial pressure or low cardiac output.

11. With the suction turned off, gently insert the catheter into the endotracheal tube or tracheostomy tube until it meets the carina or stimulates a cough reflex, then pull back the catheter by one cm. Now apply suction and withdraw the catheter by gently rotating between thumb and forefinger. The whole procedure should not take more than 10-15 seconds.
    - Inability to insert the catheter may mean that ETT or tracheostomy tube is blocked: should be investigated.
    - Rotating the catheter while withdrawing and applying suction may not be necessary with catheters having circumferential holes.
    - Prolonged suctioning will result in hypoxia and trauma.
    - In neonates, infants and in patients with bronchial stump or a lobectomy or an anastomotic line in the tracheobronchial tree, a safer practice is to pass the suction catheter till just 0.5–1.0 cm beyond the tip of endotracheal tube and apply suction.

12. Hyperoxygenate for 30 seconds before passing suction catheter again.
13. Monitor the patient.
    Continue to monitor the patient, see step 3.

14. Repeat the suction as explained above, 2-3 times only.
    Desaturation and cardiopulmonary complications increase with each successive suctioning.

15. Rinse the catheter and connecting tubing with sterile saline solution.
    Flushes the tubings and prevents the buildup of secretions and organisms in the tubings.

16. Perform nasal and/or oropharyngeal suction with a separate catheter.
    Prevents contamination of the upper airway with organisms from lower airways.

17. Discard the suction catheter and the remaining normal saline solution.
    - Decreases the incidence of infection.
    - Should be discarded in a container meant for patient's infectious waste and disposed of through standard hospital waste stream.

18. Remove gloves and wash hands.
19. Monitor the patient again before repositioning.
    See step 3.

20. Assess the outcome.

Signs indicating effective suctioning are: reduced respiratory rate, improvement in breath sounds, decreased peak inspiratory pressure, decreased airway resistance, increased tidal volume during pressure-limited ventilation, increased oxygen saturation, visible evidence of removal of secretions and absence of audible secretions in large airways.

21. Routine administration of saline into the airway to facilitate the removal of secretions is no longer recommended.

It has an adverse effect on arterial oxygen saturation, may dislodge viable bacteria from a colonized ETT into the lower airway, contributing to the development of nosocomial pneumonia, and may result in worsening of airway obstruction. Moreover, at present, there is no convincing evidence that routine instillation of saline increases recovery of secretions from the lung. Therefore, this practice should be restricted to situations where evidence of sputum retention is present after suctioning attempts without saline. A maximum of 5 ml of 0.9% sodium chloride may be used for this purpose.

B. Closed tracheal suction system

1. Procedure.

Procedure and steps are essentially the same as that for open–suction technique.

2. Present status.

- Closed suction is reported to be as effective as conventional open-suction technique in maintaining oxygenation, in clearing secretions, and is associated with fewer physiologic disturbances. Incidence of both patient and environmental contamination has been reported to be less with the use of closed suction system.
- Concerns about closed–suction system include, decreased effectiveness of suctioning, excessive negative pressure, autocontamination, catheter remaining in the airway following a suction procedure and migration of catheter into the airway between suction procedures.
- To sum up, at present, insufficient data is available to determine whether multiple–closed suction catheters are significantly different from single use catheters in terms of infection risk, oxygenation and environmental contamination.

References

1. AARC Clinical Practice Guideline. Endotracheal suctioning of mechanically ventilated adults & children with artificial airway. Respir Care 1993; 38(5): 505-504.
2. Ackerman M. The effect of saline lavage prior to suctioning. Am J Crit Care. 1993; 2:326-330.
3. Bailey C, Kattwinkel J, Teja R, Buckley T. Shallow versus deep endotracheal suctioning in young rabbits: pathologic effects on the tracheobronchial wall. Pediatrics 1988; 82(5): 746-751.

4. Brown B, Peeples D. The effects of hyperventilation and lidocaine on intracranial pressure. Heart Lung. 1991; 21:286.
5. Brucia J, Rudy E. The effects of suction catheter insertion and tracheal stimulation in adults with severe brain injury. Heart Lung 1996; 25(4): 295-303.
6. Chulay M, Graeber G. Efficacy of a hyperinflation and hyperoxygenation suctioning intervention. Heart Lung. 1988; 17:15-22.
7. Czarnik R, Stone K, Everhardt C, Pressure B. Differential effects of continuous versus intermittent suction on tracheal tissue. Heart Lung. 1991; 20:144-151.
8. Dean, E. Oxygen transport: a physiologically-based conceptual framework for the practice of cardio-pulmonary physiotherapy. Physiotherapy 1994;80(6):347-353.
9. Gallon A. Evaluation of chest percussion in the treatment of patients with copious sputum production. Respir Med 1990; 85:45-51.
10. Grap MJ, Glass C, Corley M, Parks T. Endotracheal suctioning: ventilator versus manual delivery of hyperoxygenation breaths. Am J Crit Care. 1996; 5(3): 192-197.
11. Guglielminotti J, Desmonts J, Dureuil B. Effects of tracheal suctioning on respiratory resistance in mechanically ventilated patients. Chest 1998; 113(5): 1335-1338.
12. Mancinelli-Van Atta J, Beck S. Preventing hypoxemia and hemodynamic compromise related to endotracheal suctioning. Am J Crit Care. 1991; 1(3): 62-79.
13. McCauley C, Boller L. Bradycardiac responses to endotracheal suctioning. Crit Care Med. 1986; 16:1165-1166.
14. Preusser B, Stone K, Broch K, Karl J. The effect of two methods of preoxygenation (manual versus ventilator) on mean arterial pressure, peak airway pressure and postsuctioning hypoxemia. Heart Lung. 1987; 16:317-322.
15. Rudy E, Baun M, Stone K, Turner B. The relationship between endotracheal suctioning and changes in intracranial pressure: A review of the literature. Heart Lung. 1986; 15:488-493.
16. Rudy E, Turner B, Baun M, Stone K, Brucia J. Endotracheal suctioning in adults with head injury. Heart Lung. 1991; 20:667-674.
17. Stone K, Preusser B, Grouch K, Karl J. Effect of lung hyperinflation on cardiopulmonary hemodynamics and post suctioning hypoxemia. Hurt Lung 1988; 17:309.
18. Tarnow-Mordi W. Is routine endotracheal suction justified? (editorial) Arch Dis Child 1991; 66:374-375.
19. Wain Wright SP, Gould D. Endotracheal suctioning in adults with severe head injury: a literature review. Intensive Crit Care Nurs 1996; 12(5): 303-308.

Care of Tracheal Tube Cuff 2

Introduction

- The tracheal tube cuff helps to stabilize the tube, to maintain an adequate air seal so that air moves through the tube into the lungs, and to decrease the risk of aspiration of large food particles; however, it does not protect against aspiration of liquids.
- The tracheal capillary perfusion pressure is normally 25-35 mmHg. Studies suggest a high risk for aspiration with cuff pressures less than 18 mmHg (25 cm H_2O). Based on this evidence, it seems reasonable to maintain cuff pressures at 25-35 cm H_2O (18-25 mmHg). to minimize the risk of tracheal wall injury and aspiration.
- Cuff pressure is affected by airway pressure and the required effective cuff pressure increases linearly with airway pressure. Studies show that the maximum safe cuff inflation pressure limit of 25 mmHg corresponds to a peak inflation pressure of 35.3mmHg (48 cmH_2O). Patients requiring ventilation with peak inflation pressure greater than these pressures will also require cuff inflation pressure > 25 mmHg in order to seal the trachea. Thus, patients requiring high-pressure ventilatory support remain at risk for tracheal ischaemic complications, despite the use of high volume, low-pressure ETT cuffs properly inflated to maintain a minimum occlusive pressure.
- A cuff leak may manifest in a number of ways: (a) Audible air flow through the patient's nose and mouth, (b) air-secretions mixed in the form of bubbles coming out of mouth and nose, (c) low-pressure/low-volume alarm on ventilator, (d) loss of inspiratory and expiratory volume in ventilated patients, (e) palpable leak over suprasternal notch during inspiration, (f) auscultated leak during inspiration over suprasternal notch, (g) inability to maintain cuff inflation, (h) pilot balloon deflation, and (i) patient's ability to audibly vocalize.

GUIDELINES FOR DEFLATION AND INFLATION OF CUFF

1. Wash hands.
   Reduces risk of transmission of microorganisms. Standard precaution.

2. Hyperoxygenate and suction the tracheobronchial tree before deflation.
   To clear the airway and decrease the incidence of aspiration.

3. Choose the technique.
   Two techniques have been suggested.

(a) **Minimum occlusion pressure technique.** Attach 10 mL airfilled syringe to inflating tube valve. Slowly inject air until inspiratory sounds (audible/auscultated) or palpable air leak cease over suprasternal notch during positive-pressure ventilation.

The cuff needs to seal the airway as the trachea dilates during inhalation. Cessation of (audible/auscultated/palpable) airleak indicates that the cuff is sealed against the tracheal mucosal wall.

(b) **Minimum leak technique.** Inflate the cuff till there is no leak. Slowly withdraw air (in 0.1 – 0.2 mL increments) from the cuff until a small leak is heard. Assess the leak by auscultating over the suprasternal notch.

4. Follow any of the above mentioned techniques.

Although no comparison of these approaches to cuff inflation has been reported, it appears that use of a minimal occlusion pressure technique should decrease the risk of silent aspiration of pharyngeal secretions.

GUIDELINES FOR CUFF PRESSURE MEASUREMENT

1. Wash hands.

This reduces the risk of transmission of microorganisms.

2. Measure cuff pressure every 6-8 hours and whenever tube position or cuff volume is changed.

Excessive cuff pressure is the most common problem of tracheal intubation and the best predictor of tracheolaryngeal injury.

3. Take a three-way stopcock and connect the pilot balloon to the manometer line through the stopcock (Fig. 2.1). To the third port of stopcock, attach an air-filled syringe.

Manometer line should not be attached directly to the pilot balloon because air tends to escape from the cuff to pressurize the manometer and this gives a faulty reading.

4. With the air-filled syringe, inject air into the tubing. Turn the stopcock off to the syringe. Read the cuff pressure on the manometer. It should be between 20-25 mmHg.

The method suggested here allows measurement and

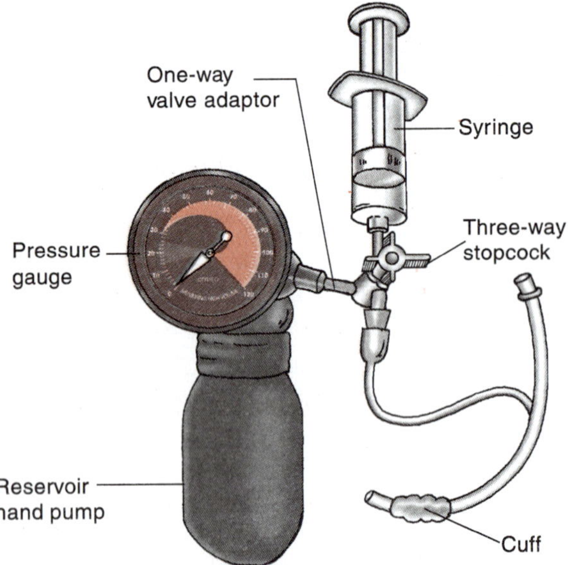

Fig. 2.1: Cuff inflator pressure gauge attached to inflating tube and syringe with a three-way stopcock.

adjustment of cuff pressure simultaneously. If pressure is not adequate, add more air and if it is already more, discard some air.

5. Turn the stopcock off to the pilot balloon. Disconnect the manometer line from the 3-way stopcock.

GUIDELINES TO SOLVE TRACHEAL CUFF PROBLEMS

1. **Assess for leak around the cuff.**
   It should be assessed every 6-8 hours and whenever there is a change either in the tube position or in the cuff volume.

2. **Leak present.**
   Add air to the cuff.

3. **No leak, assess cuff pressure.**
   - Cuff pressure < 20 mmHg – add air to the cuff.
   - Cuff pressure 20-25 mmHg – acceptable.
   - Cuff pressure > 25 mmHg – remove air from the cuff until pressure is 25 mmHg.

4. **Cuff pressure is optimal but leak present.**
   - Assess tube position – if malposition, reposition the tube.
   - Assess tube size – if smaller, change to larger size if possible.

5. **Look for any pressure loss.**
   - In case of pressure loss, add air to the cuff and clamp the pilot tube.
   (a) Presence of leak indicates ruptured cuff – change ET tube if possible.
   (b) Leak not present – connect stop cock to pilot balloon and remove clamp. Presence of leak now indicates incompetent pilot balloon-change ETT if possible or keep the pilot tube clamped.
   (c) If after connecting stop cock to pilot balloon and removing clamp no leak is present, it indicates incompetent 1-way valve – change tube if possible or use stopcock with pilot balloon.

References

1. Bernhard WN, Cottrell JE, Sivakumaran C, Patel K, Yost L, Turndorf H. Adjustment of intracuff pressure to prevent aspiration. Anesthesiology 1979; 50(4): 363-366.
2. Crimlisk JT, Horn MH, Wilson DJ, Marino B. Artificial airway: a survey of cuff management practices. Heart Lung 1996; 25:225-235.
3. Guyton D, Banner MJ, Kirgby RR. High-volume, low-pressure cuffs: are they always-low pressure? Chest 1991; 100:1076-1081.
4. Guyton DC, Barlow MR, Besselievre TR. Influence of airway pressure on minimum occlusive endotracheal tube cuff pressure. Crit Care Med 1997; 25(1): 91-94.
5. Hess DR. Managing the artificial airway. Respir Care 1999; 44(7): 759-772.
6. Pavlin EG, VanNimvegan D, Hornbein TF. Failure of a high-compliance low-pressure cuff to prevent aspiration. Anesthesiology 1975; 42(2): 216-219.

Tracheotomy/ Tracheostomy Tube Care   3

Introduction

- Tracheotomy/tracheostomy is the mainstay of airway management in critically ill patients, providing access for mechanical ventilation, clearance of secretions, and protection of the airway.
- Tracheotomy refers to an opening made in the trachea without connection to the skin surface. Tracheostomy refers to a tracheal opening with a surgical attachment to the skin. A true tracheostomy is created when some one has a laryngectomy and when a 360º tracheal mucosa is attached to the skin margin. The attachment to the skin facilitates identification of the tract and enhances patient safety.
- A percutaneous dilatation tracheotomy does not initially create a tracheostomy because there is no connection with the skin. Only after approximately two weeks, when there is a mature tract from the skin margin down to the tracheal opening, the patient has a tracheostomy.
- As compared to an endotracheal tube, a tracheostomy tube provides added benefits to the patients. These include: (a) Increased patient mobility, (b) improved airway suctioning, (c) less direct endolaryngeal injury, (d) decreased airway resistance in promoting weaning from mechanical ventilation, (e) enhanced phonation and communication, (f) increased comfort, (g) early transfer of patients from the ICU, (h) enhanced oral nutrition, (i) decreased risk of nosocomial pneumonia in patient subgroups, and (j) less requirement of sedation to maintain airway in conscious patients.
- A tracheotomy is performed either electively or as an emergency procedure for a variety of reasons. Most often, the procedure is elective. General indications for tracheotomy include: (a) Maintenance of airway patency in patients with functional or mechanical upper airway obstruction, (b) provision of airway access for suctioning of retained airway secretions in patients with poor tracheobronchial clearance mechanism, (c) prevention or limitation of aspiration in patients with glottic dysfunction, and (d) management of patients who require long-term airway access for ventilatory support.
- The existing clinical studies do not clearly establish an ideal time for tracheotomy that is applicable for all ventilator-dependent patients. One needs to individualize care, taking into consideration functional and anatomical complications associated with tracheotomy (tracheal injury) compared to translaryngeal intubation (laryngeal injury) and the differing benefits anticipated from each mode of airway support. For example, trauma patients, (who are at high risk for nosocomial pneumonia) may benefit from an earlier conversion to

tracheotomy than patients with acute exacerbation of chronic obstructive pulmonary disease. Patients requiring heavy sedation to manage hypoxic respiratory failure are less likely to benefit from the comfort advantage of tracheotomy than are mentally alert patients with respiratory failure due to neuromuscular disease. Patients with bleeding diathesis or abnormalities of cervical structure may have a greater surgical risk from tracheotomy, justifying a delay of the procedure. Similarly, a patient in the early phase of ARDS, receiving high PEEP, will be benefitted more by keeping the translaryngeal tube in place for a longer time. The decision making should also take into consideration the fact, that no data establish that 2-3 weeks is the outer limit of safety for translaryngeal intubation or, conversely, that some patients might not benefit from earlier conversion to a tracheotomy. As a general rule, the conversion to a tracheotomy should be anticipated early in the clinical course of every ventilator-dependent patient. For example, after an initial period of stabilization in a patient with respiratory failure (7-10days), patients should be assessed. Those appearing likely to be extubated within next 7-10 days may be allowed to continue with translaryngeal endotracheal tube in the absence of compelling indications (e.g. profound patient discomfort and facial or upper airway swelling that would complicate reintubation if inadvertent decannulation occurs). Conversely, those patients, whose clinical condition indicates a long-term requirement of ventilation, should be considered for tracheotomy as early as possible from this time onwards.

GUIDELINES FOR TRACHEOTOMY/TRACHEOSTOMY TUBE CARE

1. **Wash hands, wear sterile gloves.**
   This reduces the risk of transmission of microorganisms

2. **Check proper placement.**
   Proper placement should be checked by listening to breath sounds. Although displacement of the tracheostomy tube into the bronchus or carina is very rare because of the short length, it can occur with an improper selection of tube or with tracheostomy performed too low. Incorrect tube size can also place the tip of tracheotomy tube against the tracheal wall or carina. The symptoms and signs which indicate improper placement include excessive coughing, decreased chest wall motion, decreased or absent breath sounds, and expiratory wheeze.

3. **Ensure that tube is secured properly in place.**
   Tracheostomy tape should be secured around the neck, allowing sufficient space for insertion of a single finger. Tape should not be secured over gauze dressing that may later shift and loosen tube support. Suturing the tracheostomy plate /flange to the skin (although not liked by many) may decrease the risk of early extubation.

4. **Inspect and palpate for air under skin.**
   Subcutaneous emphysema occurs in less than 10% of patients undergoing

tracheostomy who are mechanically ventilated. Positive pressure escapes from the airway around an inadequately sealed tracheostomy tube cuff and decompresses into cervical tissue planes. The risk of subcutaneous emphysema is decreased by avoiding gauze packing in the tracheostomy wound. It usually gets reabsorbed spontaneously, but if it does not or it is increasing, a chest X-ray should be performed to exclude an accompanying pneumomediastinum or pneumothorax.

5. **Look for oozing of blood or frank bleeding during early postoperative period.**
    Onset of wound bleeding may be delayed into the early postoperative period when an uncontrolled blood vessel opens during patient coughing, or movement. Resolution of hypotension or dissipation of action of epinephrine may also be responsible for the bleed. Prolonged oozing that persists for longer than 2 to 3 days suggests a coagulopathy. Oozed and collected blood tends to be aspirated because of sedation secondary to anaesthesia or sedative drugs.

6. **Check cuff pressure.**
    See Chapter 2.

7. **Monitor secretions.**
    See Chapter 1.

8. **Maintain 30º head up position.**
    Minimizes the risk of aspiration and promotes oropharyngeal and nasopharyngeal drainage.

9. **Assess for presence of pain.**
    Manage, if patient complains of pain.

10. **Maintain dry, clean dressing.**
    Dressing and tapes should be changed at least once daily and whenever they get soiled. Stoma should be treated as an open wound.

11. **Remove soiled dressing with gloved hands; change gloves. Clean stomal site with swab/gauze soaked first in hydrogen peroxide and then in normal saline; pat dry the skin area surrounding the stoma site.**
    Apply clean tracheostomy dressing around stoma, under the flange of tracheostomy tube.
    Dry surface decreases the likelihood of growth of microorganisms.
    Local antibiotic should be avoided as it encourages the emergence of resistant strains.

12. **Replace inadvertent extubation.**
    - Inadvertent extubation, especially in the first 72 hours (early period) of tracheostomy placement is a potentially life-threatening complication. During this period, the stoma tract has not fully developed, and parastomal tissue can obscure tracheal opening and complicate recannulation. If tube is not easily inserted, there are increased chances of subcutaneous emphysema or bleeding.
    - Two tubes (one of the same size and one smaller) should be available at the

bedside. In a ventilator–dependent patient with early period extubation, reintubate the patient through translaryngeal route and then reinsert tracheostomy tube under controlled conditions. If emergent recannulation of tracheostomy tube is decided (without first performing intubation through translaryngeal route), then: (a) Position the patient as for surgical tracheostomy with the neck hyperextended; pull tracheal traction sutures, if present; bring the anterior wall of trachea as near to the skin as possible (to close the pretracheal fascial planes) to visulize the tracheal opening clearly; replace tracheostomy tube of same size or smaller size, or (b) thread a sterile nasogastric tube, through the tracheostomy tube placement and into the stoma to serve as a guide wire for tracheostomy tube placement, or (c) use fiberoptic bronchoscope or laryngoscope as a guiding stylet to replace tracheostomy tube. Obtain radiograph to verify position.

13. **Ensure proper humidification.**

    Presence of tracheostomy bypasses the normal mechanism within the respiratory tract for heating and humidification. Humidification prevents drying of secretions and blockage of tube.

14. **Take care of nutrition.**

    The presence of tracheostomy tube prevents the normal upward motion of larynx (during swallowing) which contributes to glottic closure. The inflated cuff can bulge posteriorly, compressing the esophagus and producing dysphagia. Therefore, before starting oral feeds, gag reflex, reflex coughing, swallowing, and oral motor strength should be evaluated. Start with ice chips followed by soft foods, such as gelatins, that do not present a problem if aspirated. Liquids are avoided at first because patients cannot effectively control fluid boluses within their mouth till they regain swallowing reflexes. Follow general guidelines to prevent regurgitation and aspiration, when feeding via nasogastric tubes (See Chapters 54 and 56).

15. **Provide an alternative method of communication.**

    With a tracheostomy tube in place, a patient is unable to talk and express himself/herself, thus leading to fear and anxiety. Some of the available methods of communication include lip reading, written communication with paper and pencil, gestural languages (i.e. yes-no responses, facial expressions, hand gestures), deflated/cuff leak methods on ventilator or T-piece, and one-way valves.

16. **Elective extubation/decannulation.** Once it is decided to remove the tracheostomy tube, the following steps may be followed:

    (a) Record basal vital signs and monitor continuously.
    (b) Wash hands, wear gloves.
    (c) Reassure the patient. Explain what is expected from him.
    (d) Check equipment, e.g. suction point and catheters, syringe, scissors, oxygen mask, and dressing for tracheostomy wound.
    (e) Cut tape securing tracheostomy tube.
    (f) Suction the airway and pharynx.

(g) Instruct the patient to take a deep breath.

(h) At the peak of a deep inspiration, deflate the balloon and remove the tube in one motion.

Alternative methods to facilitate removal of secretions while tube is removed include: (a) application of positive pressure while cuff is deflated, (b) insertion of suction catheter into tracheostomy tube (or ETT) and when patient initiates cough, deflation of the balloon and removal of tube in one motion, while applying suction.

17. After removal of tracheostomy tube, cover the stoma with a dry dressing and elastoplast.

18. Encourage the patient to take deep breaths and cough. Suction the pharynx, if required.

19. Place oxygen mask with oxygen set at 100% over patient's nose and mouth.

20. Auscultate chest, note down respiratory rate, pulse rate, blood pressure, SpO_2, chest-abdomen synchrony, stridor, bronchospasm, bleeding and effectiveness of coughing. Monitor vital signs, respiratory status and oxygenation immediately following extubation, every five minutes for 15 minutes, and every fifteen minutes for one hour.

21. Give steam inhalation.

22. Wash hands.

This reduces the risk of transmission of microorganisms.

References

1. Bach JR, Saporito LR. Criteria for extubation and tracheostomy tube removal for patients with ventilatory failure: a different approach to weaning. Chest 1996; 110(6): 1566-1571.

2. Heffner JE. Tracheotomy: Indications and Timing. Respir Care 1999; 44(7): 807-815.

3. Orringer MK. The effects of tracheostomy tube placement on communication and swallowing. Respir Care 1999; 44(7): 845-853.

4. Reibel JF. Decannulation: How and where. Respir Care 1999; 44(7): 856-859.

5. Reibel JF. Tracheotomy/Tracheostomy. Respir Care 1999; 44(7): 820-823.

6. Rumbak MJ, Graves AE, Scott MP, Sporn GK, Walsh FW, Anderson WM, Goldman AL. Tracheostomy tube occlusion protocol predicts significant tracheal obstruction to air flow in patients requiring prolonged mechanical ventilation. Crit Care Med 1997; 25(3): 413-417.

7. Stauffer JL. Complications of endotracheal intubation and tracheotomy. Respir Care 1999; 44(7): 823-843.

Introduction

- The air-entrainment mask, frequently known as the venturi mask or jet mixing mask (fig. 4.1) provides the patient with a controlled oxygen percentage at flow rates which are sufficient enough to meet the patient's peak inspiratory flow demands.
- The delivered FiO_2 depends on the size of the nozzle, size of the entrainment

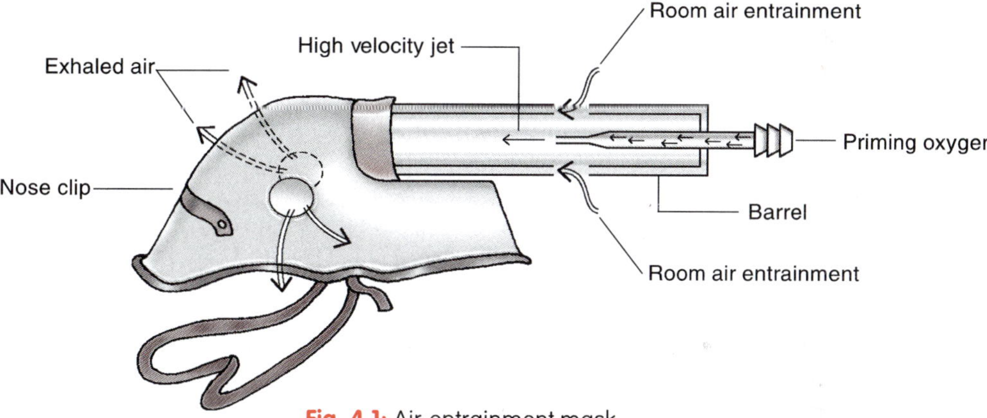

Fig. 4.1: Air-entrainment mask.

ports, and oxygen flow (Fig. 4.1).

- Two types of air-entrainment masks are available: (a) a fixed orifice variable air-entrainment mask (Fig. 4.2), and (b) a variable orifice fixed air-entrainment mask (Fig. 4.3).
- The oxygen flow rates, as suggested by the manufacturer and printed on the device, although provide the desired FiO_2, yet may not be able to meet the peak inspiratory flow demand of the patient. The total flow through the mask can be raised by increasing the oxygen flow rate. This, however, does not change the oxygen percentage significantly as

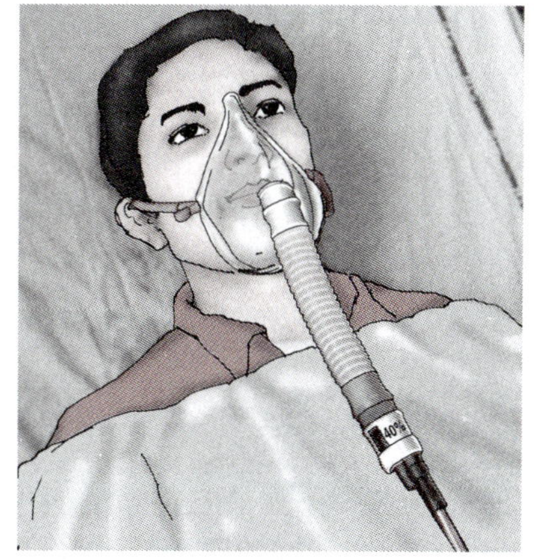

Fig. 4.2: Fixed orifice, variable air-entrainment mask, showing proper placement.

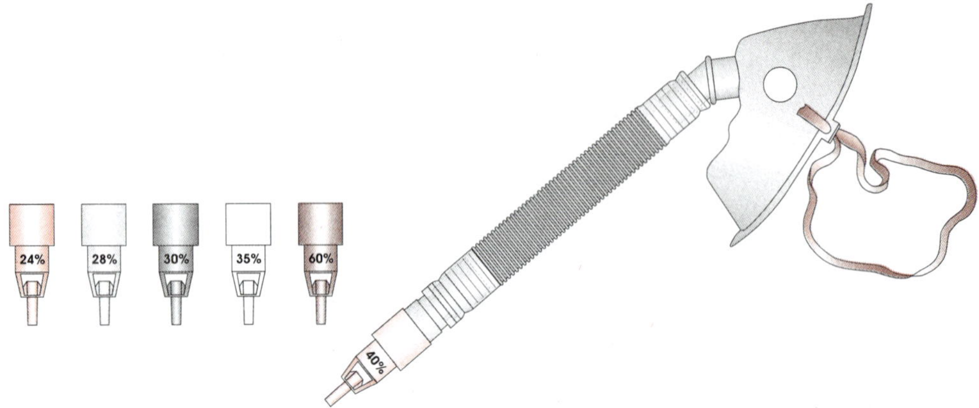

Fig. 4.3: Variable orifice fixed air-entrainment mask showing interchangeable jet orifices.

more room air is entrained to keep the ratio constant.

- An air-entrainment mask behaves like a fixed performance device for FiO_2 ≤ 0.4 with oxygen flow rate up to 12L/min in a patient with normal inspiratory flow rate. At FiO_2 more than 0.4, this mask becomes a variable performance device.
- *Humidification:* If additional humidification is required, the aerosol entrainment collar is attached to a room air aerosol system using a length of large bore tubing.
- The entrainment ratio for various desired FiO_2 are: 0.24(1:25), 0.28 (1:10), 0.30 (1:8), 0.35 (1:5), 0.4 (1:3), 0.5 (1:1.7), and 0.6 (1:1).

GUIDELINES FOR APPLYING AN AIR-ENTRAINMENT MASK

1. Wash hands.

   This reduces the risk of transmission of microorganisms.

2. Explain the procedure and goals of therapy to the patient.

   It provides reassurance to the patient.

3. Assemble the equipment. Set the desired FiO_2. Rotate the entrainment port to the desired FiO_2 or use an appropriate colour-coded jet in case of variable orifice, fixed entrainment device.

4. Attach the tubing of the mask to the oxygen flowmeter.

   Source of oxygen could be oxygen cylinder or oxygen pipeline wall outlet.

5. Set the appropriate flow of oxygen for the desired FiO_2.

   - The flow of oxygen (L/min) should be set to an extent that the total flow (after entrainment of air) through the mask meets or exceeds the patient's peak inspiratory flow rate. Measurement of the peak inspiratory flow rate is difficult in a clinical situation. However, the following points may help to ensure that the patient's flow needs are met: (a) Total flow through the mask should be at least 40 L/min in a resting patient and more if the patient is breathing rapidly, and (b) total flow provided through the mask should be at least 4–6 times the patient's minute volume.

- To provide a desired FiO_2, knowledge of the entrainment ratio helps in estimating the total flow through the mask at a given oxygen flowrate. For example, for a desired FiO_2 of 0.28, having an entrainment ratio of 1:10, oxygen flow of 6 L/min will have a total flow (through mask, after entrainment) of 6(1+10) = 66 L/min. Similarly, for a desired FiO_2 of 0.4, having an entrainment ratio of 1:3, oxygen flow rate of 10 L/min will have a total flow (after entrainment, through mask) of 10(1+3) = 40 L/min, which is just sufficient to meet peak inspiratory flow demand of the resting patient. A patient with a rapid respiratory rate having a higher peak inspiratory flow demand may require a higher total flow through the mask. This patient may need to be given 12 L/min of oxygen flow to raise the total flow (through the mask) to 48 L/min. However, this flow of 12 L/min of oxygen may not be sufficient to meet the flow demands of the patient, if desired FiO_2 is 0.5. Since the entrainment ratio for a desired FiO_2 of 0.5 is 1:1.7, the total flow through the mask (after entrainment at oxygen flow of 12 L/min) will be 12 (1+1.7) = 32.4 L/min. This flow (32.4 L/min), is inadequate to meet the inspiratory demands of a dyspnoeic patient. Patient under these circumstances (FiO_2 = 0.5, O_2 flow rate 12 L/min) may, infact, get more restless, tachypnoeic and hypoxic.

To sum up, the average oxygen flow rates recommended (to achieve an adequate total flow of at least 40 L/min) are 6, 8, 10-12 L/min to provide a desired FiO_2 of 0.30, 0.35 and 0.4 respectively (Table 4.1).

Table 4.1: Air-entrainment mask input flow versus total flow at varying FiO_2

FiO_2	Inlet oxygen flow (minimum) (L/min)	Total flow (L/min)
0.24	4	97
0.28	6	66
0.3	6	54
0.35	8	48
0.40	10–12	40–48
0.50	12	33
0.60	12	24

6. **Secure the mask on the face of the patient.**
   Place the mask over the patient's nose and mouth and secure it with the help of an adjustable, elastic band placed around the patient's head and passing above the ears. Gently pinch the soft metal at the top of the mask over the nose.

7. **Inspect the system attached to the patient as a whole.**
   Air-entrainment ports should not be covered with sheet, gown, or other material, as this may decrease air entrainment and total flow through the mask.

8. **Monitor the patient.**

9. **Wash hands.**

   This reduces the risk of transmission of microorganisms.

References

1. AARC clinical practice guidelines: oxygen therapy in the acute care hospital. Respir Care 1991; 36:1410-1413.
2. Bar ZG. Predictive equation for peak inspiratory flow. Respir Care 1985;30:766.
3. Campbell EJM. A method of controlled oxygen administration which reduces the risk of CO_2 retention. Lancet 1960;1:12.
4. Canet J, Sanchis J. Performance of a low flow O_2 venturi mask: Diluting effects of the breathing pattern. Eur J Respir Dis 1984; 65:68.
5. Scacci R. Air entrainment masks: Jet mixing is how they work; The Bernoulli and Venturi principles are how they don't. Respir Care 1979; 24:928.
6. Sills JR. Respiratory Care Certification Guide, 2 ed. St. Lowis: Mosby 1994.
7. Spearman CB, Sanders HG, Feenstra L, et al. Effects of changing jet flows on O_2 concentrations in adjustable air entrainment masks (abstract). Respir Care 1980;25:1266.
8. Woolner DF, Laniein J. An analysis of the performance of a variable venturi-type mask. Anesth Intensive Care 1980;8:44.

Incentive Spirometry

5

Introduction

- Incentive spirometry (IS), also referred to as sustained maximal inspiration (SMI), is a technique designed to mimic natural sighing or yawning manoeuvres by encouraging the patient to take long, slow, deep breaths. IS provides patients with visual feedback to quantify the depth of the breath when they inhale at a predetermined flow rate or volume and sustain the inflation for a minimum of three seconds.
- The objectives of incentive spirometry are to increase transpulmonary pressure and inspiratory volume to near-preoperative state, improve muscle performance, and to re-establish the normal pattern of periodic deep breathing.
- Incentive spirometry is thus useful in patients predisposed to the development of pulmonary atelectasis such as after upper abdominal surgery, thoracic surgery, surgery in patients with chronic obstructive pulmonary disease (COPD), immobility, abdominal binders, presence of neuromuscular disease involving the respiratory muscles, and presence of a restrictive lung defect associated with quadriplegia and/or dysfunctional diaphragm.
- Incentive spirometry is contraindicated in patients unable to deep breathe effectively (for example, with vital capacity less than about 10 mL/kg or inspiratory capacity less than about one third of predicted), and in uncooperative patients. Patient should not be tachypnoeic, and should have a respiratory rate less than 25 breaths/min to perform the procedure properly.
- Incentive spirometers are of two primary types: volume-oriented and flow-oriented. Flow-oriented devices are more commonly used (as compared to volume-oriented devices) because they are simple, less bulky and cost-effective.
- A commonly available flow-oriented device (Fig. 5.1) consists of three chambers in series, each of which contains a ball. The higher the patient's inspiratory flow, the higher is the ball raised or the greater would be the number of balls that

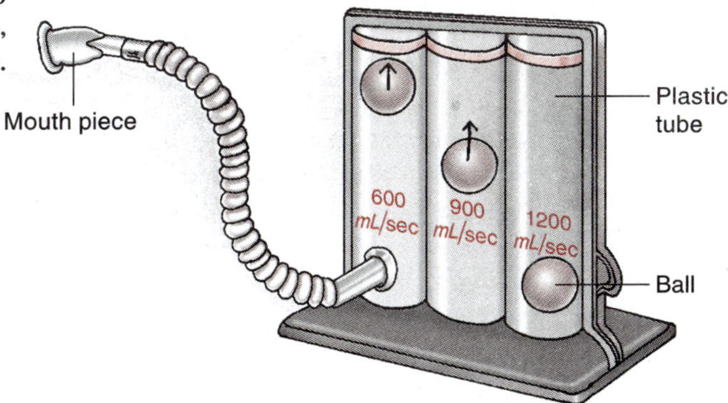

Fig. 5.1: Incentive spirometer

are raised. An inspiratory flow of 600 mL/sec raises the first ball, an inspiratory flow of 900 mL/sec is required to elevate the first and second balls, and a flow of 1200 mL/sec is required to elevate all the three balls. The longer the flow is maintained, the larger is the volume, so the patient should be encouraged to take slow deep breaths. The volume is calculated by multiplying the flow per second needed to suspend the balls by the number of seconds for which the balls are suspended. For example 600 mL/sec × 3 sec = 1800mL IC (inspiratory capacity).

- The presence of an open tracheal stoma is not a contraindication but requires adaptation of the spirometer.

GUIDELINES FOR PERFORMING INCENTIVE SPIROMETRY

1. **Wash hands.**
   This reduces the risk of transmission of microorganisms.

2. **Explain the procedure to the patient.**
   Patients need to be told the importance of deep breathing, length of time the breaths are to be held, number of breaths to be attempted in each session, and to relax in between the breaths.

3. **Manage pain, if any.**
   Presence of incisional pain and splinting may make the whole procedure painful and uncomfortable for the patient.

4. **Establish the volume goal or flow goal.**
   Set an initial IC goal at twice the patient's tidal volume, increase the goal in 200-300 mL increments as the patient tolerates a final IC goal of greater than 12 mL/kg of ideal body weight, or a forced vital capacity (FVC) goal of more than 15 mL/kg of ideal body weight.

5. **Instruct the patient to perform the following steps:**
   (a) **Assemble and place the spirometer on a flat surface in front of the patient or hold it in an upright position.**
   (b) **Place lips firmly around the mouthpiece.**
       There should be no leak around the mouthpiece.
   (c) **After a normal exhalation, inhale slowly through the mouthpiece, taking as deep a breath as possible.**
       Inhaling fast can generate high flows (with low tidal volumes) and can raise the flow indicator to target levels without the patient meeting therapeutic volume or breath-holding objectives. The patient should be instructed to raise only the first two balls as the patient's inspiratory flow will be too high if all three balls are raised.

   (d) **Hold the breath for 3–5 seconds.**
   (e) **Remove mouthpiece and exhale normally.**
   (f) **Breathe normally for several breaths.**
       Patient should be allowed to relax each time, after performing the manoeuvre.

(g) Repeat the manoeuvre for 10 breaths in each session.

6. Repeat these sessions every one to two hours while awake.

Observe and boost the morale of the patient at regular intervals, as patient's cooperation and performance of the procedure frequently and properly are important for achieving therapeutic objectives.

7. Monitor the patient.

Observe the patient's colour, heart rate, respiratory rate and compare it with basal values, taken just before the start of the procedure. Stop the procedure if patient complains of dizziness or tingling of the fingertips, or acute chest pain.

8. Assess the benefits of incentive spirometry.

Benefits could be assessed in terms of decreased respiratory rate, improved air entry in the chest on auscultation, improved $P(A-a)O_2$ gradient and increase in vital capacity and peak expiratory flows with trends towards preoperative values. The patient may bring out more sputum because of opening up of atelectatic areas and improved vital capacity.

References

1. AARC clinical practice guidelines: incentive spirometry. Respiratory Care 1991;36(12): 1402-1405.
2. Bakow ED. Sustained maximal inspiration: A rationale for its use. Respir Care 1977;22:379-382.
3. Craven JL, Evans GA, Davenport PJ, Wiolliam RHP. The evaluation of incentive spirometry in the management of post operative pulmonary complications. Br J Surg 1974;61:793-797.
4. Douce FH. Incentive spirometry and other aids to lung inflation. In:Barnes TA (ed). Core Textbook of Respiratory Care Practice. St. Louis,: Mosby, 1994, pp. 231-241
5. Fink JB. Bronchial Hygienc and lung expansion. In: Fink JB, Hunt GE (eds). Clinical practice in Respiratory Care. Philadelphia: Lippincott Williams and Wilkens. 1999, pp. 343-380.
6. Iverson L1, et al. A comparative study of IPPB, the incentive spirometer, and blow bottles: The prevention of atelectasis following cardiac surgery. Ann Thorac Surg 1978;25:197-200.
7. Krastins IRB, Corey ML, McLeod A, Edmonds J, Levison H, Moes F. An evaluation of incentive spirometry in the management of pulmonary complications after cardiac surgery in a pediatric population. Crit Care Med 1982;10:525-528.
8. Lederer DH, Van de Water J, Indech RB. Which deep breathing device should the postoperative patient use? Chest 1980;77:610-613.
9. Mang H, Obermeyer A. Imposed work of breathing during sustained maximal inspiration: Comparison of six incentive spirometers. Respir Care 1989; 34:1122-1128.
10. Sills JR. Respiratory Care Certification Guide. 2 ed. St. Louis: Mosby 1994.
11. Rau JL, Thomas L, Haynes RL. The effect of the method of administering incentive spirometry on postoperative pulmonary complications in coronary bypass patients. Respir Care 1988;33:771-778.
12. Wojciechowski WV. Incentive spirometers, secrection evacuation devices, and inspiratory muscle training devices. In:Barnes TA (ed). Textbook of Respiratory Care Practice. St. Louis,: Mosby, 1994, pp. 499-522.

Closed Chest Drainage System

6

Introduction

- Closed chest drainage systems, single-, double-, triple-or four-bottle set-ups as well as disposable units use gravity or suction or both to restore negative pressure and remove air, fluid, and blood from the pleural space, thereby restoring cardiorespiratory function by re-expansion of lung and elimination of the mediastinal shift which may cause haemodynamic instability. Chest drainage systems also prevent the entry of atmospheric air into the pleural space by using a water-seal.
- The three basic components of an effective chest drainage system are: (a) pleural tube (chest tube) to evacuate air, fluid, or blood, (b) a one-way valve, usually an underwater seal, and (c) a collection chamber for blood or pleural fluid.
- For adults, chest tubes of internal diameter (ID) 6-11 mm (sizes 26-40FG) are recommended. Connectors for joining the chest tube to the drainage tube should have an ID greater than 6 mm to prevent obstruction by blood clots.
- The optimal length of the connecting drainage tube is 1.8 m, with an ID 9.5 mm to 12mm to provide minimal resistance to drainage.
- An underwater seal creates a one-way mechanism allowing air, fluid, or blood to exit the pleural space as a result of gravity while preventing it from being drawn back into the cavity. In addition, the underwater seal produces a siphon effect which enhances drainage.
- Effective pleural drainage depends on the internal diameter of pleural tube (chest tube) and on the pressure gradient between the pleural space and the drainage collection system.
- During obstructed inspiration, large subatmospheric pressures up to -80 cm H_2O may be generated so that fluid in the collection chamber may be sucked up through the tubing into the pleural space. To prevent this, the collection chamber should always be placed 100 cm below the chest.
- In the simplest, one-bottle drainage collection system (Fig. 6.1), the drainage tube is submerged 2 cm below

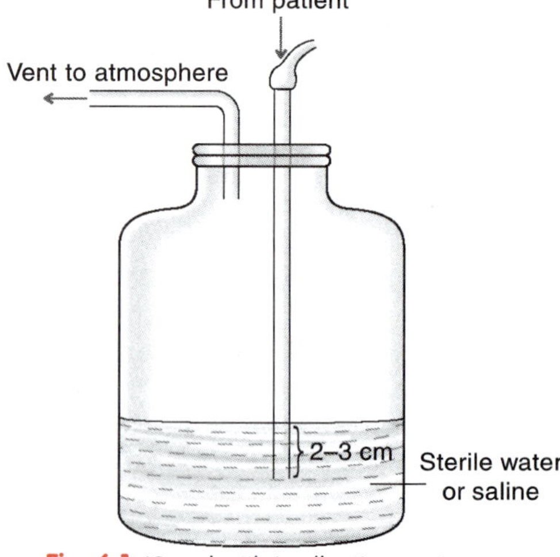

Fig. 6.1: 'One-bottle' collection system.

the level of sterile water or saline, which acts as an underwater seal. An exit vent allows the escape of pleural air to the atmosphere. One of the disadvantages of this system is that, as the collection chamber is filled with blood or fluid, the drainage tube becomes submerged to a greater depth, resulting in an increased resistance to drainage. The other disadvantage is the occurence of froth formation, which can lead to overflow and measuring problems when large volumes of air and blood are drained. If the patient has very little fluid in the intrathoracic space, one bottle system may be the system of choice.

- The disadvantages of one-bottle system may be reduced by the two-bottle system (Fig. 6.2), with the first bottle (connected to the patient) being a drainage collection chamber (fluid trap) and the second bottle acting as an underwater seal. An exit vent on the second bottle allows any pleural air to escape into the atmosphere. However, the collection chamber (fluid trap) increases the pleural dead space, impedes re-expansion of the lung and adds an extra amount of work required to expel the pleural air. In addition, the siphon effect due to the underwater seal is also lost, reducing the efficiency of drainage. Applying subatmospheric pressure to increase the pressure difference between the pleural space and the collection chamber can surmount these problems. When only gravity drainage is required, the two-bottle system is used as it is optimal for drainage of large effusions.

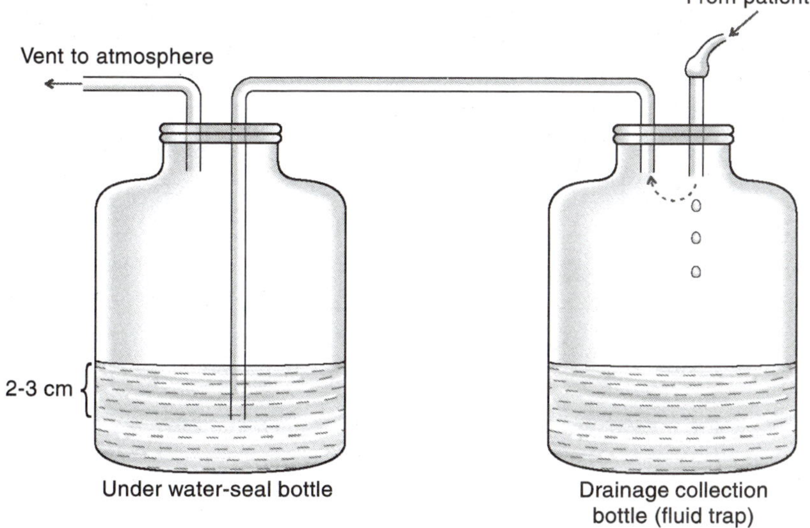

Fig. 6.2: 'Two-bottle' collection system.

- When an unregulated vacuum source (e.g. wall suction) exists and a constant negative pressure is desired, a third bottle (suction control bottle or chamber) is added between the underwater seal (second bottle) and the suction device (Fig. 6.3). It has an inlet connected to the vent of the underwater seal chamber of the two-bottle system, an outlet connected to the suction device, and a control tube, which is open to the atmosphere at one end but immersed approximately 20 cm underwater at the other end. It can be raised or lowered

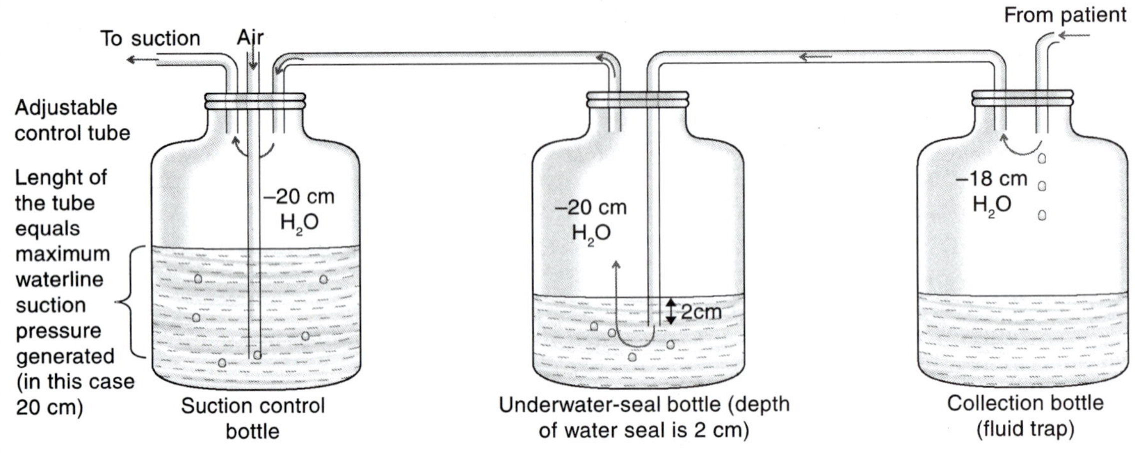

Fig. 6.3: 'Three-bottle' collection system.

to adjust its underwater depth as that determines the maximum level negative pressure the system will generate. Continuous bubbling occurs in the third bottle resulting in noise. The major disadvantages of the three-bottle system are: (a) greater complexity, (b) noise due to continuous bubbling, and (c) lack of an exit vent if suction fails. If the suction system fails, the entire system is not vented and a pneumothorax may result.

- The four-bottle suction drainage system (Fig. 6.4) consists of a fourth bottle or safety underwater seal connected to the collection chamber (fluid trap) of the three-bottle system. This will vent the entire system and relieve any pressure build-up, should there be a failure of suction.

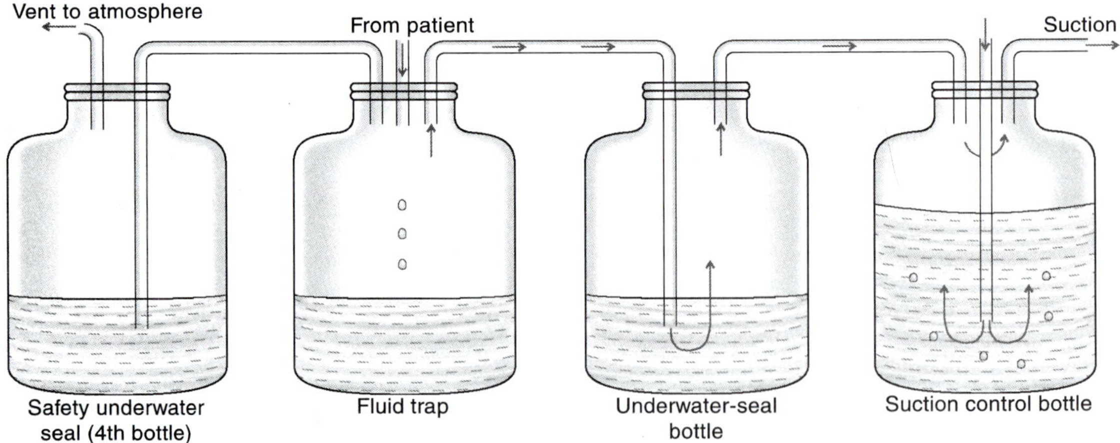

Fig. 6.4: 'Four-bottle' collection system.

- Waterless disposable chest-drainage system eliminates the need to fill any chamber. This consists of a valve which opens on expiration allowing the air to exit, and closes on inspiration to prevent atmospheric air from entering inside. These waterless variations are more compact, quieter in operation and easier to transport.

- The use of pleural drains in the post-pneumonectomy patient is controversial. On the first postoperative day, the pleural drain should be clamped and released intermittently every 2-4 hours to drain blood or fibrin. Suction of pleural drains is absolutely contraindicated, as it predisposes the patient to a mediastinal shift, which may cause cardiovascular embarrassment.

GUIDELINES FOR THE CARE OF THE PATIENT WITH CHEST DRAINAGE SYSTEM

1. **Wash hands.**

   This reduces the risk of transmission of microorganisms

2. **Assess cardiopulmonary and vital signs 2-4 hourly and as and when required.**

   Tachypnea, dyspnea, orthopnea, restlessness, cyanosis, increased heart rate, chest pain, or haemoptysis could indicate malfunctioning of chest drainage system.

3. **Assess for movement or fluctuation with respiration of the fluid level in the drainage tube of the water seal bottle or chamber, every 2-4 hours.**

   The fluctuations indicate effective communication between the pleural cavity and drainage system. The fluctuations will stop when the lung is re-expanded, and when the tubing is obstructed by a kink, a fluid-filled loop, a clot or tissue at the distal end, or when the patient is lying on the tubing.

4. **Monitor the amount and type of drainage from the chest tube by watching the collection chamber at hourly or longer intervals.**

   Decreased or absent drainage associated with respiratory distress may indicate obstruction, and that without respiratory distress may indicate lung reexpansion. Immediately after insertion of the chest tube, the fluid drained can have a bloody or pinkish tinge denoting trauma at the time of insertion. Sudden flow of dark bloody drainage on position change is often due to old blood finding its way into the chest tube. Drainage of more than 150-200 mL/hr may need to be observed for the next few hours. It should also be recorded on the chart.

5. **Keep the drainage tube free of dependent loops (Fig. 6.5).**

   Drain the drainage tube frequently. Do not allow fluid to collect in it. When fluid fills the loop, no suction is exerted on the patient and drainage becomes ineffective. The fluid in this loop acts as a clot or has the same result as does kinking of the tubing. The tubing should be coiled flat on the bed or kept in a straight line, gradually sloping to the collecting bottle. Remember, the patient needs to be able to move about in bed, therefore, do not pin or restrain the tubing in such a way that this is not possible.

6. Milk the tubing when a visible clot is present in the tubing.

    Firmly hold the chest tube (near the patient end) with left hand, pinching it off between the thumb and the fingers. Be careful not to pull away the chest tube. With the right hand pinch off the tubing just below the left hand. Slide the right hand down the tubing, pulling it tightly until the tubing between the two hands is flat, and then release the left hand and then the right hand. Continue this procedure until all of the tubing has been milked, or until the tubing is free of clots.

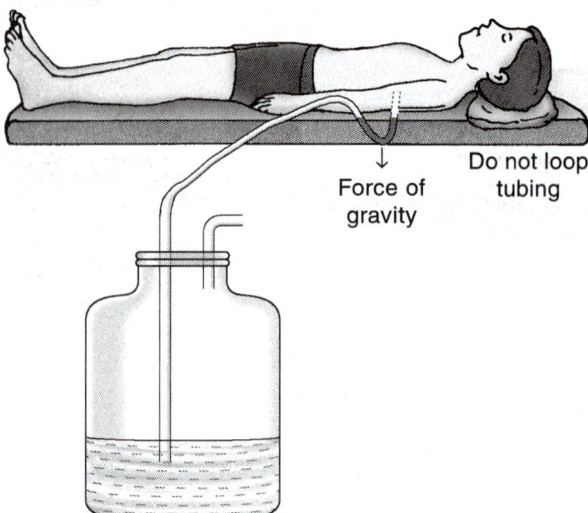

Fig. 6.5: The fluid in this loop acts as a clot or has the same result as does kinking of the tubing.

    - The purpose of milking is to keep the tubing patent and free of clots.
    - The patency of the chest tube can also be restored by momentarily disconnecting the chest tube and flushing it with 50 ml of saline (under aseptic conditions). This clears the tube by pushing the tissue or clot away from the holes in the tube. Fan-folding several sections of tubing and squeezing them has also been recommended to dislodge any clots in the tube.

7. Check and refill the saline level in the under water-seal chamber.

    This is necessary to maintain the prescribed water-seal.

8. Assess for air leaks in the system, as indicated by constant bubbling in the underwater-seal bottle or chamber.

    - No bubbling occurs when there is no collected fluid or air in the intrathoracic space or when the drainage tubing is kinked, has a clot or a high loop.
    - If no air-bubbles are seen on initial inspection of the water seal, the patient should be asked to cough and the water seal observed for bubbling. Coughing increases the patient's pleural pressure and demonstrates small air leaks into the pleural space. If air-bubbles escape through the water-seal continuously, it usually indicates a persistent air leak from the lung into the pleural space or the presence of an opening in the drainage system (i.e. around the chest tube insertion site, its connections, or in the closed drainage system itself). Locating the leaks in the system can be done by progressively clamping the tube, beginning at its exit from the chest and moving the clamp toward the drainage system. Momentary clamping will demonstrate the site of the leak-whether it is from the lung or it is at some point along the collecting system.

9. **Ask for pain at the insertion site and manage appropriately.**
    Pain produces shallow breathing, leading to atelectasis and pneumonia. Adequate pain medication and tracheobronchial toilet can prevent these complications. Instruct the patient to sit in a semi-Fowler position (unless contraindicated), to cough, take deep breaths, and to turn and change position every 2 hourly.

10. **Inspect the insertion site and change dressing when soiled or every 24-48 hours.**
    Skin integrity is altered during insertion and this can lead to infection.

11. **Obtain a drainage specimen and send it for analysis at regular intervals.**
    Pleural infection is one of the complications of tube thoracostomy. Prophylactic antibiotics are recommended for all trauma patients with chest tube drainage. The utility of prophylactic antibiotics in other situations such as in post-operative patients, and patients with spontaneous pneumothorax is yet to be evaluated.

12. **Discard all drainage tubes and other equipment as required by standard precautions.**
    Proper disposal of equipment helps prevent the spread of infection.

13. **Wash hands.**
    This reduces the risk of transmission of microorganisms.

14. **Consider removal of chest tube at an appropriate time.**
    Indications for removal are based on the reason for insertion and include the following: (a) Improved respiratory status (i.e. non-laboured respiration, decreased use of accessory muscles, respiratory rate less than 24 breaths/min, and equal breath sounds), (b) drainage reduced to 50-100 mL in 24 hours, if the tube was placed for haemothorax, empyema, or pleural effusion, (c) no air leaks, (d) absent fluctuations in the water-seal chamber, and (e) expanded lungs, as shown on chest radiograph.

References

1. Duncan C, Erickson R. Pressures associated with chest tube stripping. Heart Lung 1982; 11:166-171.
2. Fishman N. Thoracic drainage: a manual of procedures. St Louis 1983, Mosby.
3. Gongalez RP, Holevar MR. Role of prophylactic antibiotics for tube thoracostomy in chest trauma. Am Surg 1998; 64:617-620.
4. Kam AC, O'Brien M, Kam PCA. Pleural drainage systems. Anesthesia 1993; 48:154-161.
5. Kesten L. Chest-tube drainage system; indications and principles of operation. Heart Lung 1974; 3:97.
6. Miller KS, Sahn SA. Chest tubes: indications, technique, management, and complications. Chest 1987; 91(2): 258-264.
7. Nichols RL, Smith JW, Muzik AC, et al. Preventive antibiotic usage in traumatic thoracic injuries requiring closed tube thoracostomy. Chest 1994; 106:1493-1498.
8. Schmeiz JO, Johnson D, Norton JM, et al. Effects of position of chest drainage tube on volume drained and pressure. Am J Crit Care 1999; 8:319-323.

Analgesia and Sedation in Critically Ill Patients

7

Introduction

- Pain causes inadequate sleep and evokes a stress-response characterized by tachycardia, increased myocardial oxygen consumption, hypercoagulability, immunosuppression and persistent catabolism. Pain also contributes to pulmonary dysfunction by restricting movement of chest wall and diaphragm. Effective analgesia may decrease the incidence of pulmonary complications in postoperative patients.

- Pain assessment can be done either by verbal rating scale (VRS), visual analogue scale (VAS) or by numeric rating scale (NRS). NRS is a zero to ten-point scale in which a patient chooses a number that describes the pain, with ten representing the worst pain. NRS is a valid scale and correlates well with VAS. NRS may be preferable to VAS in critically ill patients because patient can complete the NRS by writing or speaking and because it is applicable in many age groups. Patients who cannot communicate should be assessed through subjective observation of pain-related behaviours (movement, facial expression, and posturing), physiological indicators (heart rate, blood pressure and respiratory rate) and the change in these parameters following analgesia therapy.

- Agitation may have a deleterious effect on patients by contributing to ventilator dyssynchrony, increase in oxygen consumption, and inadvertent removal of devices and catheters. Sedation reduces the stress response and improves the tolerance of routine ICU procedures. In patients with respiratory failure, the administration of sedatives in appropriate doses helps increase chest wall compliance, allows the manipulation of inspiratory to expiratory ratio and other variables, improves oxygenation, and improves synchronized breathing.

- Once a pain-free state is achieved, the primary goals of sedative therapy are, anxiolysis, hypnosis, and amnesia. No single analgesic or sedative or single depth of analgesia or sedation is appropriate for all patients.

- Various scales for subjective assessment of sedation have been described, e.g. the Riker Sedation-Agitation Scale (SAS), the Motor Activity Assessment Scale (MAAS), the Vancouver Interaction and Calmness Scale (VICS), the COMFORT Scale, and the Ramsay Scale. The Ramsay scale is comparatively simple to apply, has been used in many comparative sedative trials and is widely used clinically, as it is easy to remember.

- The Ramsay scale measures three levels of awake states and three levels of asleep states. The scores range from 1 to 6; 1 to 3 for awake state and 4 to 6 for asleep state. The details are as follows:

(1) Patient anxious and agitated or restless or both.
(2) Patient cooperative, oriented and tranquil.
(3) Patient responds only to commands.
(4) A brisk response, to a light glabellar tap or loud auditory stimulus.
(5) A sluggish response, to a light glabellar tap or loud auditory stimulus.
(6) No response, to a light glabellar tap or loud auditory stimulus.

- The use of any single sedation score in the ICU helps to define goals and may also be used as a uniformly understood end-point for titration of drugs, e.g. "infuse a particular drug to achieve a sedation score of 3."
- The objective assessment of sedation, (especially useful during very deep sedation or during therapeutic neuromuscular blockade), can be done with Bispectral Index Monitor (BIS). The BIS is a device that processes the raw electroencephalogram (EEG) signal into a discrete scaled number. It has a digital scale ranging from 100 (completely awake) to < 60 (deep sedation) to $\leq$ 40 (deep hypnotic state or barbiturate coma) to 0 (isoelectric EEG). Although BIS is likely to be useful when patients are deeply comatose or under neuromuscular blockade, routine use of this device cannot be recommended until its value and validity are confirmed.
- Delirium is characterized by an acutely changing or fluctuating mental status, inattention, disorganized thinking, and an altered level of consciousness that may or may not be accompanied by agitation. As many as 80% of ICU patients have delirium at some stage or the other.
- Though a continuous sedative infusion provides a more consistent level of sedation with greater level of patient comfort, it is associated with prolongation of mechanical ventilation and hospital stay, organ system failure, and higher reintubation rates as compared with no sedation or intermittent sedation strategies.

GUIDELINES FOR INITIATING THERAPY

1. Examine the patient in terms of pain, anxiety, and agitation.
    - Patient may have pain because of pre-existing disease, trauma, or invasive monitoring and therapeutic devices (such as catheters, drains, endotracheal tubes, non-invasive ventilatory device) and routine nursing care (such as dressing change, patient mobilization), airway suctioning, and prolonged immobilization.
    - Patient may have no pain, but may be anxious because of being emotionally ill and dependent on others, environment of the ICU (lighting, noise, alarms, personnel, and equipment), and inability to communicate, and sleep deprivation.
    - Agitation can be caused by multiple factors, such as extreme anxiety, delirium, adverse drug effects, pain, hypoxia, hypotension, head injury, subarachanoid haemorrhage and many stimuli common to ICU environment. A patient with neuromuscular blockade may be agitated because of lack of sedation and analgesia.

(a) Assess the patient for various clinical and physiological variables, and analgesia and sedation scales. (i.e. heart rate, blood pressure, respiratory rate, sweating, synchrony with ventilator, arterial oxygen and carbon-dioxide tensions, ECG, restricted movements of chest wall, and peak airway pressures).

(b) Record the findings.

2. **Reassure the patient**
    - Talk to your patients at least once every day, and if possible more often. Hold their hand, look into their eyes and tell them that they are going to be OK.
    - Tell your patients "we are going to do everything we can, and you will be alright very soon."
    - Remember, every patient waits for his doctor to say something to him about his progress and all that is happening to him.
    - Children may be given action oriented toys or other toys of their liking, or a few story books. Children prefer to be with their mothers.

3. **Rule out and correct reversible causes of pain, anxiety and agitation.**
    - Proper positioning of patient.
    - Stabilization of fractures.
    - Elimination of irritating physical stimulation (e.g. proper positioning of ventilator tubing to avoid traction on ETT). Reset the ventilatory settings, if required.
    - Consider pain from chest tubes.
    - Identify and treat any underlying physiological disturbances, such as hypoxaemia, hypoglycaemia, hypotension, and withdrawal from alcohol and other drugs.
    - At times, the option of early, elective tracheostomy in an agitated and difficult to wean patient can give unimaginable sense of comfort, and a boost to weaning from the ventilator.

4. **Optimize the environment.**
    - Optimize in terms of lighting (e.g. reduce the light in the night time), noise and temperature in ICU.
    - Music therapy.
    - Back massage initiates a relaxation response and increases the patient's duration of sleep.

5. **Set goals.**
    - The target is a pain free, calm patient who can be easily aroused from sleep while still maintaining the normal sleep-wake cycle (some patients may require deeper levels of sedation to facilitate mechanical ventilation).
    - Patient should be pain free. On NRS scale, the scale should be less than or equal to 2 (0 represents no pain and 10 represents worst pain).
    - An optimum level of sedation with a calm and communicative patient usually correlates with a Ramsay score of 2 or 3 and a Sedation – Agitation scale of 3 or 4. Also, there should be no discordance with the ventilator.

- Deeper levels of sedation may be required where unconventional ventilator strategies such as permissive hypercapnia, low tidal volumes, prone positioning, and pressure controlled ventilation are employed.
- In general, the best dose of sedation is that with which the patients are comfortable.

6. **Manage pain.**
   - For patients who are haemodynamically unstable:
     (a) Use fentanyl bolus 0.35-1.5 µg/kg IV every 20-30 minutes until pain is relieved. If patient requires bolus doses more frequently (every two hours or more frequently), switch over to fentanyl infusion (0.7-10 µg/kg/hr). When requirement of fentanyl is less (less frequent doses) and the patient is haemodynamically stable, switch over to morphine 0.01-0.15 mg/kg IV every 2-3 hours, OR
     (b) Use hydromorphone 0.25-0.75mg IV every 5-15 minutes until pain is relieved. Intermittent dose 10-30µg/Kg IV every 1-2 hours; infusion dose 7-15µg/kg/hr.
   - For patients who are haemodynamically stable. Use morphine bolus 0.01-0.15 mg/kg IV every 1-2 hour until pain is relieved. Continue with intermittent doses or switch over to infusion (0.07-0.5 mg/kg/hr) if boluses are required too frequently.
   - Whenever possible, use continuous regional block or epidural block.

7. **Manage agitation (start sedation only after providing adequate analgesia). Be careful in selecting the sedative agent and its dose in unintubated patients.**
   - Assess whether agitation is causing acute deterioration (e.g. hypoxia, high peak airway pressure, dyssynchrony with ventilator):
     (a) If signs of acute agitation are present: use midazolam 2-5 mg IV every 5-15 minutes until the acute event is controlled or desired sedation goal is achieved. Continue with intermittent doses of lorazepam (0.02-0.06 mg/kg every 2-6 hr) or if required too frequently, use lorazepam infusion 0.01-0.1 mg/kg/hr.
     (b) If no signs of acute agitation, start with lorazepam 1-4 mg IV every 10-20 minutes until desired sedation goal is achieved. Continue with intermittent doses or infusion as the case may be.
   - Alternatively, use propofol initially at 5 µg/kg/min and then titrate it as desired, to meet the goal. When propofol infusion is continued for more than 2 days, triglyceride levels should be monitored and total caloric intake from lipids should be included in the nutrition support orders.
   - Propofol is the preferred sedative when rapid awakening (e.g. for neurologic examination or extubation) is important.
   - Combine opioids with any one of the above drugs to get optimum results, as no single drug can achieve all the set goals for sedation and analgesia in the ICU.
   - Oral hypnotics, such as benzodiazepines or zolpidem may be used in non intubated patients to promote sleep. They should be used early in the evening.

8. Manage delirium.
   - Injection haloperidol 2-10 mg IV every 20-30 minutes until delirium is settled and then 25% of loading dose every 6 hours.
   - Haloperidol has less sedative and hypotensive effect (as compared to chlorpromazine) and is therefore the preferred agent for treatment of delirium in critically ill patients. Monitor the patient for ECG changes (prolonged QT interval and arrhythmias) when haloperidol is being given.

9. Reassess the patient every 4-6 hours, in terms of desired goals and the dose of the drug being given. Record the findings and any alteration in the drug regimen.
   - If the target goal has not been achieved, increase fentanyl infusion by 20-30 µg/hr or lorazepam infusion by 0.2 to 0.3 mg/hr or reduce by approximately the same rates, if target goal has already been achieved. In this way the level of sedation and analgesia is continuously titrated.
   - An acutely ill patient may require more frequent (every 1-2 hours) monitoring.

10. Interrupt the sedative infusions to allow the patients to "wake up" at least once a day.
    - Daily interruption of sedative infusions allows rationalizing the total dose, streamlining administration of the drugs being used, and minimizing the tendency for accumulation. This practice decreases the duration of mechanical ventilation, length of stay in the intensive care unit, need for diagnostic studies to evaluate unexplained alterations in mental status, and incidence of withdrawal symptoms in patients receiving opioids and benzodiazepines. It also improves the ability of clinicians to perform daily neurologic examinations. However, this may not be practiced in patients at high risk for myocardial infarction, and those requiring muscle paralysis, who should never be awakened from sedation until the effect of paralytic agent has worn off. For these patients daily or even twice daily interruption of neuromuscular blockade is advisable to assess the adequacy of sedation and analgesia and the ongoing need for neuromuscular blockade.
    - Interrupt the infusions until the patients are: (a) Awake and able to follow simple commands (e.g. open eyes, squeeze hand, track with eyes, stick out tongue-equivalent to Ramsay sedation scale score of 3), or (b) agitated when they are assumed to require resumption of sedation.
    - After performing "wake up" test, if it is decided to resume sedation, (because of agitation), restart at 50% of previous dose and titrate according to desired goal. In general, taper the infusion rate of benzodiazepines and opioids by 10-25% every 24hours. Keep in mind the desired goals.
    - Patients need more drug immediately following intubation and mechanical ventilation, but the infusion levels can often be reduced within a few hours, to very modest doses.

11. Taper the dose when used for longer period.
    - Patients exposed to higher doses (i.e. greater than 5 mg/24hr of fentanyl or 35 mg/24hr of lorazepam) or to more than one week of opioids or sedative

therapy may develop neuroadaptation or physiological dependence. Rapid disconnection of these agents could lead to withdrawal symptoms. Various recommendations to prevent withdrawal symptoms include:

(a) Daily dose decrements of opioids should not exceed 5-10% in high-risk patients.

(b) If the drug is administered intermittently, change the therapy to longer-acting agents.

(c) If the drug is being administered by continuous infusion, decrease the rate by 20-40% initially and make additional reductions of 10% every 12-24 hours.

References

1. American College of Critical Care Medicine, American Society of Health – System Pharmacists, American College of Chest Physicians: Clinical practice guidelines for the sustained use of sedatives and analgesics in the critically ill adult. Crit Care Med 2002; 30:119-141.

2. Boldt J, Thaler E, Lehmann A, et al. Pain management in cardiac surgery patients. Comparison between standard therapy and patient-controlled analgesia regimen. J Cardiothorac Vasc Anesth 1998; 12:654-658.

3. Brook AD, Ahrens TS, Schaiff R, Prentice D, Sherman G, Shannon W, Kollef MH. Effect of a nursing – implemented sedation protocol on the duration of mechanical ventilation. Crit Care Med 1999; 27:2609-2615.

4. Cohen D, Horiuchi K, Kemper M, et al. Modulating effects of propofol on metabolic and cardiopulmonary responses to stressful intensive care unit procedures. Crit Care Med 1996; 24:612-617.

5. De Jonghe B, Cook D, Appere-De-Vecchi C, and et al. Using and understanding sedation scoring systems: A systematic review. Intensive Care Med. 2000; 26:275-285.

6. Ibrahim EH, Kollef MH. Using protocols to improve the outcomes of mechanically ventilated patients: focus on weaning and sedation. Crit Care Clin. 2001; 17:989-1001.

7. Krachman SL, D'Alonzo GE, Criner GJ. Sleep in the intensive care unit. Chest 1995; 107:1713-1720.

8. Kress JP, Pohlman AS, Hall JB. Sedation and analgesia in the intensive care unit. Am J Respir Crit Care Med. 2002; 166:1024-1028.

9. Kress JP, Pohlman A, O'Connor MF, Hall JB. Daily interruption of sedative infusion in critically ill patients undergoing mechanical ventilation. N Eng J Med 2000; 342:1471-1477.

10. Kress JP, O'Connor MF, Pohlman AS, Olson D, Lavoie A, Toledano A, Hall JB. Sedation of critically ill patients during mechanical ventilation: a comparison of propofol and midazolam. Am J Respir Crit Care Med 1996; 153:1012-1018.

11. Kollef MH, Levy NT, Ahrens TS, Schaiff R, Prentice D, Sherman G. The use of continuous IV sedation is associated with prolongation of mechanical ventilation. Chest 1998; 114:541-548

12. Mazzeo AJ. Sedation for the mechanically ventilated patient. Crit Care Clin 1995; 11:937-955.

13. MC Collam JS, O'Neil MG, Norcross ED, et al. Continuous infusions of lorazepam, midazolam and propofol for sedation of the critically-ill surgery trauma patient: A prospective, randomized comparison. Crit Care Med 1999; 27:2454-2458.

14. Mirski MA, Muffelman B, Ulatowski JA, et al. Sedation for the critically ill neurologic patient. Crit Care Med. 1995; 23:2038-2053.

15. Mirenda J, Broyles J. Propofol as used for sedation in the ICU. Chest 1995; 108:539-548.

16. Park G, Coursin D, Ely EW, England M, Fraser GL, Mantz J, Mc Kinley S, Ramsay M, et al. Commentary: balancing sedation and analgesia in the critically ill. Crit Care Clin 2001; 17:1015-1027.

17. Pohlman AS, Simpson KP, Hall JB. Continuous intravenous infusion of larazepam versus midazolam for sedation during mechanical ventilatory support. A prospective, randomized study. Crit Care Med. 1994; 22:1241-1247.

18. Shafer A. Complications of sedation with midazolam in the intensive care unit and a comparison with other sedative regimens. Crit Care Med 1998; 26:947-956.

19. Wagner BKJ, O'Hara DA. Pharmacokinetics and pharmacodynamics of sedatives and analgesics in the treatment of agitated critically ill patients. Clin Pharmacokinet 1997; 33:425-453.

20. Watling SM, Johnson M, Yanos J. A method to produce sedation in critically ill patients. Ann Pharmacother 1996; 30:1227-1231.

21. Young C, Knudsen N, Hilton A, et al. Sedation in the intensive care unit. Crit Care Med 2000; 28:854-866.

Introduction

- Depolarization of the muscle membrane must occur for the muscle contraction to take place. Depolarizing NMBAs (neuromuscular blocking agents) have a longer duration of action than acetylcholine, therefore, after an initial contraction (fasciculation), muscles remain persistently depolarized and flaccid. Non-depolarizing NMBAs, on the other hand, prevent depolarization (by complete inhibition) of the muscle membrane and thus cause muscle paralysis.
- 70-75% of post-synaptic receptors must be occupied by non-depolarizing NMBAs before clinical blockade is detectable. Clinically relevant neuromuscular paralysis thus occurs over a narrow range of receptor occupancy (i.e. 70 100%).
- The diaphragm is the most resistant of all muscles to the action of NMBAs, requiring 1.4 to 2.0 times as much agent as the adductor policis brevis muscles for identical degree of paralysis. Most sensitive are the abdominal and peripheral muscles of the extremities.
- Neuromuscular monitoring is important while using NMBAs in the ICU because of the following reasons: (a) There is a marked variation in an individual's sensitivity to muscle relaxants, (b) the pharmacokinetics and pharmacodynamics of NMBAs varies depending on the derangement in the function of various organs (e.g. multiorgan failure) and this may lead to accumulation of the drug or its active metabolites, (c) the patient may be receiving other drugs which have significant interactions with NMBAs, (d) the presence of electrolyte and acid-base disturbances may affect the required dose of the NMBAs, and (e) studies have shown that use of peripheral nerve stimulation for monitoring the degree of blockade and adjusting drug doses in continuously paralyzed critically ill patients results in lower doses of NMBAs to maintain the desired depth of paralysis and allows a faster recovery of neuromuscular function and spontaneous ventilation.

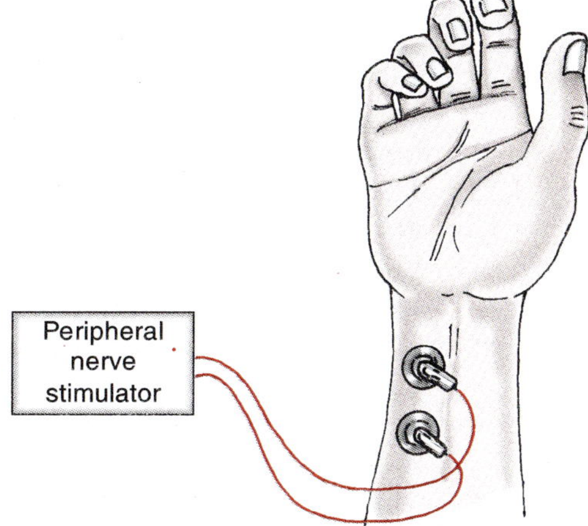

Fig. 8.1: Proper placement of stimulating electrodes on the wrist over ulnar nerve. Twitches of the adductor pollicis muscle of the thumb are felt or observed.

- Ulnar nerve (Fig. 8.1) is the most frequent site for stimulation. Three objective methods of monitoring, in common use, are:
  - (a) Mechanomyography measures the force of contraction of the appropriate muscles,
  - (b) Electromyography measures the accompanying currents over the contracting muscles, and
  - (c) Acceleromyography measures the equivalent acceleration caused by contraction of the muscles.

  The most suitable stimulation modes are train-of-four (TOF), post-tetanic count (PTC), and double-burst stimulation (DBS).
- Good correlation exists between the degree of neuromuscular blockade and the number of responses to TOF stimulation. Over the range of 75-100% blockade, the fourth, third, second, and first twitch become inappreciable, in that order. When only one response is detectable, the degree of block is 90-95%.

Table 8.1: TOF suppression and degree of neuromuscular blockade

TOF suppression	Approximate percentage of block
Four responses	0–75
Three responses	75-80
Two responses	80–90
One response	90–95
No response	100

Spontaneous recovery occurs predictably in the reverse order (Table 8.1).

- Even total elimination of the response to TOF stimulation of the ulnar nerve does not exclude movements of the diaphragm, such as hiccupping and coughing and diaphragmatic movements on tracheal suctioning. Total elimination of the response to facial nerve stimulation, however, normally means that diaphragm is paralyzed.
- In critically ill patients, there is approximately a 10% incidence of prolonged neuromuscular weakness of varying duration, following the use of NMBAs. The prolonged weakness could be because of overdose of the NMBAs, hepatic and renal dysfunction prolonging the effect of the drug or its active metabolite, electrolyte disorders (e.g. hypocalcaemia, hypermagnesaemia, hypophosphataemia, or hypokalaemia) acting alone or in combination with NMBAs, and concurrent use of drugs potentiating neuromuscular blockade, e.g. clindamycin, aminoglycosides, metronidazole, furosemide, antiarrhythmic agents, local anaesthetics, xylocaine, magnesium, calcium channel blockers, and lithium carbonate.
- The likelihood of weakness is also increased by the concurrent administration of corticosteroids. The incidence of myopathy may be as high as 30% in patients receiving corticosteroids and NMBAs. Risk of myopathy increases further with higher doses of steroids (e.g. more than one gm of methylprednisolone) and when steroids are used for longer than one or two days. Therefore, every effort

should be made to discontinue NMBAs as soon as possible, more so, when used with corticosteroids. Corticosteroids may have the following effects: (a) Increase in the number of post synaptic acetylcholine receptors, (b) interaction with inflammatory mediators in sepsis, or (c) potentiate injury of the motor end plate, by prolonged denervation of the neuromuscular junction in association with NMBAs.

- In view of the above, NMBAs should be used as a last resort when various combinations of sedatives and analgesics have failed to achieve the desired results, and if used, they should be stopped as early as possible.

- Succinylcholine is the only available depolarizing NMBA. It has a rapid onset and a short duration of action. In the ICU, it is used more often for rapid control of airway rather than for long term use. In patients with denervation injuries, administration of succinylcholine can lead to life-threatening hyperkalaemia because of a massive increase in the number of extrajunctional nicotinic acetylcholine receptors. Direct muscle injury, extensive burns, and a recent history of chronic administration of nondepolarizing NMBAs are other contraindications for the use of succinylcholine.

- The commonly used non- depolarizing compounds belong to one of two groups: the amino steroid compounds (e.g. pancuronium, vecuronium, pipecuronium, and rocuronium) and the benzylisoquinolinium compounds (D-tubocurarine, metocurine, atracuruim, mivacurium, and cisatracurium).

- Pancuronium is a long acting and vagolytic NMBA (more than 90% of ICU patients will have an increase in heart rate of $\geq$ 10 beats/min) thus limiting its use in those patients who cannot tolerate an increase in heart rate. In patients with renal or hepatic failure, its effects are prolonged due to an increase in the elimination half-life and decrease in the clearance of 3-hydroxypancuronium metabolite which has one-third to one-half the activity of pancuronium.

- Vecuronium is an intermediate acting non-vagolytic muscle relaxant. Its action is prolonged in patients with renal and hepatic insufficiency because of its dependence on renal and biliary excretion and because of an increase in the concentration of 3-desacetyl-vecuronium metabolite, which has 50% of the pharmacological activity of the parent compound. When compared with other NMBAs, it has been reported to be more commonly associated with prolonged blockade once discontinued.

- Rocuronium is an intermediate acting drug with a rapid onset of action. Its metabolite, 17-desacetylrocuronium, has only 5%-10% of activity when compared with the parent compound.

- Atracurium is an intermediate acting drug with nominal cardiovascular adverse effects and is associated with histamine release at higher doses. It is inactivated in plasma by ester hydrolysis and Hofmann elimination so that renal or hepatic dysfunction does not affect the duration of blockade. It has no active metabolite. Recovery of normal neuromuscular activity usually occurs within one to two hours after stopping the infusion and is independent of organ function. Atracurium has also been reported to be associated with persistent neuromuscular weakness, like other NMBAs.

GUIDELINES FOR USING NMBAs IN ICU

1. **Consider preconditions for the use of NMBAs.**
   - Patients should be receiving mechanical ventilatory support.
   - Patients should be free of pain and adequately sedated (Ramsay score $\geq$ 5) so that they are not consciously aware of their surroundings.
   - Adequately trained medical staff to look after the patient and the ventilator should be available all the time in the ICU. At no time the patient should be left unattended. The staff should preferably have appropriate anaesthetic experience.
   - The ventilator should be equipped with alarms, which should be on at all times. Hypoxaemia may result from emptying of oxygen cylinder (when not running on pipeline), loss of airway, disconnection from the ventilator, or ventilator malfunction.
   - Provision to suction the airway as and when required should be available round-the-clock.

2. **Consider indications.**
   NMBAs should be used only as a last resort when a patient cannot be managed by any other available modality. The suggested indications for use of NMBAs in the ICU are:
   (a) To facilitate the following short procedures under general anaesthesia: (i) Tracheal intubation, and (ii) surgical procedures, e.g. tracheotomy, emergency thoracotomy, bronchoscopy, and gastrointestinal endoscopy.
   (b) To facilitate mechanical ventilation with the following objectives in mind: (i) Increasing chest wall compliance, (ii) preventing patient-ventilator dyssynchrony, (iii) reducing peak airway pressure, (iv) reducing the risk of barotrauma, (v) allowing optimal gas exchange, and (vi) facilitating inverse ratio ventilation and permissive hypercapnia. NMBAs may be used in the above conditions when it is critical to maintain oxygenation despite the adequate use of sedation and analgesia.
   (c) To manage increased intracranial pressure, by preventing coughing and patient—ventilator dyssynchrony. However, there have been no controlled studies evaluating the role of NMBAs in the routine management of increased ICP.
   (d) To facilitate treatment of status epilepticus or tetanus. Muscle relaxants, however, should never be used as a substitute for rapid and effective anti-convulsive medication.
   (e) To decrease respiratory muscle oxygen consumption in patients with increased respiratory muscle work, when myocardial function is impaired or when oxygenation is critical. Studies have shown that although the use of neuromuscular blockade improves respiratory compliance, it does not alter intramucosal pH, oxygen consumption, oxygen delivery, or oxygen extraction ratio. Sedative drugs alone are usually adequate in this situation since the evidence for achieving this objective by neuromuscular blockade is not strong.

3. **Consider analgesics and sedatives.**
    See Chapter 7.
    Any patient receiving NMBAs must be sedated adequately to ensure unconsciousness, and the sedation used must be appropriate to meet this objective. Opioids alone cannot be relied upon to produce unconsciousness.

4. **Choose NMBA.**
    - There is no evidence of superiority of any one NMBA over the other but there is enough evidence in literature to show that pancuronium may be as good or better than other NMBAs, whenever indicated.
    - In patients where increase in heart rate is to be avoided (e.g. those with cardiovascular disease), other NMBAs may be used.
    - Atracurium is recommended for patients with significant hepatic or renal disease because of its unique metabolism.

5. **Decide the mode of delivery.**
    - Bolus administration of NMBAs offers potential advantages for controlling tachyphylaxis, monitoring for accumulation, analgesia and amnesia, limiting complications related to prolonged or excessive blockade and improving economics. However, NMBAs may also be administered by continuous infusion.
    - Atracurium, although can be given as repeated bolus injections, is usually administered by continuous infusion in an ICU setting.

6. **Use repeated bolus injections or a continuous infusion.**
    The doses for bolus or intermittent injections are:
    Pancuronium – 0.1 mg/kg every 90 minutes
    Vecuronium – 0.1 mg/kg every 35-40 minutes
    Rocuronium – 0.6 – 1.0 mg/kg every 25-30 minutes
    Atracurium – 0.4 – 0.5 mg/kg every 25-30 minutes.

    The doses for continuous infusion are:

	Loading dose (mg/kg)	Maintenance dose (μg/kg/min)
Pancuronium	0.06-0.1	1-2
Vecuronium	0.08-0.1	0.8-1.2
Rocuronium	0.6-1.0	10-12
Atracurium	0.4-0.5	4-12

    Reduce maintenance dose by half in case of renal or liver failure.

    - **Titrate the rate of infusion.**
      Titrate to minimum effective dose. For example, for pancuronium, decrease the dose by 0.35 μg/kg/min (= 0.02 mg/kg/hr) every 2 to 3 hours until the patient breathes above the preset ventilatory rate; then, increase the infusion rate by 0.02 mg/kg/hr.

7. **Monitor the response.**
    (a) Monitor clinically every 2-4 hours.

(b) With each change in dose of neuromuscular blocking agent, perform TOF every 1-2 hours until desired goal is achieved.

(c) Once a dose is standardized, monitor TOF every 12 hours.

- The response can be monitored clinically by observing skeletal muscle movement, patient-ventilator dyssynchrony, or by noting the respiratory efforts of the patient on ventilator (e.g. comparing the total respiratory rate on the ventilator with the set mandatory ventilatory breaths).
- When the purpose is to control the ventilation, complete paralysis is seldom required.
- When repeated bolus injections are used, one should aim at either small amounts of spontaneous movements or one and preferably two or three responses in TOF being present, before giving the next bolus.
- With continuous infusion, the goal should be to adjust the infusion rate to achieve one or two twitches in TOF stimulation. This is usually adequate for controlling respiration.
- If deeper blockade is necessary, for example in patients with raised intracranial pressure, PTC can be used when there is no TOF response. Almost complete PTC suppression may be needed to prevent diaphragmatic movement on tracheal suction. The block should be allowed to wear off at least twice a day until one or two twitches are present in TOF.

8. **Stop NMBAs at least once, every day.**

 Stopping NMBAs daily may decrease the incidence of myopathy. Discontinuation of NMBA administration should occur at least once in every 24 hours (until forced to restart them based on the patient's condition) as this decreases the incidence of complications, helps prevent overdose or accumulation of active metabolites, and allows early recognition of prolonged blockade.

9. **Adopt general measures.**

 General care includes prophylactic eye care (methylcellulose drops, ophthalmic ointment, taping the eyelids shut to ensure complete closure), prevention of soft tissue injury and pressure necrosis, prophylaxis for deep venous thrombosis, and physical therapy to maintain joint mobility.

References

1. Bevan DR. Neuromuscular blockade: Inadvertent extubation of the partially paralyzed patient. Anesthesiol Clin North Am 2001; 19(4): 913-922.
2. Bolton CF. Neuromuscular complications of sepsis. Intensive Care Med 1993; 19:558-563.
3. Elliot JM, Bion JF. The use of neuromuscular blocking drugs in intensive care practice. Acta Anaesthesiol Scand Suppl 1995; 106:70-82.
4. Ford EV. Monitoring neuromuscular blockade in the adult ICU. Am J Crit Care 1995; 4:122-130
5. Freebairn RC, Derrick J, Gomersall CD, et al. Oxygen delivery, oxygen consumption, and gastric intramucosal pH are not improved by a computer-controlled, closed-loop, vecuronium infusion in severe. Crit Care Med 1997; 25:72-77.

6. Hansen-Flaschen J H, Brazinsky S, Basile C, Lanken PN. Use of sedation drugs and neuromuscular blocking agents in-patient requiring mechanical ventilation for respiratory failure. A national survey. JAMA 1991:226:2870-2875.

7. Hoyt JW. Persistent paralysis in critically ill patients after the use of neuromuscular blocking agents. New Horiz 1994; 2:48-55.

8. Lopez DM, Singer LP, Weingarten-Arams JS, et al. Use of neuromuscular blocking agents and sedation in pediatric patients and associated prolonged neuromuscular weakness. Pharm Ther 1999; 24:290-296.

9. Luer JM. Sedation and chemical relaxation in critical pulmonary illness: suggestions for patient assessment and drug monitoring. AACN Clin Issues 1995; 6:333-343.

10. Martin R, Bourdua I. Theriault S, et al. Neuromuscular monitoring: does it make a difference? Can J anesth 1996; 43:585-588.

11. Murray MJ, Coursin DB, Scuderi PE, et al. Double blind, randomized, multicenter study of doxacurium vs. pancuronium in intensive care unit patients who require neuromuscular blocking agents. Crit Care Med 1995;23;450-458.

12. Murry MJ et al. clinical practice guidelines for sustained neuromuscular blockade in the adult critically ill patient. Developed through the task force of ACCM, SCCM, and ASMP. Crit Care Med 2002; 30(1): 142-156.

13. Pino RM. Neuromuscular blocker studies of critically ill patients. Intensive Care Med 2002; 28:1695-1697.

14. Rudis MI, Sikora CP, Angus E, et al. A prospective, randomized, controlled evaluation of peripheral nerve stimulation versus standard clinical dosing of neuromuscular blocking agents in critically ill patients. Crit Care Med 1997; 25:575-583.

15. Shapiro BA, Warren J, Egol AB, et al. Practice parameters for sustained neuromuscular blockade in the adult critically ill patient: an executive summary. Crit Care Med 1995; 23:1601-1605.

16. Strange C, Vaughan L, Franklin C, et al. Comparison of train-of-four and best clinical assessment during continuous paralysis. Am J Resp Crit Care Med 1997; 156:1556-1561.

17. Tavernier B, Rannou JJ, Vallet B. Peripheral nerve stimulation and clinical assessment for dosing of neuromuscular blocking agents in critically all patients. Crit Care Med 1998; 26:804-805.

18. Viby-Mogensen J. Monitoring neuromuscular function in the intensive care unit. Intensive Care Med 1993:19:S75-S79.

19. Watling SM, Dasta JF. Prolonged paralysis in intensive care unit patients after the use of neuromuscular blocking agents: a review of the literature. Crit Care Med 1994; 22:884-893.

20. Wong KC. Narcotics are not expected to produce unconsciousness and amnesia. Anesth Analg 1983:62:625-626.

Arterial Puncture and Cannulation

Introduction

- Analysis of the arterial blood provides an evaluation of the patient's oxygenation, ventilation, and acid-base status.
- Indications for arterial cannulation include haemodynamic monitoring in high risk patients, frequent (3 or more per day) arterial blood gas (ABG) sampling, arterial administration of drugs such as thrombolytics, and the use of intra aortic balloon pump.
- Radial artery is the preferred site for puncture and cannulation as it is superficial and easily accessible, is not adjacent to large veins, and has potentially good collateral circulation from the ulnar artery. Ulnar artery provides an adequate flow in approximately 92% cases of total occlusion of the radial artery.
- Presence of collateral flow to the area distal to the site of arterial cannulation should be evaluated before cannulation. For radial arterial lines, a modified Allen's test is performed.
- For simple arterial puncture, modified Allen's test need not be performed routinely in adults, as there is no report of total occlusion of the radial artery after puncture for ABG.
- Contraindications to using radial artery include absent ulnar circulation, impaired circulation (e.g. Raynaud's disease or Buerger's disease), and an arteriovenous fistula for dialysis.
- If a radial artery is not accessible, dorsalis pedis, posterior tibial, superficial temporal (in infants), brachial, and femoral arteries are the suitable alternatives. Radial and femoral catheters constitute more than 90% of all the catheterizations.
- Arterial catheters can be safely left in place for upto 4 days without the risk of increase in the incidence of infection. The site of insertion does not appear to be an important factor for the incidence of infection.
- Complications associated with arterial cannulation include thrombosis, embolization, haematoma, haemorrhage, ischaemia, and infection.

GUIDELINES FOR ARTERIAL PUNCTURE AND FOR ARTERIAL CATHETER INSERTION

1. Check whether the blood gas analyser is ready. (if the puncture is being made for drawing a sample).

    Before drawing an arterial sample, make sure that the analyzer is working, has been calibrated, and a competent person, who knows how to use it, is available.

2. **Fill in the 'request form' accurately.**
   The 'request form' should accurately mention the patient's inspired oxygen concentration. This is essential for interpretation of the results.

3. **Wash hands.**
   This reduces the risk of transmission of micro-organisms.

4. **Reassure the patient.**
   Explain to the patient, the procedure to be performed and allay his anxiety.

5. **Perform modified Allen's test (Figs. 9.1–9.4).**
   The test is performed to assess the patency of the ulnar artery and intactness of the superficial palmer arch.

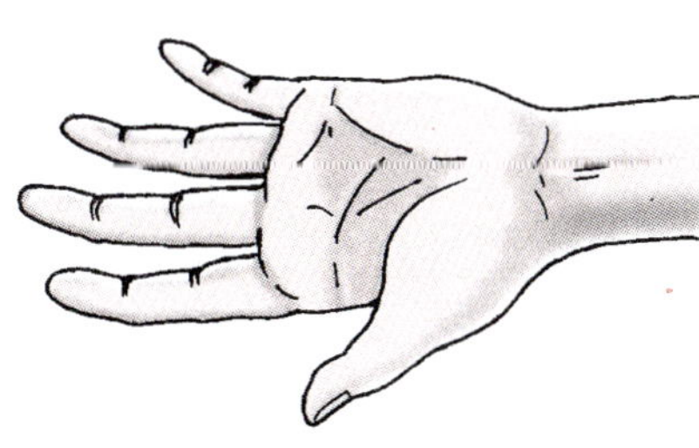

Fig. 9.1: Hand at rest.

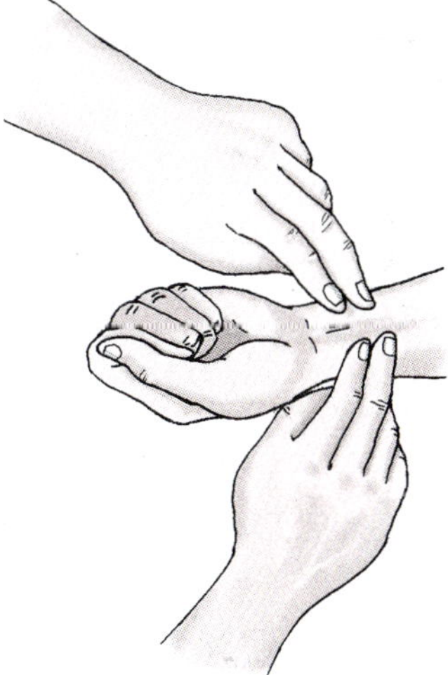

Fig. 9.2: Patient clenches his fist and a pressure is applied over the radial and ulnar arteries.

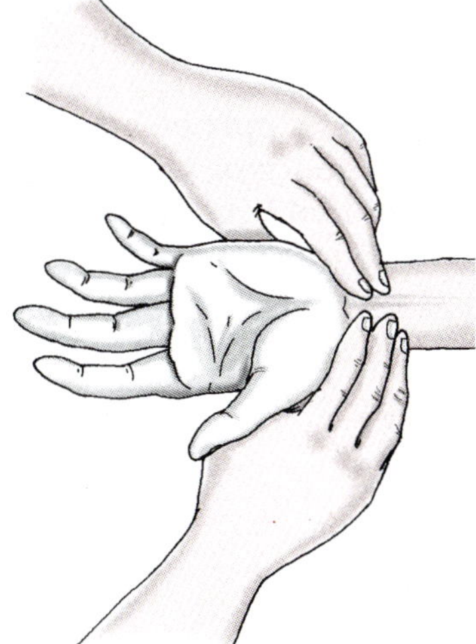

Fig. 9.3: With compression of the arteries the hand becomes pale.

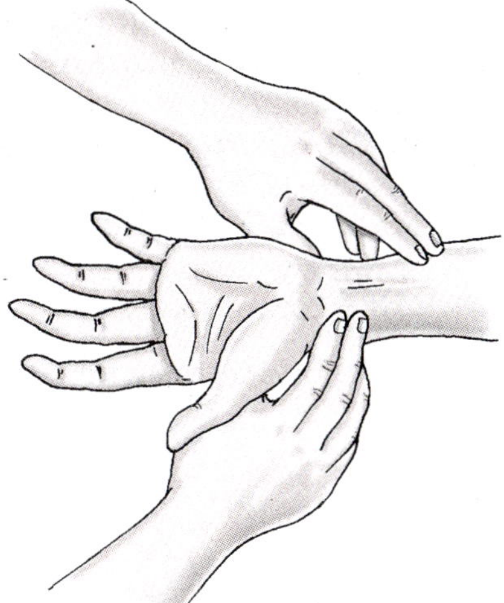

Fig. 9.4: Ulnar artery compression is released. The distinct pink coloration of the palm indicates good ulnar circulation.

(a) Hold the patient's hand with the palm facing upwards.

(b) Occlude ulnar and radial arteries while the patient rapidly closes and opens the hand a few times and then finally clenches his fist tightly.

   This manoeuvre forces blood out of the hand.

(c) Ask the patient to open the hand.

   Observe palm and fingers for blanching.

(d) If the area is blanched, release the pressure on the ulnar artery.

   Watch for the return of colour. Return of colour within 7 seconds indicates patency of the ulnar artery and an intact superficial palmer arch. If the colour returns between 8 and 14 seconds, the test is considered equivocal. If it takes 15 seconds or more for the colour to return, the test is considered negative. If the test is negative, perform the test on the opposite hand.

6. Wash hands and wear gloves.

   This reduces the risk of transmission of micro-organisms.

7. Place the patient in a semi-recumbent or supine position on the bed with the selected, non-dominant arm hyperextended and supported on a pillow. Extend the wrist by (20º-30º) with a rolled towel, to move radial artery into a more superficial position.

   This provides an optimal position for arterial puncture.

8. Prepare the site.

   Use povidone-iodine followed by alcohol.

9. Drape the area around the site with sterile towels.

   It minimizes transmission of micro-organisms.

10. Anaesthetize the puncture site with plain xylocaine (1%) using a 25G needle. Inject sufficient volume (approximately 0.2 –0.3 mL solution for an adult) to raise a wheal.

   - It reduces discomfort to the patient and consequent hyperventilation and prevents arterial spasm.
   - Pain and anxiety, in the absence of local analgesia, may be associated with breath holding which may lead to altered blood gas values. Thirty-five seconds of breath holding in normal subjects has been associated with a fall in PaO_2 by 50 mmHg and pH by 0.07 and a rise in $PaCO_2$ by 10 mmHg.
   - EMLA cream may be used as an alternative to intradermal xylocaine.

Follow steps 11-16 for arterial puncture and steps 17-20 for arterial catheter insertion.

11. Locate the artery. Using the index and middle fingers of the non-dominant hand, palpate the artery to locate a point where the strongest pulse is found (Fig. 9.5).

12. Take a heparinized syringe and a needle (22G) to perform the puncture.

   - Glass syringe is preferable as plastic syringe is much more permeable to oxygen than glass. Diffusion of oxygen through the walls of plastic syringes

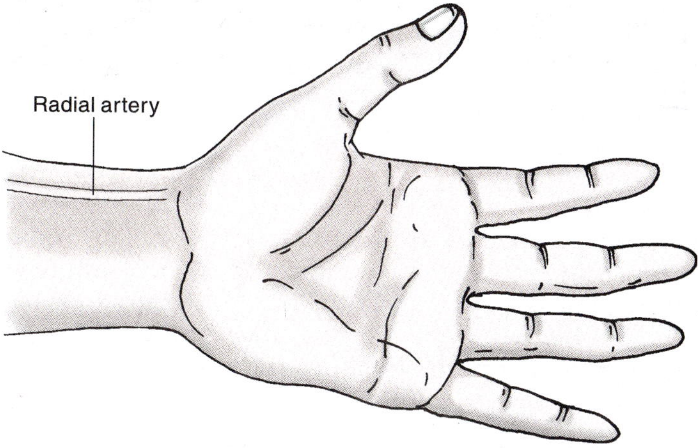

Fig. 9.5: Surface anatomy of the radial artery.

may lead to a false reduction in the measured PaO_2, particularly in samples with high oxygen tension.

- The syringe should only be *rinsed* with heparin. PaO_2 and HCO_3^- show an inverse relationship to the volume of heparin used, especially if the volume exceeds 10% of the sample volume. Also, heparin 5000 IU/mL is acidic and may influence the pH reading as well.

13. For performing a puncture, hold the syringe with the needle at an angle of 45º, with the bevel of the needle facing the flow of blood (bevel up) (Fig. 9.6). Advance the needle slowly towards the artery.

    When the artery is punctured, blood from the artery should pulsate into the syringe. It should not be necessary to aspirate or pull back the plunger to fill

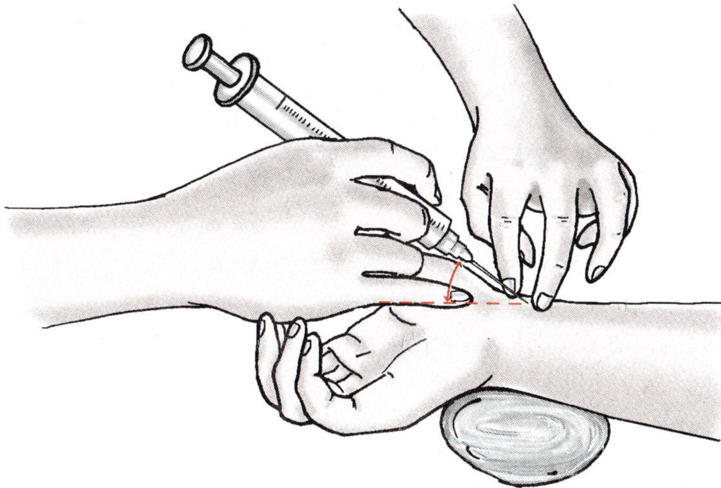

Fig. 9.6: Inserting needle into the radial artery, bevel facing upwards, at an angle of 45° to the skin.

the syringe. If the needle goes through the artery, slowly withdraw the needle until it re-enters the artery. If the attempt is unsuccessful, withdraw the needle to the level of the subcutaneous tissue and redirect it.

14. Obtain a sample and withdraw the needle. Express any air bubble, cap the sample immediately, and roll the syringe between both the palms for 5-15 seconds. Apply firm pressure on the puncture site for at least 5 minutes.
    - PO_2 of air in the room is approximately 150 mmHg and PCO_2 is negligible. When large air bubbles (more than 0.5-1% of sample volume) are mixed with arterial blood, PaO_2 and the $PaCO_2$ will diffuse in or out of the sample from the bubbles, thereby altering the results.
    - Rolling is done to mix the heparin and the blood.

15. Analyse the sample as soon as possible.
    Any sample that cannot be measured in less than 10 minutes must be sealed, packed in ice and measured within 1 hour, as the $PaCO_2$ rises approximately 3 to 10 mmHg/hr in an un-iced specimen, causing a fall in pH. There is also a fall in PaO_2 which can be substantial in patients with leukaemia and/or thrombocytosis.

16. If the sample cannot be obtained, ask for help.
    It is better to seek help than to try repeatedly. As taking sample is painful, it makes the patient hyperventilate, and this means the result one gets is not truly representative of the patient's condition.

17. For cannulation, take a 20G, 2 inch, non-tapered, PVC/Teflon catheter over needle.
18. Once the artery is punctured as in step 13, slowly advance both catheter and needle. Change (reduce) the angle and bring the catheter and needle closer/near to skin. Advance the catheter over the needle with a steady rotatory action.
    - At times it becomes difficult to advance the catheter over the needle. Replacing the needle and slightly advancing catheter and needle into the artery can solve the problem.
    - An alternative approach is to go through the posterior wall of the vessel. The needle is then removed and the catheter pulled back until a spurt of arterial blood is noted. The needle is then inserted partially into the catheter and the catheter is advanced over the needle with a steady rotatory motion.

19. Fix the catheter to the skin with a suture, attach to the transducer tubing, and apply a dry sterile dressing.
    Fixing reduces chances of accidental dislodgement.

20. Dispose of the needle according to the policy of the hospital.
    This reduces the risk of transmission of micro-organisms

21. Remove gloves and wash hands.

References

1. Adems AP, Morgan-Hyghes JO, Sykes MK. pH and blood gas analysis: Methods of measurement and sources of error using electrode systems. Anaesthesia 1967; 22:575.
2. Bloom SA, Canzanello VJ, Strom JA, et al. Spurious assessment of acid-base status due to dilutional effect of heparin. Am J Med 1985; 79:528.
3. Cerveri I, Zoia MC, Fanfulla F, et al. Reference values of arterial oxygen tension in the middle-aged and elderly. Am J Respir Crit Care Med 1995;152:934.
4. Curley FJ, Irwin RS. Disorders of temperature control,: Hyperthermia. J Intens Care Med 1986;1:5s, 270.
5. Giner J, Casan P, Belda J, et al. Pain during arterial puncture. Chest 1996;110:1443.
6. Gronbeck C, Miller EL. Non physician placement of arterial catheters: Experience with 500 insertions. Chest 1993;104:1716.
7. Gwinnutt C. How to take an arterial blood gas sample. In: Driscol P, Brown T, Gwinnutt C, Wardle T (eds). A simple guide to blood gas analysis, 2 ed. BMJ Publishing Group, 2000, pp, 1-14.
8. Hansen JE, Simmons DH. A systematic error in the determination of blood PCO_2. Am Rev Respir Dis 1977;115:1061.
9. Martin L. All you really need to know to interpret arterial blood gases. Philadelphia: Lippincott, Williams & Wilkins, 2 ed., 1999, pp 218-223.

Central Venous Pressure   10

Introduction

- Central venous pressure (CVP) is the pressure of blood in the right atrium or the vena cava. Because the tricuspid valve is open during diastole, CVP also represents the end-diastolic pressure in the right ventricle (RVEDP) and reflects preload for the right ventricle. CVP can also reflect left heart filling pressure in young patients with no hypertension, cardiac disease, or pulmonary disease.
- Conditions causing increased CVP include elevated vascular volume, increased intrathoracic pressure, constrictive pericarditis, cardiac tamponade, pulmonary hypertension, right heart failure, venoconstriction, pulmonary embolism, tricuspid regurgitation, pulmonary stenosis and infusion of solution into the CVP line.
- Conditions causing decreased CVP include hypovolaemia, spontaneous inspiration, vasodilatation (by drugs or hyperthermia), placement of transducer or zero level of the water manometer above the patient's right atrial level and air bubbles or leaks in the pressure line.
- While interpreting the measured central venous pressure, vascular tone should also be taken into account. For example, when venous tone is high (prolonged sympathetic stimulation, heart failure), a normal blood volume may result in a venous pressure so high that pulmonary edema is produced. Conversely, when venous tone is low (sympathetic paralysis, barbiturate overdosage), a normal blood volume may still result in such a low venous pressure that cardiac filling is inadequate and cardiac output low. Therefore, venous pressure should be interpreted in conjunction with the physical signs of vasoconstriction or vasodilatation.
- Central venous pressure measurements are best made and compared at the same point in the ventilatory cycle – usually end-expiration. When positive end-expiratory pressure (PEEP) is applied, the positive pressure is transmitted through the right atrium, causing a decrease in venous return and a rise in CVP. The magnitude of this effect of PEEP on CVP varies with pulmonary compliance and blood volume.
- A single reading of CVP is not significant. Monitoring trends in CVP readings is more meaningful.
- Understanding a, c, and v waves is necessary. The 'a' wave reflects right atrial contraction and occurs during ventricular diastole. The 'c' wave reflects the closure of the tricuspid valve. The 'v' wave reflects the right atrial filling during ventricular systole when the AV valve is closed.

- CVP may be obtained using a transducer system or a water manometer. Water manometer usually overestimates transducer – determined mean CVP. This is because water does not fall to the mean pressure in each cardiac cycle and also because location of the tip cannot be verified as the individual waves cannot be seen and wide fluctuations of the water column do not occur even when the catheter is located in the right ventricle. When changing from one system to the other, it is important to know that the values will be different. Water manometer measures centimeters of water pressure, whereas transducer measures mmHg (1 mmHg = 1.36 cm H_2O).
- Normal CVP: < 6 mmHg by transducer; < 12 cm H_2O by water manometer.

GUIDELINES FOR CVP MEASUREMENT

Water Manometer System

1. **Wash hands.**
   This reduces the risk of transmission of micro-organisms.

2. **Confirm the position of CVP catheter.**
   Look for the following:
   - Free-flowing intravenous fluid.
   - Ability to easily aspirate a blood sample from the CVP catheter.
   - A rapidly falling water column when the pressure is obtained.
   - Small oscillations at the top of the water column indicating changes in CVP during the cardiac cycle.
   - Larger oscillations occurring with respiration.
   - X-ray verification of the tip of the catheter (if possible).

3. **Position the bed so that the patient is supine with the head of the bed flat or elevated, no more than 60º.**
   Intracardiac pressures may be accurate for patients in the supine position with the head of the bed elevated to 60º or less. A uniform atrial reference point for prone and lateral positions has not been identified.

4. **Locate the phlebostatic axis.**
   The phlebostatic axis is defined as "the junction between the transverse plane of the body passing through the fourth intercostal space at the lateral margin of the sternum, and a frontal plane of the body passing through the midpoint of a line from the outermost point of the sternum to the outermost point of the posterior chest", or more simply stated, the mid-chest level at the fourth intercostal space. The reference point recommended for the lateral decubitus position is the fourth intercostal space midsternum, although further studies are required to support this.

5. **Mark the atrial reference point on the patient's skin with an indelible marker.**
   It will ensure that future readings are taken at the same location.

6. Use a carpenter's level to match the zero level of the manometer with the phlebostatic axis.

    This permits accurate measurements.

7. Turn the water manometer stopcock open to the IV fluid bag and open the IV tubing roller clamp so that fluid flows from the IV fluid bag into the water manometer (Fig. 10.1, System A).

    This ensures that there are no air bubbles in the manometer. Fill two-thirds of the manometer or fill it above the level of the expected CVP measurement. Overfilling will cause contamination, and underfilling will result in an inaccurate measurement.

8. Close the roller clamp on the IV tubing.

9. Turn the water manometer stopcock open to the patient and closed to the IV solution (Fig. 10.1, System B).

    The fluid column in the manometer will fall faster initially and then gradually to the point where fluid column equalizes with the right atrial pressure. Oscillations in the water column occurring with respiration can be seen.

10. Measure the CVP reading.

    The CVP measurement should be recorded at end-expiration.
    - For an awake and alert patient—ask the patient to stop breathing for a few seconds at end-expiration.
    - For a patient who cannot follow commands and is not on PEEP or on low PEEP—disconnect the ventilator for a few seconds.

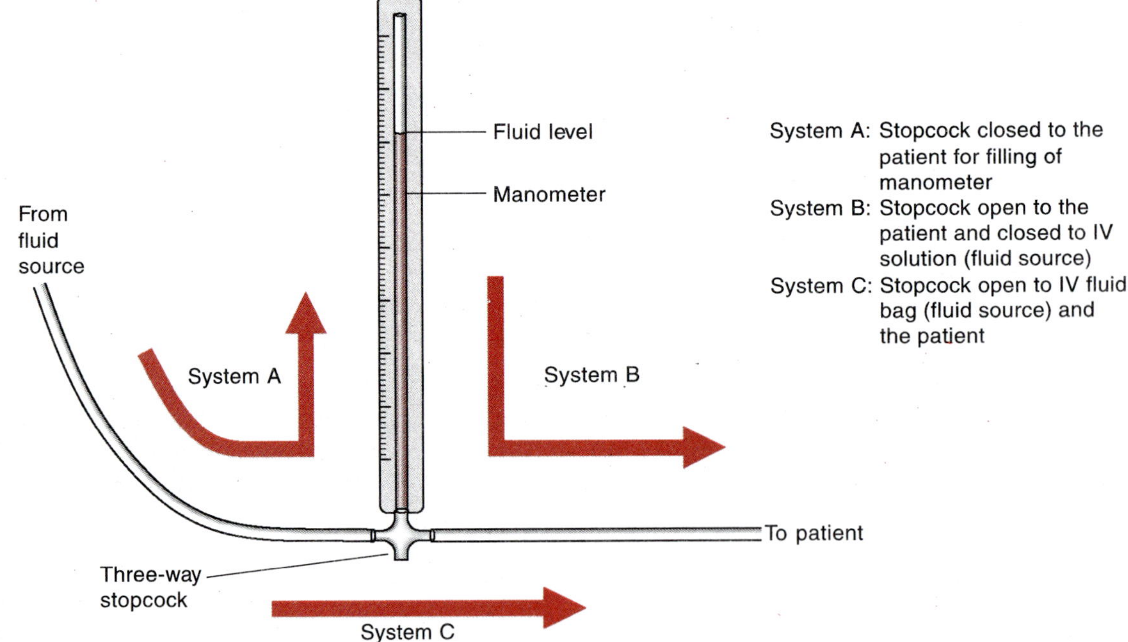

Fig. 10.1: Central venous pressure measurement.

- For a patient on mechanical ventilation with high PEEP—DO NOT disconnect the ventilator from the patient as it may cause acute haemodynamic changes, induce stress, and promote pulmonary edema, especially in patients whose extravascular lung water content is high and whose PEEP level is more than 10 cm H_2O. In these patients, an esophageal probe can be inserted to estimate transthoracic pressure. Subtracting the transthoracic pressure from the CVP provides transmural pressure, which is a better estimate of right atrial pressure in the presence of elevated transthoracic pressure.

11. Turn the water manometer stopcock open to the IV fluid bag and to the patient (Fig. 10.1, System C).

Adjust the rate of fluid to prevent clotting of the catheter.

12. Wash hands.

References

1. Brisman R, Parks IC, Benson DW. Pitfalls in the clinical use of central venous pressure. Arch Surg 1967; 95:902.
2. Chapin JC, Downs JB, Douglas ME, et al. Lung expansion, airway pressure transmission, and positive end-expiratory pressure. Arch Surg 1979; 114:1193-1197.
3. Davidson R, Parker M, Harrison RA. The validity of determinations of pulmonary wedge pressure during mechanical ventilation. Chest 1978; 73:352.
4. DelGuercia LRM, Cohn JD. Monitoring: methods and significance. Surg Clin North Am 1976; 56:977.
5. Krider SJ. Invasively monitored hemodynamic pressures. In: Wilkins RL, Krider SJ, Scheldon RL (eds). Clinical assessment in respiratory care, 4 ed. St. Louis: Mosby. 2000, pp. 331-371.
6. Pinsky MR. The influence of positive-pressure ventilation on cardiovascular function in the critically ill. Crit Care Clin 1985; 1:699.
7. Rajacich N et al. Central venous pressure and pulmonary capillary wedge pressure as estimates of left atrial pressure: effects of positive end-expiratory pressure and catheter tip malposition. Crit Care Med 1989; 17:7.

11

Fluid Challenge

Introduction

- Hypovolaemia is not only the primary mechanism of shock but can also complicate cardiogenic, distributive and obstructive types of shock. Therefore, volume replacement represents the single, most important therapeutic intervention in the management of shock. However, overzealous fluid administration may result in cardiac decompensation and pulmonary edema, especially in older patients and those with compromised cardiac function.
- Since, CVP (central venous pressure) and PCWP (pulmonary capillary wedge pressure) reflect both, the vascular volume and the ability of the ventricle to pump, these pressures can be used to guide fluid challenge. A fluid challenge can help assess both volume deficits and pump failure.
- Large volume of fluid may be safely administered, utilizing the simple "5-2" and "7-3" rules of fluid challenge. The fluid challenge is repeated until measurements indicate that adequate volume expansion has occured. The fluid challenge is discontinued as soon as haemodynamic signs of shock are reversed or signs of cardiac decompensation are evident.

GUIDELINES FOR FLUID CHALLENGE IN ADULTS

1. **Monitor the filling pressure.**
   Fluid challenge can be guided either by CVP or by PCWP.

2. **Select the volume of fluid to be given as a fluid challenge.**
   - If CVP is < 8 cmH$_2$O (or PCWP is < 12 mmHg): Select a fluid challenge volume of 200 mL.
   - If CVP is 8-14 cmH$_2$O (or PCWP is 12-16 mmHg): Select a fluid challenge volume of 100mL.
   - If CVP is >14 cmH$_2$O (or PCWP is >16 mmHg): Select a fluid challenge volume of 50mL.

3. **Infuse selected fluid challenge volume over 10 minutes.**
   Monitor CVP/PCWP continuously while infusion is going on. If rise in pressure is more than 5 cmH$_2$O in CVP or more than 7 mmHg in PCWP: Stop the infusion and continue to monitor.

4. **Continue to monitor after the selected fluid volume is infused.**
   Immediately after challenge:

- If rise in CVP is less than 2 cmH_2O (or in PCWP is < 3 mmHg): Repeat the challenge.
- If rise in CVP is 2-5 cmH_2O (or in PCWP is 3-7 mmHg): Wait for 10 minutes. Continue to monitor.

10 minutes after challenge:

- If rise in CVP is ≤ 2 cmH_2O (or in PCWP ≤ 3 mmHg): Repeat the challenge.
- If rise in CVP is > 2 cmH_2O (or in PCWP > 3mmHg): Stop the infusion, continue to monitor.

5. Fluid administration is continued until either the haemodynamic signs of shock are corrected or the CVP "5-2" rule or the PCWP "7-3" rule is violated.

GUIDELINES FOR FLUID CHALLENGE IN CHILDREN

1. Monitor the filling pressure.

    Fluid challenge can be guided by either CVP or by PCWP (pulmonary capillary wedge pressure).

2. Select the volume of fluid to be given as a fluid challenge.
    - If CVP is < 10 cmH_2O (or PCWP is < 15 mmHg): Select a fluid challenge volume of 4mL/Kg.
    - If CVP is ≥ 10 cmH_2O (or PCWP is ≥ 15 mmHg): Select a fluid challenge volume of 2 mL/kg.

3. Infuse selected fluid challenge volume over 10 minutes.

    Monitor CVP/PCWP continuously while infusion is going on. If rise in pressure is more than 4 cmH_2O in CVP or more than 7 mmHg in PCWP: Stop the infusion and continue to monitor.

4. Continue to monitor after the selected fluid volume is infused.

    Immediately after challenge:

    - If rise in CVP is less than 2 cmH_2O (or in PCWP is < 3 mmHg): Repeat the challenge.
    - If rise in CVP is 2-4 cmH_2O (or in PCWP is 3-7 mmHg): Wait for 10 minutes. Continue to monitor.

    10 minutes after challenge:

    - If rise in CVP is ≤ 2 cmH_2O (or in PCWP ≤ 3 mmHg): Repeat the challenge.
    - If rise in CVP is > 2 cmH_2O (or in PCWP >3 mmHg): Stop the infusion, continue to monitor.

5. Fluid administration is continued, keeping the above guidelines in mind.

References

1. Krider SJ. Invasively monitored hemodynamic pressures. In: Wilkins RL, Krider SJ, Sheldon RL (eds). Clinical assessment in respiratory care, 4ed. St. Louis: Mosby, 2000, pp 358-360.

2. Raphachy RC, Browning RA. The role of preload in the manipulation of the failing circulation. In: Swenlow DB, Raphaely RC, eds. Cardiovascular problems in pediatric critical care. New York: Churchill Livingstone, 1986.
3. Rubenstein JS, Hageman JR. Monitoring of crtically ill infants and children. Crit Care Clin 1988;4:621.
4. Weil MH, Henning RJ. New concepts in the diagnosis and fluid treatment of circulatory shock. Anaesth Analges 1979:58(2):124-131.

Defibrillation 12

Introduction

- Cardiac arrest in adults is not uncommon and those who can be saved from the cardiac arrest are mostly the individuals who developed ventricular fibrillation (VF) or pulseless ventricular tachycardia (VT). These disturbances of rhythm are most commonly caused by coronary artery disease and are usually associated with myocardial infarction. Electrical defibrillation provides the single, most important therapy for the treatment of these patients.
- Defibrillation refers to the delivery of electrical current to the heart muscle either directly through open chest, or indirectly through the chest wall, to terminate VF and VT. The goal is to restore co-ordinated electrical and mechanical pumping action, resulting in adequate cardiac output, tissue perfusion, and oxygenation.
- The greatest chances of survival result when the interval between the start of VF and the delivery of defibrillation is as brief as possible, and when cardiopulmonary resuscitation is administered during the arrest-shock interval.
- The defibrillator contains a capacitor which (on charging) accepts a charge, stores the energy and delivers it to the patient in a short controlled pulse. Typical duration of the defibrillator pulse is three to nine milliseconds, but it can vary with the defibrillator model.
- A number of factors, patient related or operational, can affect the defibrillation outcome. Patient factors include the duration of pre-shock VF (longer than 10 minutes is associated with low survival rate), the functional state of the myocardium, acid-base balance, hypoxia, early initiation of adequate CPR (may improve the chances of defibrillation success), and administration of certain drugs like epinephrine. Operational factors include paddle position, energy level, and transthoracic impedance.
- External defibrillation has been effective for over 40 years with two types of monophasic waveforms: damped sinusoidal and truncated exponential. Recently, biphasic waveforms have become available in external defibrillation. Since efficacy of defibrillation is a function of both the waveform and the shock dose used for that waveform, implementation of different waveforms at similar dose, or similar waveforms at different doses, may result in different clinical efficacies (Fig. 12.1).
- Biphasic waveforms have higher defibrillation efficiency per unit energy and are affected to a lesser degree by transthoracic impedance, when compared to monophasic waveforms. In other words, when compared with monophasic

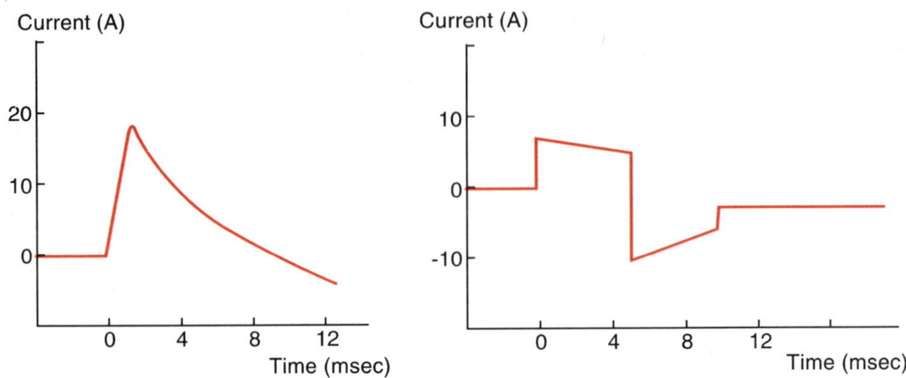

Fig. 12.1: Defibrillation waveforms. Left, monophasic waveform. Right, biphasic waveform.
Monophasic waveforms deliver current in one direction. Biphasic waveforms, in contrast, deliver current that flows in a positive direction for a specified duration. The current then reverses and flows in a negative direction for the remaining milliseconds of the electrical discharge.

shocks, biphasic shocks are equally effective and use less delivered energy which may result in less post-shock myocardial dysfunction.

- The ideal sequence of energy settings for biphasic defibrillators, in the management of VF/pulseless VT is presently not clear. Although low (150-200 Joules) energy biphasic waveforms appear to be as effective as high energy (200-360 Joules) monophasic shocks, it is not known whether higher energy biphasic shocks are more effective than low energy biphasic shocks.
- One of the suggested recommendations, until clear evidence is available, is that biphasic energy settings for the treatment of VF/pulseless VT may be similar to traditional monophase shock settings (200, 200–300, 360 J followed by triplets of 360 J). This recommendation is based upon: (a) The paucity of guiding evidence, (b) the possibility that high energy biphasic shock is more effective than low energy shock, and (c) the expectation that most rescuers will wish to escalate energy settings to the maximum available in the case of VF/VT refractory to low energy shocks.

GUIDELINES FOR EXTERNAL DEFIBRILLATION

1. **Prepare the patient.**
   Preparation of the patient includes positioning the patient supine, removing loose dentures, initiating basic life support if immediate defibrillation is not available, oxygenating the patient, removing clothings from upper half of body, removing excessive hair from the electrode/paddle site, cleaning the skin, and drying it with towel or gauze. Do not apply alcohol or tincture of benzoin to the skin.

2. **Wash hands.**
   This reduces the risk of transmission of micro-organisms.

3. **Switch on the defibrillator and place it in the defibrillation mode.**
    Make sure that the defibrillator is not in the synchronized mode. In this mode the defibrillator will not fire in the absence of a QRS complex.

4. **Apply conductive gel to the paddle electrodes or on the patient's chest. Gel should be evenly distributed on the defibrillator paddles.**
    Skin is a poor conductor of electricity. Therefore, a conductive interface material (gel) is required to reduce impedance at the junction between the skin and the paddles. Use only defibrillation or ECG gel or paste, since ultrasonic gel or any other lubricant may not be sufficiently conductive and may increase the transthoracic impedance.

5. **Ensure that the defibrillator cables are positioned to allow for adequate access to the patient.**

6. **Switch on the ECG recorder for continuous printout.**
    This provides a permanent record of the response to defibrillation.

7. **Select the energy to be delivered and charge the defibrillator.**
    The energy selected should be enough to generate sufficient current flow through the heart (transmyocardial current) to achieve defibrillation while causing minimal electrical injury to the heart. In adults, there is no definite relationship between body size and energy requirement for defibrillation. In children, the recommended sequence is 2, 2, and 4 J/kg, followed by subsequent shocks at 4 J/kg. Recommended energy levels for adults are 200 J, 200-300 J, 360 J, followed by subsequent shocks at 360 J.
    The intent of this escalating energy dosage protocol is to maximize shock success (termination of VF) while minimizing shock toxicity.
    In patients with an implanted pacemaker, no adjustments in defibrillation energy are necessary.

8. **Place the paddles on the chest (Fig. 12.2).**
    *   The paddles should be so placed that the heart (primarily the ventricles) is

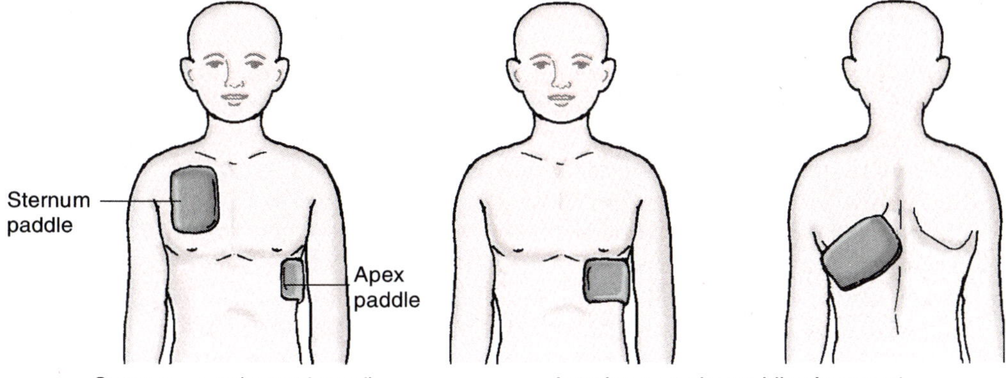

Fig. 12.2: Proper positions for anterolateral and anterior-posterior paddle placement.

in the pathway of the current. Bone is not a good conductor of electricity; therefore, paddles should not be placed over the sternum. Two positions for paddles placement have been recommended: (a) antero-lateral position – the anterior paddle is placed on the patient's upper right chest, to the right of the sternum below the clavicle. The apex paddle is placed on the patient's lower left chest, to the left of the nipple with the center of the paddle on the mid-axillary line. Avoid placement over a woman's breast to reduce transthoracic impedance. (b) anterior-posterior position – the anterior paddle is placed over the apex of the heart just to the left of the left sternal border. The posterior paddle is placed on the patient's back (posterior chest) beneath the left scapula and lateral to the spine.

- Antero-lateral position is used more frequently because of the ease of placement of paddles.
- In patients with an implanted pacemaker, placing the paddles in the anterior-posterior reduces the potential for pacemaker damage.
- For internal defibrillation, place one paddle over the apex of the left ventricle and the other over the base of the right ventricle.
- Do not permit gel to accumulate between the paddle electrodes on the chest wall. This will cause defibrillating energy to arc between paddles (causing burns) and will reduce the amount of energy delivered to the heart.

9. **Apply appropriate pressure to each paddle against the chest wall.**

    Appropriate pressure (approx. 12 kg per paddle) improves contact between the skin surface and the paddles, and reduces the transthoracic impedance. Remember, air pockets between the skin and paddles can cause skin burns.

10. **Ensure that all the personnel are clear of contact with the patient, and the bed.**

    It maximizes safety because electric current can be conducted from the patient to another person, if contact occurs.

11. **Verify that the patient is still in VF or pulseless VT.**

12. **Press both the buttons on paddles simultaneously, and release after defibrillator fires.**

    - Since air is a poor conductor of electricity, transthoracic impedance is decreased when shocks are delivered during end-expiration as compared to inspiration.
    - Normal response to the electrical charge is a 'jerk' or a 'jump' in the patient's body. If it is not visible, there could be many possibilities: the electrical charge may not have been delivered; or if the charge was delivered, the response may be diminished or absent due to prolonged cardiac arrest, drugs such as sedatives and anaesthetics, hypothermia, drug overdose, and size and general condition of the patient's musculature.

13. **Observe/monitor for conversion of dysrhythmia.**

14. **If successful, turn the defibrillator off, clean the paddles thoroughly, prior to storing them.**

15. Continue to monitor the patient after defibrillation.

- Monitor blood pressure, heart rate, and rhythm immediately after defibrillation and every 5-10 minutes until stable.
- Monitor electrolytes, ABG.
- Initiate antiarrhythmic therapy, as indicated, if not already started. Dysrhythmias may develop again after successful defibrillation.

16. If unsuccessful, repeat the shock and if third attempt is unsuccessful, initiate ACLS (advanced cardiac life support).

- Epinephrine 1 mg IV, repeated every 3-5 minutes or Vasopressin 40 units IV as a single dose, one time only. If no response for 5-10 minutes after a single dose of vasopressin, resume epinephrine 1 mg IV, every 3-5 minutes.
- Resume attempts to defibrillate (360 J).
- Consider antiarrhythmics (only fair evidence supports possible benefit of antiarrhythmics for shock-refractory VF/VT).
- Sodium bicarbonate 1mEq/kg IV, when indicated.
- Resume defibrillation attempts: Use 360 J shock after each medication or after each minute of CPR. Acceptable patterns include: CPR-drug-shock (repeat) or CPR-drug-shock-shock-shock (repeat).
- Antiarrhythmic agents: (a) Amiodarone 300 mg IV push. If VF/VT recurs, consider second dose of 150 mg IV. Maximum cumulative dose 2.2 g over 24 hours, (b) Xylocaine 1.0 – 1.5 mg/kg IV push. Consider repeat in 3 to 5 minutes to a maximum cumulative dose of 3 mg/kg. A single dose of 1.5 mg/kg in cardiac arrest is acceptable, (c) Magnesium sulphate 1 to 2 g IV in polymorphic VT (torsades de pointes) and suspected hypomagnesaemic state.
- Sodium bicarbonate is indicated in the following situations: (a) If patient has known, pre-existing hyperkalaemia, (b) if known, pre-existing bicarbonate-responsive acidosis, (c) in tricyclic anti-depressant overdose, (d) in intubated and ventilated patients with long arrest interval, and (e) to alkalinize urine in drug overdose.

References

1. Advanced Cardiovascular Life Support: Defibrillation. Resuscitation 2000;46:109-113.
2. Bayes de Luna A, Coumel P, Leelereq JF. Ambulatory sudden cardiac death: mechanisms of production of fatal arrhythmia on the basis of data from 157 cases. Am Heart J 1989;117:151-159.
3. Calle PA, Monsieurs KG, Buylaert WA. Equivalence of the standard monophasic waveform shocks delivered by automated external defibrillators? Resuscitation 2002;53:41-46.
4. Cummins RO, Chesemore K, White RD, et al. Defibrillator failures: Causes of problems and recommendations for improvement. JAMA 1990; 264:1019-1025.
5. Cummins RO, Hazinski MF, Kerber RE, Kudenchuk P, Becker L, Nichol G, Malanga B, Aufderheide TP, Stapleton EM, Kern K, Ornato JP, Sanders A, Valenzuela T, Eisenberg M. Low-energy biphasic waveform defibrillation: evidence-based review applied to emergency cardiovascular care guidelines: a statement for healthcare professionals from the American Heart Association Committee on Emergency Cardiovascular Care and the Subcommittees on Basic Life Support, Advanced Cardiac Life Support and Pediatric Resuscitation. Circulation. 1998;97:1654-1667; 2000;102(Suppl I):142-1157.

6. Cummins RO, Ornato JP, Thies WH, Pepe PE. Improving survival from sudden cardiac arrest: the 'chain of survival' concept: a statement for health professionals from the Advanced Cardiac Life Support Subcommittee and the Emergency Cardiac Care Committee, American Heart Association. Circulation 1991;244:510-511.

7. Cummins RO. From concept to standard-of-care? Review of the clinical experience with automated external defibrillators. Ann Emerg Med 1987;18:1269-1275.

8. Dalzell GW, Adgey AA. Determinants of successful transthoracic defibrillation and outcome in ventricular fibrillation. Br Heart J 1991;65:311-6.

9. DeSilva RA, Graboys TB, Podrid PJ, et al. Cardioversion and defibrillation. Am Heart J. 1980; 100:881-895.

10. Fain E, Sweeney M, Fraaz M. Improved internal defibrillation efficacy with a biphasic waveform. Am Heart J 1989;117:358-364.

11. Kerber R, Becker L, Bourland J, et al. Automatic external defibrillators for public access defibrillation: recommendations for specifying and reporting arrhythmia analysis, algorithm performance, incorporating new waveforms, and enhancing safety. Circulation 1997;95:1677-1682.

12. Kerber RE, Grayzel J, Hoyt R, Marcus M, Kennedy J. Transthoracic resistance in human defibrillation. Influence of body weight, chest size, serial shocks, paddle size and paddle contact pressure. Circulation 1981;63:676-682.

13. Kerber RE, Jensen SR, Gascho JA, et al. Determinants of defibrillation: Prospective analysis of 183 patients. Am J Cardiol 1983; 52:739-745.

14. Kerber RE, Martins JB, Kelly KJ, Ferguson DW, Kouba C, Jensen SR, Newman B, Parke JD, Kieso R, Melton J. Self-adhesive preaplied electrode pads for defibrillation and cardioversion. J Am Coll Cardiol 1984;3:815-820.

15. Kleiger R, Lown B. Cardioversion and digitalis II. Clinical studies. Circulation 1966; 33:878-887.

16. Mittal S, Ayati S, Stein KM, et al. Comparison of a novel rectilinear biphasic waveform with a damped sine wave monophasic waveform for transthoracic ventricular defibrillation. J Am Coll Cardiol 1999;34:1595-1601.

17. Mittal S, Ayati S, Stein KM, et al. Transthoracic cardioversion of atrial fibrillation: comparison of rectilinear biphasic versus damped sine wave monophasic shocks. Circulation 2000;101:1282-1287.

18. Mosesso VN, Davis EA, Auble TE, Paris PM, Yearly DM. Use of automated external defibrillators by police officers for treatment of out-of-hospital cardiac arrest. Ann Emerg Med 1998;32:200-207.

19. Page RL, Kerber RE, Russell JK, et al. Biphasic vs monophasic shock waveform for conversion of atrial fibrillation: the results of an international randomized, double-blind multicenter trial. J AM Coll Cardiol 2002;39:1956-63.

20. Rogrove HJ, Hughes CM. Defibrillation and cardioversion. Critical Care Clinics 1992; 8(4):839-863.

21. Schneider T, Martens PR, Paschen H, et al. Multicenter, randomized, controlled trial of 150-J biphasic shocks compared with 200-to 360-J monophasic shocks in the resuscitation of out-of-hospital cardiac arrest victims. Circulation 2000;102:1780-1787.

22. Shuster M, Keller JL. Effect of fire department first responder automated defibrillation. Ann Emerg Med 1993;4:721-727.

23. Sirna SJ, Ferguson DW, Charbonnier F, et al. Factors affecting transthoracic impedance during electrical cardioversion. Am J Cardiol 1988; 62:1048-1052.

24. The automatic external defibrillator: Key Link in the Chain of Survival. Resuscitation 2000;46:73-91.

25. Walker RG, Melnick SB, Chapman FW, et al. Comparison of six clinically used external defibrillators in Swine. Resuscitation 2003;57:73-78.

26. Weaver WD, Cobb LA, Hallstrom AP, et al. Factors influencing survival after out-of-hospital cardiac arrest. J Am Coll Cardiol 1986; 7:752-757.

27. White RD. Maintenance of defibrillators in a state of readiness. Ann Emerg Med 1993;22:302-306.

13

Cardioversion

Introduction

- Cardioversion refers to the electrical conversion of rhythms other than ventricular fibrillation.
- Synchronized cardioversion is recommended for termination of unstable paroxysmal supraventricular tachycardia, atrial fibrillation, atrial flutter, and unstable ventricular tachycardia with a pulse. The unstable condition, however, must be related to the tachycardia. Rate related signs and symptoms may occur at any rates, but seldom at a rate less than 150/min. The signs and symptoms may include chest pain, shortness of breath, decreased level of consciousness, low blood pressure, shock, pulmonary congestion, congestive heart failure, and acute myocardial infarction.
- Elective cardioversion may be used to convert haemodynamically stable atrial fibrillation or atrial flutter into normal sinus rhythm, in cases where antiarrhythmic medication has not been successful.
- When used to convert atrial fibrillation/atrial flutter, especially of more than 48 hours duration, anticoagulation should be considered for a period of 3 weeks prior to cardioversion to decrease the risk of thromboembolism. In case, early cardioversion is to be considered: Begin IV heparin at once, get transesophageal echocardiography to exclude atrial clot, then consider cardioversion within 24 hours followed by anticoagulation for 4 weeks to cover up the possibility of delayed embolism.
- Synchronized cardioversion differs from defibrillation. During ventricular fibrillation (when defibrillation is performed) there are no identifiable P, Q, R, S, or T waves and no identifiable vulnerable period. But other arrhythmias (when synchronized cardioversion is performed) have identifiable waveforms and vulnerable period. Synchronized cardioversion aims to avoid firing during this vulnerable period so as to avoid inducing ventricular fibrillation. This

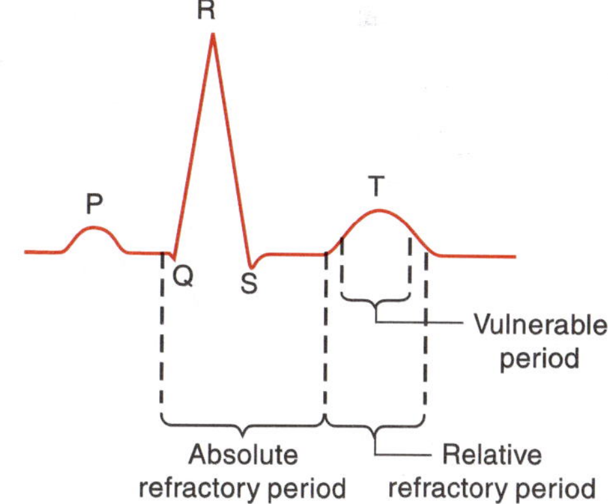

Fig. 13.1: Vulnerable period. Period near the peak through the downslope of the T wave corresponds to vulnerable period. Impulses occurring during the vulnerable period can spread in a disorganized wave of depolarization, commonly known as the "R on T" phenomenon.

synchronization occurs a few milliseconds after the highest part of the R wave but before the vulnerable period associated with the T wave (Fig. 13.1).

- Obtain serum potassium, magnesium, digitalis levels, and arterial blood gas analysis because electrolyte imbalances, acid-base disturbances, and digitalis toxicity, significantly contribute to electrical instability and may increase the incidence of post-conversion arrhythmias. Cardioversion in the presence of digoxin toxicity is relatively contraindicated, as ventricular arrhythmias may be precipitated; however, with serum levels in the therapeutic range, cardioversion can be attempted with little increased risk.

GUIDELINES FOR CARDIOVERSION

1. **Prepare the patient.**

   Preparation of the patient includes: (a) Reassuring the patient, obtaining informed consent, (b) nil orally for at least six hours prior to the procedure, (c) establishing intravenous access, (d) positioning the patient supine, (e) removing loose-fitting dentures, (f) oxygenating the patient, maintaining an airway, (g) removing clothes from upper half of the body, (h) removing all metallic objects from the patient, and (i) administering sedation and analgesia to provide amnesia and to decrease pain during the procedure. Diazepam, midazolam, or ketamine with or without morphine, pethidine or fentanyl may be used.

2. **Wash hands.**

   This reduces the risk of transmission of micro-organisms.

3. **Switch on the defibrillator and attach the patient cable and ECG electrodes to monitor the patient's ECG.**

   Place ECG electrodes away from paddle sites.

4. **Select a lead, which provides a tall R wave.**

   Synchronized cardioversion must sense the R wave to deliver the current outside the heart's vulnerable period. A synchronized countershock delivers energy during ventricular depolarization (QRS complex on ECG). The monitor searches for certain criteria such as slope and amplitude that distinguish R wave from other parts of ECG such as the P or T wave, and when the R wave is detected, the monitor places a flag of "sync marker" on that R wave. The marker may appear as a line or highlighted triangle, oval or square on the ECG display (Fig. 13.2).

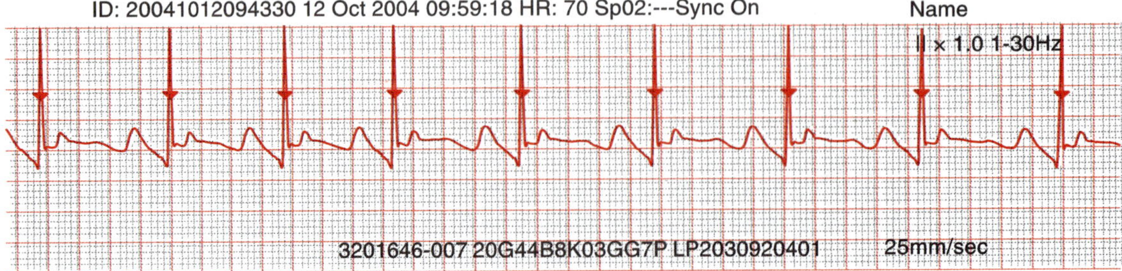

Fig. 13.2: Sync marker on the R wave.

5. Place the defibrillator in synchronization mode.

   Synchronization prevents the random delivery of an electric charge, especially during the vulnerable period, which may trigger ventricular fibrillation.

6. If defibrillator is unable to distinguish between the peak of the QRS complex and the peak of the T wave, because of wide, complex and variable forms, as in polymorphic ventricular tachycardia, proceed with unsynchronized cardioversion (defibrillation).

   Under these circumstances, there is a greater chance of a synchronized discharge occurring on T wave than a random unsynchronized discharge. Therefore, defibrillation may be safer in this situation. Thus, a patient who is pulseless, unconscious, hypotensive, or in severe pulmonary edema, should receive unsynchronized shock to avoid the delay associated with attempts to synchronize.

7. Apply conductive gel to the paddle electrodes or on the patient's chest. Gel should be evenly distributed on the defibrillator paddles.

   See Chapter 12.

8. Ensure that the defibrillator cables are positioned to allow for adequate access to the patient.

9. Switch on the ECG recorder for a continuous print out.

   This provides a permanent record of the response to cardioversion.

10. Select the energy to be delivered and charge the defibrillator.

    Recommended energy levels for synchronized cardioversion are:

	Initial shock energy (Joules)	Subsequent shock energy (Joules)
Atrial fibrillation	100	200, 300, 360
Ventricular tachycardia	100	200, 300, 360
Atrial flutter	50	100, 200, 300, 360
Paroxysmal supra-ventricular tachycardia	50	100, 200, 300, 360

11. Place the paddles on the chest.

    See Chapter 12.

12. Disconnect oxygen source during actual cardioversion.

    This decreases the risk of combustion in the presence of electric current.

13. Apply appropriate pressures to each paddle against the chest wall.

    See Chapter 12.

14. Reconfirm that the sync markers are properly located.

15. Ensure that all personnel are clear of contact with the patient and the bed.

    See Chapter 12.

16. Press both buttons on paddles simultaneously and hold until defibrillator fires.

    There will be a short delay before the charge is fired. The monitor first tells the defibrillator that an R wave has been detected and then defibrillator fires.

17. Observe monitor for conversion of dysrhythmia.

18. When successful, turn the defibrillator off, clean the paddles thoroughly, prior to storing them.

19. Continue to monitor the patient after cardioversion.
    - Monitor blood pressure, heart rate and rhythm immediately after cardioversion and every 5-10 minutes until stable.
    - Monitor electrolytes, ABG.
    - Initiate antiarrhythmic therapy, as indicated, if not already started.
    - Remember, dysrhythmias may develop again after successful cardioversion

20. If unsuccessful, repeat the shock.
    Increase the energy according to the electrical cardioversion algorithm.

References

1. Advanced Cardiovascular Life Support: Defibrillation. Resuscitation 2000;46:109-113.

2. Bayes de Luna A, Coumel P, Leelereq JF. Ambulatory sudden cardiac death: mechanisms of production of fatal arrhythmia on the basis of data from 157 cases. Am Heart J 1989;117:151-159.

3. Calle PA, Monsieurs KG, Buylaert WA. Equivalence of the standard monophasic waveform shocks delivered by automated external defibrillators? Resuscitation 2002;53:41-46.

4. Cummins RO, Chesemore K, White RD, et al. Defibrillator failures: Causes of problems and recommendations for improvement. JAMA. 1990; 264:1019-1025.

5. Cummins RO, Hazinski MF, Kerber RE, et al. Low-energy biphasic waveform defibrillation: evidence-based review applied to emergency cardiovascular care guidelines: a statement for healthcare professionals from the American Heart Association Committee on Emergency Cardiovascular Care and the Subcommittees on Basic Life Support, Advanced Cardiac Life Support, and Pediatric Resuscitation. Circulation. 1998;97:1654-1667; Circulation 2000;102(Suppl I):1142-1157.

6. Cummins RO, Ornato JP, Thies WH, Pepe PE. Improving survival from sudden cardiac arrest: the 'chain of survival' concept: a statement for health professionals from the Advanced Cardiac Life Support Subcommittee and the Emergency Cardiac Care Committee, American Heart Association. Circulation 1991;244:510-511.

7. Cummins RO. From concept to standard-of-care? Review of the clinical experience with automated external defibrillators. Ann Emerg Med 1987;18:1269-1275.

8. Dalzell GW, Adgey AA. Determinants of successful transthoracic defibrillation and outcome in ventricular fibrillation. Br Heart J 1991;65:311-3/6.

9. DeSilva RA, Graboys TB, Podrid PJ, et al. Cardioversion and defibrillation. Am Heart J 1980; 100:881-895.

10. EwaldGA, Rogers JG. Heart failure, cardiomyopathy, and valvular heart Disease. In: The washington mannual of medical Therapeutics, editors – Ahya SN, Flood K, Paranjothi S. Lippincott, Williams & Wilkins, Philadelphia 2001, 30th edn, pp 131-152.

11. Fain E, Sweeney M, Fraaz M. Improved internal defibrillation efficacy with a biphasic waveform. Am Heart J 1989;117:358-364.

12. Kerber R, Becker L, Bourland J, et al. Automatic external defibrillators for public access defibrillation: recommendations for specifying and reporting arrhythmia analysis, algorithm performance, incorporating new waveforms, and enhancing safety. Circulation 1997;95:1677-1682.

13. Kerber RE, Grayzel J, Hoyt R, Marcus M, Kennedy J. Transthoracic resistance in human defibrillation. Influence

of body weight, chest size, serial shocks, paddle size and paddle contact pressure. Circulation 1981;63:676-82.

14. Kerber RE, Jensen SR, Gascho JA, et al. Determinants of defibrillation: Prospective analysis of 183 patients. Am J Cardiol 1983; 52:739-745.

15. Kerber RE, Martins JB, Kelly KJ, et al. Self-adhesive preapplied electrode pads for defibrillation and cardioversion. J Am Coll Cardiol 1984;3:815-820.

16. Kleiger R, Lown B. Cardioversion and digitalis II. Clinical studies. Circulation 1966; 33:878-887.

17. Mittal S, Ayati S, Stein KM, et al. Comparison of a novel rectilinear biphasic waveform with a damped sine wave monophasic waveform for transthoracic ventricular defibrillation. J Am Coll Cardiol 1999;34:1595-601.

18. Mittal S, Ayati S, Stein KM, et al. Transthoracic cardioversion of atrial fibrillation: comparison of rectilinear biphasic versus damped sine wave monophasic shocks. Circulation 2000;101:1282-1287.

19. Mosesso VN, Davis EA, Auble TE, Paris PM, Yearly DM. Use of automated external defibrillators by police officers for treatment of out-of-hospital cardiac arrest. Ann Emerg Med 1998;32:200-207.

20. Page RL, Kerber RE, Russell JK, et al. Biphasic vs monophasic shock waveform for conversion of atrial fibrillation: the results of an international randomized, double-blind multicenter trial. J AM Coll Cardiol 2002;39:1956-1963.

21. Rogrove HJ, Hughes CM. Defibrillation and cardioversion. Critical Care Clinics 1992; 8(4):839-863.

22. Schneider T, Martens PR, Paschen H, et al. Multicenter, randomized, controlled trial of 150-J biphasic shocks compared with 200- to 360-J monophasic shocks in the resuscitation of out-of-hospital cardiac arrest victims. Circulation 2000;102:1780-1787.

23. Shuster M, Keller JL. Effect of fire department first responder automated defibrillation. Ann Emerg Med 1993;4:721-727.

24. Sirna SJ, Ferguson DW, Charbonnier F, et al. Factors affecting transthoracic impedance during electrical cardioversion. Am J Cardiol 1988; 62:1048-1052.

25. The automatic external defibrillator: Key Link in the Chain of Survival. Resuscitation 2000;46:73-91.

26. Walker RG, Melnick SB, Chapman FW, et al. Comparison of six clinically used external defibrillators in Swine. Resuscitation 2003;57:73-78.

27. Weaver WD, Cobb LA, Hallstrom AP, et al. Factors influencing survival after out-of-hospital cardiac arrest. J Am Coll Cardiol 1986; 7:752-757.

28. White RD. Maintenance of defibrillators in a state of readiness. Ann Emerg Med 1993;22:302-306.

Automated External Defibrillation

14

Introduction

- An automated external defibrillator (AED) is a highly sophisticated, microprocessor-based device, that recognizes various cardiac rhythms, distinguishes between those that require defibrillation and those that do not, and delivers a series of preprogrammed electric shocks, without requiring interpretation of the rhythm by medical personnel.

- The rationale for use of AED is based on the following observations : (a) Most adults with sudden, witnessed, non-traumatic cardiac arrest are found to be in VF, (b) for those victims the time from collapse to defibrillation is the single greatest determinant of survival, (c) survival from VF cardiac arrest declines by approximately 7% to 10% for each minute without defibrillation, and (d) AED, by eliminating the need for training in recognition of rhythm, makes early defibrillation possible by first responding personnel (who may be minimally trained).

- Early defibrillation refers to shock delivery within 5 minutes of receiving a call in the community, and to shock delivery with a collapse-to-shock interval of less than 3 minutes in areas of the hospital and ambulatory care facilities.

- Use of AED in infants and children less than 8 years of age and less than approximately 25 kg body weight is not recommended.

- AEDs should be placed in the analysis mode only when full cardiac arrest has been confirmed and only when all movement, particularly patient transport, has ceased. AED should be applied only to unresponsive, non-breathing, and pulseless patients.

- Although AEDs are not programmed to deliver synchronized shocks, they will deliver asynchronous shocks to rapid monomorphic and polymorphic ventricular tachycardia with rates greater than the specified cut-off rates. Assuming that the AED has been appropriately attached to an unconscious, apnoeic, and pulseless patient, this shock of a patient in nonperfusing ventricular tachycardia is appropriate under current ACLS guidelines.

- Use of AED is not a substitute for cardiopulmonary resuscitation. CPR should be started and continued till AED is put in function. CPR will help to keep the patient in a rhythm able to be defibrillated for a longer time, increasing the chance that defibrillation will be effective.

- It should also be understood that in the management of VF/unstable VT cardiac arrest, the use of an AED by first responding personnel is likely to be less effective than manual defibrillation delivered by a skilled operator. Manual defibrillation allows more rapid shock delivery, with minimum delays in the institution and performance of CPR.

GUIDELINES FOR AUTOMATED EXTERNAL DEFIBRILLATION

1. **Turn the power on. Press the "on".**
   Most AEDs require a short period for a self-check of their circuit. Some AEDs can be turned on simply by lifting the monitor cover or screen to the "up" position.

2. **Attach electrode pads.**
   - The AED uses the electrode pads to monitor and to deliver shock. Place the pads on the upper-right sternal border (directly below calvicle) and lateral to the left nipple, with the top margin of the pad a few inches (approx. 7 cm) below the axilla. For defibrillation purposes, the polarity of the pads is interchangeable. Do not place an AED pad directly over an implanted device as this may reduce the effectiveness of defibrillation. Instead, place the pad at least 1 inch (2.5cm) away from the power source of the pacemaker or internal cardiac defibrillator.
   - If the victim has a hairy chest, the electrode pads may not have effective contact with the skin of the chest, causing high transthoracic impedance, leading to a "check electrodes" or "check electrode pads" message from the AED. To correct this problem, one of the following methods may be effective: (a) Press firmly on each pad, (b) remove the original pads (this will remove the hair under the pad), and apply a second set of electrodes, or (c) shave the chest in the area of pads, apply another set of pads.

3. **Press the "Analyze" button to analyze the patient's rhythm.**
   The machine needs to analyze the rhythm to determine the need for defibrillation. To prevent artifactual errors, avoid CPR, transport, or any contact with the patient while rhythm is being analyzed. It usually takes 5-15 seconds, depending on the brand of AED. If VF is present and defibrillation is required, the device will announce it through an audio or a visual message.

4. **Clear the victim and press the shock button.**
   Before pressing the shock button, ensure that no one is touching the victim. Any body touching the patient during the delivery of shock may also receive that shock. The shock will produce a sudden contraction of the patient's musculature (like that seen with a conventional defibrillator).

5. **Reanalyze the rhythm.**
   The rhythm is analyzed to determine if another shock is indicated. In some models, if VF persists, the AED will indicate it, and the "shock indicated" and "charging" sequence will repeat for a second and, if needed, third shock automatically. The purpose for this is to treat a shockable rhythm as quickly as possible.
   After a gap of three shocks, AEDs are programmed to pause for 1 minute for

CPR. During this time look for signs of circulation and resume CPR.

6. **After the third shock, or if a "no shock advised" message occurs, check the pulse.**
Checking the pulse determines whether the last shock restored a rhythm with a pulse and determines the need for continued CPR. If no pulse, resume CPR.

7. **Repeat the step 3 to 6, if so advised until ACLS facilities available.**
Three "no shock indicated" messages with no signs of circulation indicate that there is a low probability of the rhythm being successfully defibrillated. Continue CPR until ACLS facilities available.

8. **If "no shock message" is received and the patient has a pulse, check for breathing.**
If signs of circulation are present, check for breathing. If the patient is breathing adequately, place him in a recovery position.

9. **Monitor vital parameters.**
Even after successful resuscitation, the AED should always be left attached. If VF recurs, most AEDs will prompt the rescuer to check for signs of circulation. If at any time patients lose their pulse, begin again at step 3.

References

1. Advanced Cardiovascular Life Support: Defibrillation. Resuscitation 2000;46:109-113

2. Cummins RO, Eisenberg MS, Bergner L, Hallstrom A, Hearne T, Muray JA. Automatic external defibrillation: evaluation of its role in the home and in emergency medical services. Ann Emerg Med 1984;13(9 pt 2): 798-801.

3. Cummins RO, Eisenberg MS, Litwin PE, et al. Automatic external defibrillators used by emergency medical technicians: A controlled clinical trial. JAMA 1987;257:1605-1610.

4. Cummins RO. From concept to standard-of-care? Review of the clinical experience with automated external defibrillators. Ann Emerg Med 1989;18:1269-1275.

5. Early Defibrillation. An Advisory Statement by the Advanced Life Support Working Group of the International Liaison Committee on Resuscitation Bossaert L, Callanan V, Cummins RO. Resuscitation 34: (1997);113-114.

6. Mancini M, Kaye W. In-hospital first-responder automated external defibrillation: what critical care practitioners need to know. Am J Crit Care 1998;7:314-319.

7. Physio-Control Corporation. Defibrillation: What you should know. Crockett et al (eds). Washington: Redmond 1996.

8. Recommended guidelines for uniform reporting of data from in hospital cardiac arrest. Prepared by a Task Force of Representatives from the European Resuscitation Council, American heart Foundation, Heart and Stroke Foundation of Canada, Australian Resuscitation Council. Resuscitation Council of South Africa. Resuscitation 1997.

9. Recommended guidelines for uniform reporting of data from out of hospital cardiac arrest: the Utstein style. Prepared by a Task Force of Representatives of the European Resuscitation Council, American Heart Association, Heart and Stroke Foundation of Canada, Australian Resuscitation Council. Resuscitation 1991;22:1-26.

10. The automatic external defibrillator: Key Link in the Chain of Survival. Resuscitation 2000;46:73-91.

11. Weisfeldt ML, Kerber RE, McGoldrick RP, et al. AHA medical/scientific statement. Task Force Report. Public access defibrillation: a statement for health care professionals from the American heart Association Task Force on automatic external defibrillation. Circulation 1995;92:2763.

Rhabdomyolysis 15

Introduction

- Rhabdomyolysis is a clinical syndrome caused by injury to skeletal muscle that results in release of its contents into the extracellular fluid and the circulation.
- The causes of rhabdomyolysis can be divided broadly into two categories: traumatic and non-traumatic. Traumatic rhabdomyolysis may be caused by burns or crush injuries. Non-traumatic rhabdomyolysis may occur due to (a) Metabolic or electrolyte disorders (hyperglycaemia, hypokalaemia, hypophosphataemia), (b) excessive muscular activity (heat stroke, seizures, vigorous exercise), (c) immobilization and passive compression, (d) infections (clostridium, staphylococcus, legionella, typhoid, viral), (e) drugs (alcohol, cocaine, heroin, and amphetamines), and (f) muscle ischaemia (vascular occlusion, compartment syndrome).
- Although classically described as associated with trauma and crush injuries, majority of the cases of rhabdomyolysis are non-traumatic, developing as complications of alcohol abuse, passive muscle compression from immobilization, and seizures.
- Despite a variety of diseases causing rhabdomyolysis, the final common pathway of injury involves damage to the sarcolemma. The damage may be the result of a direct mechanical or toxic insult to the membrane (sarcolemma), or due to an inability to maintain ionic gradients across the membrane (because of ATP depletion either because of a mismatch between energy supply and demand or due to a defect in energy use).
- The damage to sarcolemma with loss of its intrinsic function results in: (a) Influx of calcium, leading to rise in intracellular calcium concentration, and (b) liberation of intracellular contents, such as myoglobin, aldolase, aspartate transaminase, lactate dehydrogenase, creatinine kinase, potassium, uric acid, and phosphorus. Elevated intracellular calcium leads to a greater activity of intracellular proteases, phospholipases and other proteolytic enzymes, which then cause further cell damage and destruction.
- With the release of myoglobin, levels of free plasma myoglobin rise. Excess myoglobin is filtered by the kidneys and enters the urine. Myoglobin accumulation, coupled with hypovolaemia and acidosis, can precipitate and cause blockage to renal tubular flow. The clinical picture may be subtle, or severe and obvious.
- Symptoms and signs of a compartment syndrome include pain, a hard swollen limb, poor distal perfusion indicated by prolonged capillary return, cold

extremities, etc. If compartment syndrome is suspected pressure should be measured in all the suspected compartments. Normal pressure is less than 15 mmHg. If pressure is above 35 mmHg, if there is circulatory compromise, or if compartmental pressures within 30 mmHg of the diastolic blood pressure are noted, urgent surgical intervention (fasciotomy) should be performed.

- Treatment of rhabdomyolysis is aimed at: (a) Appropriate management of airway, breathing and circulation, (b) correction of the underlying cause, (c) correction of biochemical abnormalities e.g. potassium, phosphate, uric acid, (d) early detection and management of any compartment syndrome, (e) prevention of acute renal failure, and (f) wherever possible, keeping the limb elevated.

GUIDELINES FOR THE MANAGEMENT OF RHABDOMYOLYSIS

1. Take history and examine the patient clinically.
   - Have high index of suspicion in patients at risk.
   - History should include any recent trauma or compression, excessive exertion, envenomations, infections, electrical shock, extremes of temperature, or use of alcohol or illicit drugs. Family history of muscle dysfunction or disease may also be important.
   - Symptoms may include cramping pain in the involved muscles, frequently the calves and lower back, progressive weakness, paraesthesias and brown to cola-coloured urine. These typical or characteristic symptoms are present only in a small group of patients.
   - Physical examination may reveal fever, volume depletion (due to reduced extracellular fluid volume) and respiratory insufficiency (due to diffuse muscle injury, resulting in weakened respiratory efforts). The muscles involved may demonstrate swelling, tenderness and a firm or doughy consistency. Haemorrhagic discolouration of overlying skin may be noted. But again, these signs are often absent or present minimally.

2. Laboratory evaluation.
   (a) Urine analysis (myoglobinuria)
   - Urinalysis typically shows brown urine with a large amount of blood on dipstick evaluation but few if any red blood cells (RBCs) on microscopic evaluation. This occurs because the various dipstick tests cannot distinguish myoglobinuria from haematuria or haemoglobinuria. Brown casts and renal tubular epithelial cells may also be found. Radioimmunoassay is the best method to measure urine myoglobin.
   (b) Creatinine kinase (CK, CPK) levels.
   - It is a more sensitive method than myoglobin testing.
   - CK is present in the serum immediately after injury. Peak CK levels occur within 24-36 hours after injury and diminish by approximately 39% per day. Failure of levels to decrease in this manner suggests an ongoing injury. CK level greater than five times the normal value is diagnostic. The CK subtype present in skeletal muscle is MM. There appears to be a clear relationship between CK level and severity of disease.

(c) **Serum potassium.**
- Hyperkalaemia is due to intracellular potassium release because of muscle necrosis and decreased renal excretion.

(d) **Serum phosphate.**
- Hyperphosphataemia is due to leakage of phosphorus from injured muscles.

(e) **Serum calcium.**
- Hypocalcaemia is noted in the acute stage and is due mainly to deposition of calcium in the damaged muscles. While hypocalcaemia may be noted acutely in rhabdomyolysis and during oliguric myoglobinuric renal failure, hypercalcaemia may be noted during diuretic phase of resolution of renal failure. It is considered secondary to mobilization of calcium previously deposited in injured muscles.

(f) **Serum uric acid.**
- Hyperuricaemia is due to release of purines from damaged muscles and subsequent hepatic conversion to uric acid.

(g) **Arterial blood gases.**
- There is usually anion gap acidosis. It could be because of increased release of sulphur-containing proteins during injury. Hydrogen and sulphate loads could overwhelm renal excretory mechanisms, resulting in acidosis. Other causes include lactic acidosis from ischaemia and the acidosis of uraemia.

(h) **Serum creatinine, blood urea.**
- Serum creatinine is often elevated out of proportion to the BUN concentration and may rise more than usual 1mg/dL/day. A BUN/creatinine ratio lower than 10 may suggest the presence of rhabdomyolysis.

(i) **Prothrombin time, platelet count, fibrinogen levels, fibrin degradation products.**
- DIC (disseminated intravascular coagulation) may complicate rhabdomyolysis (activation of the clotting cascade by components released from the damaged muscle). There may be prolongation of PT and PTT, hypofibrinogenaemia, thrombocytopenia, and increased FDPs in serum or urine. Therapy with platelets, vitamin K, and fresh frozen plasma may be required.

3. **Maintain urine flow rate at 200 mL/hr or more.**

   Early intervention and administration of large volumes of saline to titrate to a high urine output is the mainstay of therapy. Use half-isotonic saline. Avoid potassium-containing fluids due to the risk of rhabdomyolysis associated hyperkalaemia.

4. **Monitor at regular intervals – SpO_2, CVP, PAP, serum electrolytes, ABG, ECG.**

   Monitor CVP or pulmonary artery pressure, electrolytes and pulmonary status of the patient. Patient may require upto 20 L fluid in the first 24 hours to achieve the desired urinary output.

5. **Alkalinize the urine. Check urine pH hourly.**
- Alkalinization of urine probably adds to the beneficial effect of high urine flow but prospective, randomized, controlled trials are required to determine the clinical relevance.

- Keep urinary pH > 6.5.
- If urinary pH is 7, add 1 ampoule of sodium bicarbonate to each liter of half-isotonic saline.
- If the serum pH < 7.4 and urine pH < 7, add 2 ampoules of sodium bicarbonate to each liter of half-isotonic saline.
- If the serum pH > 7.45 and urine pH still < 7, add acetazolamide (upto 4 hourly).

6. **Add mannitol.**

   Mannitol may be used to encourage diuresis. The exact role of mannitol is yet to be studied in controlled trials. Care must, however, be exercised if oliguric ARF develops, because mannitol or sodium bicarbonate therapy can precipitate pulmonary edema. Loop diuretics should be avoided wherever possible because they tend to acidify the urine. Furosemide may be used if there is no response to saline infusion, alkalinization and mannitol.

7. **Maintain urinary output, alkalinization, and mannitol (if required).**

   Continue therapy until the underlying cause has resolved, the creatinine kinase (CK) levels are falling and the urine has been negative for myoglobin for twenty four hours. If the serum CK levels does not fall by 50% over 48 hours, careful search should be made for evidence of increased tissue pressures in the involved muscle group (compartment syndrome).

8. **Consider dialysis.**

   Dialysis should be considered if, inspite of therapy, serum potassium is rising, there is persistent acidosis, or oliguric renal failure with fluid overload develops. Dialysis may be necessary for the treatment of hyperkalaemia well before there are other indications for dialysis.

References

1. Chugh KS, Nath IV, Ubroi HS, et al. Acute renal failure due to non-traumatic rhabdomyolysis. Postgrad Med J 1979;55:386.
2. Gabow PA, Kaehny WD, Kelleher SP. The spectrum of rhabdomyolysis. Arn J Med 1982; 61:141-152.
3. Hiran S et al. Rhabdomyolysis due to multiple honey bee stings. Postgrad Med J 1994; 70:937.
4. Poels PJE, Gabreels FJM. Rhabdomyolysis: a review of the literature, Clin Neurol Neurosurg 1993;95:175.
5. Slater MS, Mullins RJ. Rhabdomyolysis and myoglobinuric renal failure in trauma and surgical patients: a review. J Am Coll Surg 1998;186:693.
6. Vanholder R et al. Rhabdomyolysis. J Am Soc Nephrol 2000;11(8).

Effective Use of Blood and Blood Components

16

Introductions

- Both haemoglobin concentration and blood loss, should be taken into consideration when assessing a patient, as both can interfere with oxygen transport. Chronic anaemia is better tolerated than acute anaemia, as oxygen delivery is facilitated through increases in 2, 3-diphosphoglycerate levels in RBCs. In patients with chronic anaemia, cardiac output usually does not change until the haemoglobin concentration falls below 7 g/dL. In acute anaemia, reductions in arterial oxygen content are well tolerated because of compensatory increase in cardiac output. This compensatory mechanism, however, may be affected by several factors, e.g. left ventricular dysfunction, β-blockade, calcium channel blockade, drugs like anaesthetics, hypnotics, and body temperature.

- Transfusion is rarely indicated when the haemoglobin concentration is more than 10 g/dL and is always indicated when it is less than 6 g/dL, especially when anaemia is acute. Whether intermediate haemoglobin concentrations (6-10 g/dL) justify transfusion should be based on the patient's risk for complications of inadequate oxygenation. In young, healthy patients with good cardiovascular reserve, with slow blood loss, or chronic anaemia, haemoglobin levels may be allowed to drop between 6-8 g/dL. Patients with a higher risk should be transfused to attain haemoglobin concentrations between 8 and 10 g/dL, and closer to 10 g/dL when the risk is highest. Conditions which increase the risk include atherosclerotic disease (cerebrovascular, cardiovascular, peripheral, renal), cardiac disease, pulmonary disease, and increased oxygen consumption (affected by body temperature, drugs, sepsis, muscular activity). When hypovolaemia is suspected in a rapidly bleeding patient, transfusion may be indicated even when the haemoglobin is between 10 and 12 g/dL.

- In the resuscitation of hypotensive patients after haemorrhage, haemoglobin and haematocrit measurements are unreliable. Following acute haemorrhage, the haematocrit may not reflect true red cell losses for upto 72 hours. Clinical assessment of circulatory status, including monitoring of pulse, blood pressure, respiratory rate, urinary output, CVP, and mental status, is essential.

- Microvascular bleeding refers to diffuse bleeding from wound edges, mucous membranes, and insertion sites of vascular cannulae.

- Albumin represents only 50% of the total gram weight of the protein present in the plasma, but because of its relatively low molecular weight, it accounts for a large number of molecules and therefore, accounts for approximately 75-80% of the plasma oncotic pressure in normal individuals. The distribution of albumin is predominantly extravascular, with only 35 – 40% of albumin residing intravascularly, and it exerts a colloid oncotic pressure (COP) of 21.8 mmHg at the vascular/interstitial interface. Apart from plasma volume expansion and restoration of COP, albumin is a protein carrier for many substances, a scavenger of oxygen radicals, and may play a role in preserving microvascular integrity.

GUIDELINES FOR EFFECTIVE USE OF BLOOD/BLOOD COMPONENTS

1. **Whole blood.**
    - Whole blood can correct combined deficits in oxygen carrying capacity and blood volume and is therefore, potentially indicated in trauma and massive surgical bleeding when the blood type of the patient has been determined.
    - If available, whole blood is preferable to packed RBCs for massive transfusion therapy, because the former contains not only red cells but fibrinogen and other stable coagulation factors also. Further, volume-expanding effect of plasma may be an advantage in a hypovolaemic patient. Use of whole blood also minimizes the use of red blood cells and plasma from different donors, thus decreasing the risk of transfusion-transmitted infectious diseases.

2. **Packed red blood cells (pRBCs).**
    - Packed RBCs are manufactured by removal of the majority of plasma from a unit of whole blood. pRBCs have a volume of approximately 250-300 mL and a haematocrit of 65 – 80%.
    - pRBCs are indicated in the treatment of anaemia with symptomatic deficits of oxygen-carrying capacity and in haemorrhagic shock, when administered with volume expanders.
    - pRBCs impose less volume load per dose of red cells, so they are safer if the patient is normovolaemic.
    - One unit of pRBCs should raise the haemoglobin of an average adult by 1g/dL and the haematocrit by 3%. For pediatric patients, the usual dose is 3mL/kg to raise the haemoglobin by 1gm/dL and the haemotocrit by 3%.
    - If both red cells and plasma are required in a particular patient, then the patient is exposed to more donors.

3. **Fresh frozen plasma (FFP). Dose 10 –15 mL/kg body weight.**
    - Fresh frozen plasma (FFP) is prepared by simple centrifugation and freezing of a single donor's plasma within 6 hours of collection. One unit of plasma is defined as the amount of plasma obtained from centrifugation of one unit of whole blood and usually contains 180–300 mL. Before transfusion, FFP must be thawed at 37°C, which can take up to 35-45 minutes. It contains all soluble coagulation factors and one unit of plasma should raise coagulation factor levels by approximately 2–3%. ABO compatible FFP should be used; however, compatibility testing is not a must.

- Indications for FFP include: (a) Coagulopathies (liver disease, congenital factor deficiencies, warfarin induced, dilution induced, and disseminated intravascular coagulation), (b) replacement of other factor(s) (plasma infusion or exchange in thrombotic thrombocytopenic purpura, haemolytic uraemic syndrome, HELLP syndrome, and fluid replacement in therapeutic plasma exchange).
- FFP is contraindicated for volume expansion, immunoglobulin replacement, nutritional support, reconstitution of pRBCs, and wound healing.
- Warfarin-induced coagulopathy: complete reversal of warfarin-induced coagulopathy occurs within 48 hours after discontinuation of the oral anticoagulant, within 12-18 hours after vitamin K administration, and immediately after the administration of FFP. A single FFP infusion at a dose of 15–20 mL/kg is usually sufficient to normalize haemostasis rapidly.
- Dilutional coagulopathy: FFP administration, in patients with massive transfusion is indicated (a) for correction of microvascular bleeding in the presence of elevated (1.5 – 1.8 times the normal) PT or PTT, and (b) for correction of microvascular bleeding secondary to coagulation factor deficiency in patients transfused with more than one blood volume and when PT and PTT cannot be obtained in a timely fashion. There is no justification for the prophylactic use of FFP in the massively transfused patient.

4. Cryoprecipitate: One unit of cryoprecipitate per 10 kg body weight raises plasma fibrinogen concentration by approximately 50 mg/dL in the absence of continued consumption or massive bleeding.

- Cryoprecipitate is produced by the controlled thawing of FFP. Before administration, cryoprecipitate is thawed in a water bath at 30°C-37°C for approximately 5-10 minutes, and several bags are pooled to a single container to ensure sterility of the product. Cryoprecipitate must be transfused within 4 hours if it is pooled.
- Cryoprecipitate contains factor VIII, fibrinogen, fibronectin, von Willebrand's factor, and factor XIII. Cryoprecipitate contains no RBCs and only a small amount of isohaemagglutinins (e.g., anti–A, anti –B); therefore, compatibility and Rh testing are not required before its use in adults.
- Cryoprecipitate is indicated for (a) prophylaxis in non-bleeding perioperative or peripartum patients with congenital fibrinogen deficiencies or von Willebrand's disease unresponsive to DDAVP, (b) bleeding patients with von Willebrand's disease, and (c) correction of microvascular bleeding in massively transfused patients with fibrinogen concentrations less than 80-100mg/dL (or when fibrinogen concentrations cannot be measured in a timely fashion).

5. Platelet concentrate: The post-transfusion increment after administration to an adult of 1 unit of platelet concentrate is about $5 – 8 \times 10^9$/L. An average adult dose is approximately 1 unit for each 10 kg of body weight or 6 units per transfusion episode. A platelet count should be done 10 minutes to 1 hour after transfusion, and again in 16 to 24 hours.

- Normal platelet count is $130\text{-}400 \times 10^9$/L (130,000-400,000/mm³).

- Platelet concentrate is separated from platelet-rich plasma which is produced by the centrifugation of whole blood just after collection. Each unit of platelet concentrate comes from a single donor. An individual unit contains approximately $5\text{-}10 \times 10^{10}$ platelets in 30–70 mL of plasma, whereas an apheresis unit contains $3\text{-}5 \times 10^{11}$ platelets in 200–400mL of plasma. A temperature of 20°C–24°C with the use of agitation is ideal for storage.

- Prophylactic platelet transfusion is rarely indicated in surgical patients when the platelet count is greater than $100 \times 10^9/L$ and is usually indicated when the count is below $50 \times 10^9/L$. Between the range of $50 \times 10^9/L$ to $100 \times 10^9/L$, platelet transfusion should be guided by the risk of bleeding. The risk of spontaneous haemorrhage increases as the count drops below $20 \times 10^9/L$. In patients receiving platelet concentrate for massive acute blood loss, the platelet count should be maintained greater than $50 \times 10^9/L$ (see Chapter 18). However, there is no indication for routine administration of platelets for a predetermined number of units of blood transfused.

- Platelet transfusion may be indicated despite an apparently adequate platelet count if the patient has a known platelet dysfunction and microvascular bleeding.

- Prophylactic platelet transfusion in the management of acute leukaemia should be considered if the platelet count is below $5 \times 10^9/L$. In the presence of fever, infection or drugs that may be associated with platelet dysfunction, prophylactic platelet transfusions may be indicated at a higher platelet count, that is, below $10 \times 10^9/L$.

- Patients with thrombocytopenia secondary to sepsis often require platelet transfusions, although their response is often suboptimal because of continued platelet destruction.

- Thrombocytopenia caused by massive splenomegaly responds poorly to transfusion, as the transfused platelets become sequestered in the spleen.

6. Albumin.
   (a) Albumin preparations are sterile, nonpyrogenic, free of preservatives and coagulation factors, are balanced to physiologic pH, and contain approximately 145 ± 15 mEq/L of sodium and approximately 2 mEq/L of potassium.
   (b) Albumin is commercially available as 5% and 25% solutions.
   (c) Plasma protein fraction is a 5% solution containing 12.5 g protein per 250 mL, of which 83% is albumin, and 17% is α, β, and γ globulins.
   - Albumin is extracted from pooled plasma through Cohn fractionation and is pasteurized at 60°C for 10 hours to ensure viral inactivation, and has an approximate plasma half life of 16 hours. The 5% solution exerts an oncotic pressure of 20 mmHg, and produces a 100% volume expansion effect. The 25% solution exerts an oncotic pressure of 100 mmHg and produces a 300% volume expansion effect. Albumin preparations are stored at room temperature without extreme temperature fluctuations.
   - The concentration of the albumin solution administered is dictated by the

underlying disease and by the oncotic stress of the patient. For example, 5% albumin is used as volume replacement in therapeutic plasma exchange, whereas 25% albumin is beneficial in promoting extravascular fluid mobilization in nephrotic syndrome.

- The conditions in which albumin is indicated include: (a) Following large volume paracentesis, (b) nephrotic syndrome resistant to potent diuretics, and (c) volume/fluid replacement in plasmapheresis. Compared to conventional diuretic therapy, large volume paracentesis (4–6 L/24 hr) when combined with intravenous administration of albumin is associated with fewer complications, such as hepatic encephalopathy, renal impairement, and hyponateraemia. However, when less than 4L of ascites are removed per day, albumin may be unnecessary, and haemodynamic stability can usually be maintained with crystalloids. In nephrotic syndrome 25% albumin with diuretic therapy is a clinically beneficial approach only in patients resistant to diuretic therapy. A 5% albumin solution is the replacement fluid most frequently used in therapeutic plasma exchange. Although partial or full volume replacement with hydroxyethyl starch (HES) may be a cost-effective alternative to albumin, it is associated with more frequent untoward reactions (e.g. allergic reactions, coagulopathy).
- Albumin is also recommended from the beginning when burn injuries exceed 50% of body surface , and from 8 hours to 24 hours post-injury for burns between 15% and 50% of body surface in adults. The goal is to restore COP and not to normalize serum albumin. Other conditions in which albumin may be useful include: (a) Treatment of shock when membrane permeability has been restored and when hypoproteinemia prevents reversal of tissue oedema, as well as when renal dysfunction precludes the use of non-protein colloids. If sodium restriction is required, 25% albumin offers the additional benefit of a lower sodium load, (b) during cardiopulmonary bypass for pump or for perioperative plasma volume expansion in pediatric cardiac surgery, (c) liver transplant surgery, and (d) in conjunction with transfusion for the treatment of neonatal hyperbilirubinemia, owing to its in vivo bilirubin-binding capacity.
- The University Hospital Consortium guidelines for albumin, non-protein colloid, and crystalloid solutions state that (a) the effectiveness of colloid solution in the treatment of sepsis has not been shown in clinical trials, (b) crystalloids are considered the initial resuscitation fluid of choice for haemorrhagic shock, (c) colloids should be used in thermal injury after the first 24 hours if crystalloids fail to correct hypovolaemia, and (d) there is inconclusive published supportive evidence for using albumin for patients with severe hypoalbuminaemia.

References

1. American College of Physicians. Practice strategies for elective red blood cell transfusion. Ann Intern Med 1992;116:403-406.

2. American Society of Anesthesiologists Task Force on Blood Component Therapy Practice Guidelines for Blood Component Therapy, Anesthesiology 1996;84:732-742.
3. Beutler E. Platelet transfusions: the 20,000/ml, trigger. Blood 1993;81:1411-1413.
4. Bucur SZ, Berkman EM, Hillyer CD. Transfusion of Plasma Derivatives: Fresh-Frozen Plasma, Cryoprecipitate, Albumin, and Immunoglobulins. In: Hoffman R, Benz E, Shattil SJ, et al (eds). Hematology: Basic Principles and Practice, 3/ed.. Philadelphia: Churchill Livingstone, 2000, pp. 2266-2268.
5. Ciavarella D, Reed RL, Counts RB, et al. Clotting factor levels and the risk of diffuse microvascular bleeding in the massively transfused patient. Br J Haematol 1987;67:365-368.
6. Cochrane Injuries Group Albumin Reviewers. Human albumin administration in critically ill patients: systematic review of randomized controlled trials. BMJ 1998;317:235-40.
7. Collins JA, Simmons RL, James PM, Bredenberg CE, Anderson RW, Heisterkamp CA III. Acid base status of seriously wounded combat casualties: II. Resuscitation with stored blood. Ann Surg 1971;173:6-18.
8. Consensus Development Conference. Platelet transfusions. JAMA 1987;257:1777-1780.
9. Development Task Force of the College of American Pathologists: Practice parameters for the use of fresh-frozen plasma, cryoprecipitate and platelets. JAMA 1994;271:777.
10. ELY EW, Bernard GR. Transfusions in Critically Ill patients. N Engl J Med. 1999;340(6):467-468.
11. Gattinoni L, Brazzi L, Pelosi P, et al. A trial of goal-oriented hemodynamic therapy in critically ill patients. N Engl J Med 1995;333:1025-32.
12. Gines P, Arroyo V, Quintero E, et al. Comparison of paracentesis and diuretics in the treatment of cirrhotics with tense ascites. Results of a randomized study. Gastroenterology 1987;93:234-241.
13. Goodnough LT, Brecher ME, Kanter MH, Aubuchon JP. Transfusion medicine: Blood transfusion. N Engl J Med 1999;340(6):438-446.
14. Goodnough LT, Brecher ME, Kanter MH, Aubuchon JP. Transfusion Medicine: Blood Conservation. N Engl J 1999;340(7):525-532.
15. Hebbert PC, Wells G, Blajchman MA et al. With the Transfusion Requirements in Critical Care Trials Group. A multicentre, randomized controlled clinical trial of transfusion requirements in critical care. N Engl J Med 1999;340:409-417.
16. Hebert PC, Wells G, Marshall J, et al. Transfusion requirements in critical care: a pilot study. JAMA 1995;273:1439-1444 (Erratum, JAMA 1995;274:944.).
17. Hebert PC, Wells G, Martin C, et al. A Canadian survey of transfusion practices in critically ill patients. Crit Care Med 1998;26:282-287.
18. Heckman K. Weiner GJ, Strauss RG, et al. Randomized evaluation of the optimal platelet count for prophylactic platelet transfusion in patients undergoing indiction therapy for acute leukemia (abstract). Blood 1993;82(suppl 1):192a.
19. Humphries JE. Transfusion therapy in acquired coagulopathies. Transfus Med 1994;8:1181.
20. Linko K, Saxelin I. Electrolyte and acid-base disturbances caused by blood transfusions. Acta Anaesth Scand 1986;30:139-144.
21. Linko K, Tigerstedt I. Hyperpotassemia during massive blood transfusions. Acta Anaesth Scand 1984;28:220-221.
22. McClelland B. Albumin: don't confuse use with the facts. Editorial. Br Med J 1998;317:829-30.
23. Murray DJ, Olson J, Strauss R, Tinker JH. Coagulation changes during packed red cell replacement of major blood loss. Anesthesiology 1988;69:839-845.
24. Practice parameter for the use of fresh-frozen plasma, cryoprecipitate and platelets. Fresh-Frozen Plasma, Cryoprecipitate and Platelets Administration Practice Guidelines Development Task Force of the College of American Pathologists. JAMA 1994;271:777-781.

25. Reed RI II. Ciavarella D, Heimbach DM, et al. Prophylactic platelet administration during massive transfusion. A prospective, randomized, double-blind clinical study. Ann Surg 1986;203:40-48.

26. Reed RL II, Heimbach DM, Counts RB, et al. Prophylactic platelet administration during massive transfusion: a prospective, randomized, double-blind clinical study. Ann Surg 1986;203:40-48.

27. Shearer MJ, Barkhan P. Vitamin K and therapy of massive warfarin overdose, Lancet 1979; 1:266.

28. Soni N. Human albumin administration in critically ill patients. Validity of review methods must be assessed. Br Med J 1998;317:883-884.

29. Valeri CR, Khabbaz K, Khuri SF, et al. Effect of skin temperature on platelet function in patients undergoing extracorporeal bypass. J Thorac Cardiovasc Surg 1992;104:108-116.

30. Vermeulen LC Jr, Ratko TA, Erstad BL, Brecher ME, Matuszewski KA. A Paradigm for consensus: The University Hospital Consortium guidelines for the use of albumin, nonprotein colloid, and crystalloid solutions. Arch Intern. Med 1995;155:373-379.

31. Wallace EL, Churchill WH, Surgenor DM, Cho GS, McGurk S. Collection and transfusion of blood and blood components in the United States, 1994. Transfusion 1998;38:625-36.

32. Yim JM, Vermeulen, LC, Erstad BL, et al: Albumin and nonprotein colloid solution use in US academic health centers. Arc Intern Med 1995; 155:2450.

Administration of Blood and Blood Component 17

Introduction

- It may be useful to remember that a transfusion is a transplant with its inherent risks. Therefore, transfusion should only be ordered when the benefits outweigh the risks for a particular patient.
- "Blood cold chain" refers to the system of storing and transporting of blood and blood products so that they are at the correct temperature at all times, from the time of collection from the donor till the administration to the patient.
- Whole blood and red cells must always be stored at a temperature between +2 and +6°C. Temperatures above 6°C favour the growth of bacteria while temperatures below 2°C can haemolyse the RBCs. If this blood is transfused, the presence of cell membrane fragments and free haemoglobin can cause fatal bleeding problems or renal failure.
- Whole blood and red cells should be issued from the blood bank in a blood transport box or insulated box that helps keep the temperature below 10°C. This is necessary when blood has to be kept at a room temperature greater than 25°C or if there is a possibility that the blood will not be transfused within 30 minutes.
- If transfusion cannot be started within 30 minutes, blood should be stored in a refrigerator specifically designed for blood storage at a temperature between 2°C and 6°C. The temperature inside the refrigerator should be monitored at regular intervals to maintain temperature within this range. If a domestic refrigerator is used, blood should not be stored in the door, where the temperature is normally higher than inside the refrigerator or near the freezer compartment.
- Platelet concentrates should never be placed in a refrigerator.
- No medication or intravenous solution should be added to blood or blood components, with the exception of 0.9% sodium chloride (normal saline). Dextrose solutions can lyse the red cells. Any solution containing additives such as calcium can cause citrated blood to clot. Moreover, if there is an adverse reaction during the transfusion, it may be impossible to determine whether it is due to the blood, or to the added drug, or to an interaction between the two.

GUIDELINES FOR BLOOD AND BLOOD COMPONENT ADMINISTRATION

1. Explain the procedure and reason for administration of blood/blood component to the patient and/or family.

   Decreases anxiety.

2. **Record the baseline vital signs. Ask for history of transfusion in the past and the severity of transfusion reaction, if any.**

   Record temperature, pulse, blood pressure, breath sounds, fluid balance, and if applicable CVP and PAP/PCWP. Ensure that monitoring continues during and after transfusion in order to detect any adverse event as early as possible.

3. **Check/match the information on the patient's case sheet, blood bag label and on the compatibility label.**
   - Verifying this information reduces the chances of administration of an incompatible blood/blood component.
   - The checked/matched parameters should include: (a) Patient's name (exact spelling), (b) patient's hospital MRD/reference number, (c) patient's ward/operation theatre, (d) patient's blood group. Any discrepancy between the ABO group, Rh type, unit number, expiry date on blood bag and compatibility label should be checked.
   - After matching/checking the blood, the doctor should sign on the compatibility label.

4. **Examine the blood bag for any signs of deterioration (Fig. 17.1).**

   Look for any damage or for any leak in the bag. If time allows, mix the blood and let it settle until one can see the colour of the plasma layer, check for the following: (a) any sign of haemolysis in the plasma, (b) any sign of haemolysis on the line between red cell and plasma, (c) any sign of contamination, such as a change of colour in the red cells, which often look darker or purple/black when contaminated, and (d) any clots, which may mean that the blood was not mixed properly with the anticoagulant when it was collected. Any bag which shows signs of leakage, or has pink or red plasma, or the red cells look purple or black, should not be transfused.

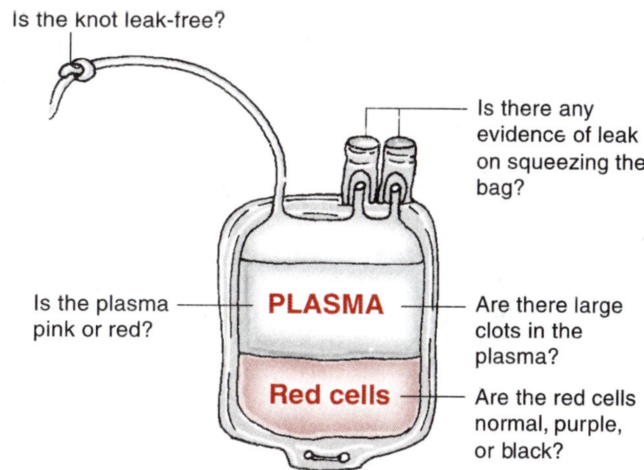

Fig. 17.1: Checking for signs of deterioration in blood or plasma.

5. **Consider the total time the blood/blood component has been out of correct storage conditions.**
   - There is a risk of bacterial proliferation or loss of function of blood products once they have been removed from the correct storage conditions.
   - The administration of whole blood or red cells should be started within 30 minutes of removing the bag from the storage temperature of 2°C to 6°C. It should be completed within 4 hours of starting the transfusion.

- Platelet concentrates should be administered as soon as they are received and each concentrate should be completely infused within 20 minutes.
- Fresh frozen plasma should be infused as soon as possible after thawing, to avoid loss of labile clotting factors and the infusion should be completed within 20 minutes.
- Any bag which has been (or may have been) out of the refrigerator for longer than 30 minutes should not be used.

6. **Wash hands.**
   This reduces the risk of transmission of micro-organisms.

7. **Establish or ensure the patency of intravenous line.**
   Use an 18G, (minimum 20G) cannula, as the flow of blood at high pressures (if required to be transfused fast) through a smaller-gauge cannula may damage the red cells. If necessary, flush the line with normal saline solution before transfusion.

8. **Consider if warming of blood is required.**
   When infusion is slow, there is no need to warm the blood. Warming is more commonly required when large volume/rapid transfusion is required (i.e. adults: greater than 50 mL/kg/hr, children greater than 15 mL/kg/hr) or during exchange transfusion in infants. Blood should only be warmed in a blood warmer and not in a bowel of hot water, as this could lead to the haemolysis of the red cells and liberation of potassium, both of which could be life threatening.

9. **Prepare the administration set. Spike the unit of blood/blood component. Prime the drip chamber (making sure that the filter is covered) and the remaining length of the administration set tubing.**
   All blood/blood components should be administered through a set containing an integral 170-200 microns filter. The set should be changed at least 12 hourly during blood/blood component infusion.

10. **Connect the administration set to the IV cannula under aseptic conditions.**
11. **Adjust the rate of infusion to 10-15 drops per minute for the first 15 minutes.**
    Ensures that the patient receives a small amount of blood/blood component, which can help detect a transfusion reaction.

12. **If there is no transfusion reaction, adjust the rate to complete transfusion within the prescribed time limit or according to the condition of the patient.**
    Likelihood of a bacterial contamination increases beyond the prescribed hang time.

13. **In case of suspected transfusion reaction, take the necessary steps.**
    - Stop blood transfusion immediately.
    - Do not discard the blood bag and administration set.
    - Obtain a urine sample and get it examined for the presence of red blood cells or free haemoglobin.
    - Obtain the blood sample.
    - Recheck the blood bag label, compatibility label and the patient's case sheet. Fill in the specific form for transfusion reaction.

- Return the blood bag, samples and the form to the blood bank.
- Treat the patient with antihistaminics, steroids, oxygen, fluid resuscitation, vasopressors, mannitol, antipyretics, and adrenaline, as and when required.
- Monitor hourly urine output in addition to the monitoring prescribed for blood transfusion.

14. On completion of the transfusion, remove the empty bag and start a primary fluid infusion at the prescribed rate.
15. Discard the bag and administration set. Wash hands.

    This reduces the risk of transmission of micro-organisms.

16. Monitor the patient.

    Monitor the patient at the following stages: (a) Before starting the transfusion, (b) as soon as transfusion is started, (c) continuously for the first 15 minutes, (d) at 15 minute intervals during the first hour, (e) at least every hour after the first hour, (f) on completion of transfusion, and (g) 4 hours after completing the transfusion.

17. Record the observations.

    Documentation should include: (a) Time of starting and completing the transfusion, (b) volume and type of the product transfused, (c) baseline and serial vital sign measurements, and (d) any untoward reactions/effects.

References

1. American College of Physicians. Practice strategies for elective red blood cell transfusion. Ann Intern Med 1992;116:403-6.
2. American Society of Anesthesiologists Task Force on Blood Component Therapy Practice Guidelines for Blood Component Therapy. Anesthesiology 1996;84:732-742.
3. Beutler E. Platelet transfusions: the 20,000/ml, trigger. Blood 1993;81:1411-1413.
4. Bucur SZ, Berkman EM, Hillyer CD. Transfusion of Plasma Derivatives: Fresh-Frozen Plasma, Cryoprecipitate, Albumin, and Immunoglobulins. In: Hoffman R, Benz E, Shattil SJ, et al, eds. Hematology: Basic Principles and Practice, 3/ed. Philadelphia: Churchill Livingstone, 2000, pp 2266-2268.
5. Ciavarella D, Reed RL, Counts RB, et al. Clotting factor levels and the risk of diffuse microvascular bleeding in the massively transfused patient. Br J Haematol 1987;67:365-368.
6. Cochrane Injuries Group Albumin Reviewers. Human albumin administration in critically ill patients: systematic review of randomized controlled trials. BMJ 1998;317:235-240.
7. Collins JA, Simmons RL, James PM, Bredenberg CE, Anderson RW, Heisterkamp CA III. Acid base status of seriously wounded combat casualties: II. Resuscitation with stored blood. Ann Surg 1971;173:6-18.
8. Consensus Development Conference. Platelet transfusions. JAMA 1987;257:1777-1780.
9. Development Task Force of the College of American Pathologists: Practice parameters for the use of fresh-frozen plasma, cryoprecipitate and platelets. JAMA 1994;271:777.
10. ELY EW, Bernard GR. Transfusions in Critically Ill patients. N Engl J Med. 1999;340(6):467-468.
11. Gattinoni L, Brazzi L, Pelosi P, et al. A trial of goal-oriented hemodynamic therapy in critically ill patients. N Engl J Med 1995;333:1025-1032.
12. Gines P, Arroyo V, Quintero E, et al. Comparison of paracentesis and diuretics in the treatment of cirrhotics with tense ascites. Results of a randomized study. Gastroenterology 1987;93:234-241.

13. Goodnough LT, Brecher ME, Kanter MH, Aubuchon JP. Transfusion medicine: Blood transfusion. N Engl J Med 1999;340(6):438-446.

14. Goodnough LT, Brecher ME, Kanter MH, Aubuchon JP. Transfusion medicine: Blood conservation. 1999;340(7):525-532.

15. Hebbert PC, Wells G, Blajchman MA et al. With the Transfusion Requirements in Critical Care Trials Group. A multicentre, randomized controlled clinical trial of transfusion requirements in critical care. N Engl J Med 1999;340:409-417.

16. Hebert PC, Wells G, Marshall J, et al. Transfusion requirements in critical care: A pilot study. JAMA 1995;273:1439-19944. (Erratum JAMA 1995;274:944).

17. Hebert PC, Wells G, Martin C, et al. A Canadian survey of transfusion practices in critically ill patients. Crit Care Med 1998;26:282-287.

18. Heckman K. Weiner GJ, Strauss RG, et al. Randomized evaluation of the optimal platelet count for prophylactic platelet transfusion in patients undergoing indiction therapy for acute leukemia (abstract). Blood 1993;82(suppl 1):192a.

19. Humphries JE. Transfusion therapy in acquired coagulopathies. Transfus Med 1994;8:1181.

20. Linko K, Saxelin I, Electrolyte and acid-base disturbances caused by blood transfusions. Acta Anaesth Scand 1986;30:139-144.

21. Linko K, Tigerstedt I. Hyperpotassemia during massive blood transfusions. Acta Anaesth Scand 1984; 28:220-221.

22. McClelland B. Albumin: don't confuse use with the facts. Editorial. Br Med J 1998;317:829-30.

23. Murray DJ, Olson J, Strauss R, Tinker JH. Coagulation changes during packed red cell replacement of major blood loss. Anesthesiology 1988;69:839-845.

24. Practice parameter for the use of fresh-frozen plasma, cryoprecipitate and platelets. Fresh-Frozen Plasma, Cryoprecipitate and Platelets Administration Practice Guidelines Development Task Force of the College of American Pathologists. JAMA 1994;271:777-781.

25. Reed RI II. Ciavarella D, Heimbach DM, et al. Prophylactic platelet administration during massive transfusion. A prospective, randomized, double-blind clinical study. Ann Surg 1986;203:40-48.

26. Reed RL II, Heimbach DM, Counts RB, et al. Prophylactic platelet administration during, massive transfusion: a prospective, randomized, double-blind clinical study. Ann Surg 1986;203:40-48.

27. Shearer MJ, Barkhan P. Vitamin K and therapy of massive warfarin overdose, Lancet 1979; 1:266.

28. Soni N. Human albumin administration in critically ill patients. Validity of review methods must be assessed. Br Med J 1998;317:883-884.

29. Valeri CR, Khabbaz K, Khuri SF, et al. Effect of skin temperature on platelet function in patients undergoing extracorporeal bypass. J Thorac Cardiovasc Surg 1992;104:108-116.

30. Vermeulen LC Jr, Ratko TA, Erstad BL, Brecher ME, Matuszewski KA. A Paradigm for consensus: The University Hospital Consortium guidelines for the use of albumin, nonprotein colloid, and crystalloid solutions. Arch Intern Med 1995;155:373-379.

31. Wallace EL, Churchill WH, Surgenor DM, Cho GS, McGurk S. Collection and transfusion of blood and blood components in the United States, 1994. Transfusion 1998;38:625-36.

32. Yim JM, Vermeulen, LC, Erstad BL, et al. Albumin and nonprotein colloid solution use in US academic health centers. Arc Intern Med 1995; 155:2450.

Management of a Patient with Massive Transfusion 18

Introduction

- Massive transfusion refers to: (a) Replacement of a patient's entire blood volume in a 24-hour period, (b) transfusion of more than 10 units of whole blood or 20 units of packed red blood cells, or (c) replacement of more than 50% of the circulating blood volume in 3 hours or less.
- The purpose of transfusion is to: (a) Restore circulation, (b) achieve adequate oxygen carrying capacity, (c) normalize haemostasis, (d) achieve optimum oncotic pressure, and (e) maintain normal plasma biochemistry.
- The pathophysiological changes associated with massive transfusion may be related to the patient's underlying condition or injury, a consequence of haemorrhagic shock (i.e. tissue hypoperfusion, acidosis, and hypoxia), or may result from the transfused blood components.
- Adverse effects of massive transfusion include coagulopathy, citrate toxicity, derangement of acid-base balance, platelet abnormalities, hypothermia, transfusion reactions, and changes in potassium and coagulation factors.
- The haemostatic abnormalities (coagulopathy) associated with massive transfusion occur either because of a dilutional effect of massive transfusion or due to the patient's underlying condition (e.g. consumption due to DIC). Dilutional effects occur because the stored whole blood does not contain viable platelets and the labile coagulation factors V and VIII. Probably, the more important pathophysiological process contributing to the coagulopathy associated with massive transfusion, is consumption of coagulation elements due to DIC. In a patient with massive haemorrhage requiring massive blood transfusion, tissue perfusion and oxygen-carrying capacity are often inadequate, and a cycle of hypotension, tissue injury or ischaemia, and acidosis results in release of tissue factors into the circulation. This results in a systemic activation of the coagulation system. The resulting pathological process of DIC is characterized by coagulation factor and platelet activation and consumption, intravascular thrombi formation, and activation of the fibrinolytic system. This leads to thrombocytopenia, depletion of plasma coagulation factors and fibrinogen, and elevated levels of fibrinogen/fibrin degradation products (FDPs). Circulating FDPs interfere with normal clot formation and thus exacerbate the haemostatic defect. Other factors contributing to the development of coagulopathy are dilutional effect of crystalloids/colloids and hypothermia.
- Routine administration of calcium, bicarbonate and prophylactic transfusion of fresh frozen plasma following massive transfusion is contraindicated.

- Patients receiving massive transfusion who develop microvascular bleeding unrelated to hypothermia are best treated with platelet concentrates, which provide clotting factors in addition to platelets. Platelet concentrates contain a significant amount of all clotting factors except factor VIII, which is often released as part of the acute phase reaction.

GUIDELINES FOR MANAGING A PATIENT WITH MASSIVE TRANSFUSION

1. Monitor the patient's vital signs every 5–15 minutes, as indicated. Once the patient becomes more stable, the frequency of monitoring can be decreased (every 15–30 minutes) until the blood pressure remains stable for more than 2 hours.
   - Although the volume of blood transfused may lead to a variety of potentially serious problems, both, the duration and severity of shock appear to be more significant determinants of physiologic derangements than the transfusion of blood itself.
   - Gives early information about transfusion reactions, if any.

2. Assess the patient's core temperature every 15 – 30 minutes.
   - Patients in severe shock have impaired thermogenesis. This, in combination with rapid infusion of inadequately warmed (often cold) fluids, old age, debilitated condition, and the nature of surgery (thoracotomy or laparotomy), very commonly leads to hypothermia. Further, not only is systemic temperature important, but the temperature at which the wound is expected to coagulate is critical. It is not uncommon during surgery to find a patient's bladder or rectal temperature at 35°C and the wound edge (where coagulation is expected to take place) at 27–28°C. At that temperature coagulation is dysfunctional. Hypothermia (a) increases the affinity of haemoglobin for oxygen, (b) impairs platelet function, (c) induces coagulopathy (below core temperature of 35°C), even if the levels of clotting factors and platelets are normal, apparently because of decreased enzymatic activity, (d) increases the potential for hypocalcaemia, as a cold liver cannot metabolize citrate as well, and (e) can induce fatal arrhythmias, if blood is being transfused through a central line with the tip near the sinoatrial node.
   - Hypothermia can be prevented by (a) warming intravenous fluids and blood before administration (should not be heated to more than 40°C), (b) warming the inspired gas, (c) insulating the patient's head and extremities (especially in infants and small children), and (d) keeping the resuscitation room or operating room heated to approximately 30°C.

3. Assess the integrity of IV sites every 15 minutes.
   IV sites under pressure are at a higher risk for extravasation. Lines may be pulled out during change of position or other similar manoeuvres. IV sites should be clearly visible, especially in neonates and infants as they tend to get hidden under drapes.

4.　Assess haemodynamic parameters every 15–30 minutes.
　　Gives a complete picture of the patient.

5.　Assess urine output every 30–60 minutes.
- If urine output is less than 0.5 mL/kg/hr, it is presumed that the kidneys are not being perfused, and it is possible that other major viscera are also not being perfused.
- Direct trauma to the urinary tract may interfere with accurate assessment of urine output, as clots may block the drainage of urine and laceration of ureters may result in extravasation of urine into the peritoneum.
- Output might decrease after a major transfusion reaction.

6.　Draw blood samples for haemoglobin, haematocrit, platelet count, prothrombin time (PT), partial thromboplastin time, thrombin time, fibrinogen levels, and/or whole blood TEG, in the intraoperative as well as in the postoperative period.

- Determines presence of ongoing blood loss and coagulopathies.
- Any massively transfused patient, whose haematocrit falls for an unknown reason, or who develops fever or jaundice, should be suspected of having a haemolytic reaction, which can occur even hours to days after a blood transfusion.
- Probably the most common cause of bleeding in a massively transfused patient is hypothermia, although depletion of platelets and coagulation factors depletion may occasionally be contributory. The primary treatment of microvascular bleeding associated with massive transfusion includes correction of shock and hypothermia. There is no demonstrated role of prophylactic platelet or FFP transfusion in a patient receiving blood transfusion. It is appropriate to monitor the platelet count and delay platelet therapy until coagulopathy and thrombocytopenia actually coexist (see Chapter 16). Generally, dilutional thrombocytopenia should be anticipated after a blood volume replacement of 150% and in order to secure haemostasis, the platelet count should be maintained above 50×10^9/L. If the platelet count falls below 50×10^9/L, platelets should be administered even in the absence of microvascular bleeding, because this degree of thrombocytopenia has historically been considered the lower limit for adequate surgical haemostasis. If microvascular bleeding persists despite a platelet count of at least 90×10^9/L to 100×10^9/L, either platelet dysfunction (e.g. due to hypothermia or FDPs) or coagulation factor abnormalities can be presumed. The next step at this juncture is to look for fibrinogen levels. If the fibrinogen level is less than 80–100 mg/dL, cryoprecipitate transfusion is indicated. It should be noted that severe hypofibrinogenemia (i.e. less than 50–75 mg/dL) can result in prolongation of the PT and PTT independent of the levels of other coagulation factors. Furthermore, a prolonged thrombin time in the presence of a fibrinogen level greater than 100 mg/dL indicates the presence of a circulatory coagulation inhibitor (e.g. FDP or heparin). When the thrombin time is normal, and fibrinogen level is greater than 100 mg/dL and PT and/or PTT

are prolonged (more than 1.5 times control), it is an indication for the transfusion of FFP. Generally transfusion of 2–6 units of FFP may be required at this stage.

7. **Draw arterial sample for blood gases.**

    Although stored packed RBCs have an acidic pH (about 6.3), massive transfusion usually result in alkalosis (because sodium citrate in the anticoagulant is converted to sodium bicarbonate in the liver). Therefore, routine prophylactic administration of bicarbonate is not indicated. Presence of metabolic acidosis in a patient of shock, is usually due to anaerobic conversion of glucose to lactate, and provides a marker for additional resuscitation and efforts to improve perfusion to major organs.

8. **Draw sample for calcium and potassium.**

    - Transient hypocalcaemia due to citrate anticoagulant binding ionized calcium can arise after massive transfusion. But this problem is significant only in neonates and if hypothermia is present. Treatment with 10% calcium gluconate should be given only if clinical or electrocardiographic evidence of hypocalcaemia exists in the form of hypotension, narrowed pulse pressure, elevated left ventricular end-diastolic, pulmonary artery and central venous pressures, and prolonged QT interval on the ECG.
    - Stored blood has increased concentration of potassium, and theoretically, there is a possibility of hyperkalaemia with massive transfusion. In clinical practice, with transfusion rates not exceeding 100–150 mL/minute, this is rarely a problem.
    - Hypokalaemia may also occur during massive transfusion and is related to metabolic disturbances such as hypotension, alkalosis, and catecholamine release, causing reentry of potassium into the red cells. Since potassium levels depend on many coexisting factors and are unpredictable, potassium levels should be monitored closely in massively transfused patients.

9. **Continue to monitor the patient at regular intervals.**

    It takes time (24-72 hr) for a patient with shock who has received massive transfusion to become stable.

References

1. Collins JA. Massive blood transfusion. Clin Haematol 1976;5:201-222.
2. Iserson KV, Huestis DW. Blood warming: current applications and techniques. Transfusion 1991;31: 558-571.
3. Lim RC Jr, Olcott C, Robinson AJ, Blaisdell FW. Platelet response and coagulation changes following massive blood transfusion. J Trauma 1973;13:577-582.
4. Lovric V. Alterations in blood components during storage and their clinical significance. Anaesth Intensive Care 1984;12:246-251.
5. Michelsen T, Salmela I, Tigerstedt I, Makelainen A, Linko K. Massive blood transfusion: is there a limit? Crit Care Med 1989;17:699-700.

6. Mikisalo HJ, Soini HO, Nordin AJ, Haekerstedt KAV. Effects of bicarbonate therapy on tissue oxygenation during resuscitation of haemorrhagic shock. Crit Care Med 1989;17:1170-1174.

7. Patterson A. Massive transfusion. Int Anesthesiol Clin 1987;25:61-74.

8. Rutledge R, Sheldon GF, Collins ML. Massive transfusion. Crit Care Clinics 1986;2:791-805.

9. Valeri CR. Feingold H, Cassidy G, Ragno G, Khuri S, Allschule MD. Hypothermia-induced reversible platelet dysfunction. Ann Surg 1987;205:175-181.

10. Wilson RF, Binkley LE, Sabo FM Jr, et al. Electrolyte and acid-base changes with massive blood transfusions. Am Surg 1992;58:535-545.

11. Wudel JH, Morris JA Jr, Yates K, Wilson A, Bass SM. Massive transfusion: outcome in blunt trauma patients. J Trauma 1991;31:1-7.

Management of Acute Hyperkalaemia

19

Introduction

- Hyperkalaemia is defined as serum potassium levels exceeding 5 mmol/L. It may be associated with high, normal or low potassium stores.
- Pseudohyperkalaemia, an in vitro phenomenon, results from potassium release from cells in the test tube during sampling of blood. It can also be seen in patients with extreme leukocytosis (leukocyte count > 200,000/mm^3) or thrombocytosis (platelets >750,000/mm^3).
- Hyperkalaemia may produce serious side effects when the serum potassium is greater than 6 mmol/L. The correlation between the serum potassium and untoward effects (arrhythmias) is not reliable. In general, the rate at which hyperkalaemia develops is as important as its degree in determining its overall threat to the patient. Hyperkalaemia endangers life by provoking cardiac arrhythmias. Mortality and ECG studies support the contention that a level of 7 mmol/L is a critical value for potassium.
- In patients on digitalis, calcium must be given cautiously and slowly over 20-30 minutes (with dilution in 100 mL of saline) as hypercalcaemia can potentiate digitalis cardiotoxicity. If hyperkalaemia is a manifestation of digitalis toxicity, calcium is contraindicated; magnesium sulfate 2 g IV bolus may instead be given, used over 20 minutes followed by a continuous infusion of 1–2 g/hr to maintain serum magnesium levels of 4–5 mEq/L.

GUIDELINES FOR MANAGEMENT OF ACUTE HYPERKALAEMIA

1. **Is the hyperkalaemia real?**

   Pseudohyperkalaemia is due to cell rupture or depolarization of cell membranes during withdrawal of blood. It may occur because of excessive fist clenching, improper technique of drawing blood and lysis of blood cells. To minimize the error, draw two blood samples simultaneously – one from the arm by the usual technique and the other, from the femoral vein or an artery using a fresh heparinized syringe. Both reports should differ by less than 0.2 – 0.3 mmol/L. Moreover, pseudohyperkalaemia is not associated with ECG changes.

2. **Define the urgency.**

   There is no specific level of serum potassium that indicates a life-threatening situation. In general, hyperkalaemia is better tolerated if it develops slowly (chronic) and in the very young. The factors pointing towards the possibility of an arrhythmia are changes in the ECG, a sudden rise in the level of serum potassium, likelihood of potassium being released into the extracellular fluid (cell lysis and recovery from an ileus, especially if oral potassium was given), and the continued use of drugs like β-blockers which may worsen the hyperkalaemia.

If the danger of arrhythmia appears to be small, go slow, stop potassium intake, make a diagnosis and proceed accordingly.

3. **When urgency is established (ECG changes are present) or there is a high risk of arrhythmias:**
   - Give calcium gluconate 10%, 10 mL IV over 2-5 minutes. Onset of action is within 1-3 minutes and lasts for 30-60 minutes. It may be repeated once, if there is no response to the first dose. It works by antagonizing the cardiac effects of hyperkalaemia.
   - Shift potassium into cells with insulin (avoid hypoglycaemia). Give 10 U regular insulin diluted in 500mL of 10% Dextrose at the rate of 150-200 mL/hr. Action starts within 20 minutes and lasts for 4-6 hours. It decreases the potassium level by 1mmol/L for 1-2 hours. If acidaemia is present (bicarbonate < 15 mmol/L) and if there is no heart failure, give 50 mmol of $NaHCO_3$. Intravenous salbutamol (4 mcg/kg in 5 ml water) or nebulised salbutamol (2.5-5.0 mg) given over 15-20 minutes also acts rapidly to lower serum potassium levels.
   - Stop potassium intake; avoid drugs that predispose to hyperkalaemia (ACE inhibitors, β-blockers, NSAIDS, succinylcholine, potassium sparing diuretics, and heparin).
   - Promote urinary potassium loss - use loop diuretics, e.g. furosemide. Restore the ECF volume if it is contracted (e.g. infuse saline).
   - Bind potassium in the GI tract – give potassium exchange resins (kayexalate, Na^+ polystyrene sulphonate), orally or by enema. Enema acts faster. 100 g of resin is given in as little water as is needed to dissolve it (say, 200 mL) and kept in the colon for as long as possible.
   - Haemodialysis – action is immediate and it is the most effective method of lowering serum potassium.

4. **Assess the cause and manage.**
   After the treatment of the actue phase, a long-term plan should be implemented to prevent recurrence of the hyperkalaemia.

References

1. Blumberg A, Weidmann P, Gnadinger M. Effect of various therapeutic approaches on plasma potassium and major regulating factors in terminal renal failure. Am J Med 1988; 85:507-512.
2. Don BR, Sebastian A, Cheitlin M, et al. Pseudohyperkalemia caused by fist clenching during phlebotomy. N Eng J Med 1990; 322:1290-1293.
3. Rasterger A, Soleimani M. Hypokalaemia and hyperkalaemia. Postgrad Med J 2001; 77:759-764.

Introduction

- Hypokalaemia is defined as serum potassium levels less than 3.5 mmol/L.
- The urgency of replacement is dictated by a number of factors like (a) Intake of drugs (e.g. digitalis) or presence of heart disease, which may increase the likelihood of cardiac arrhythmias, (b) the possibility that potassium will shift into the cells (e.g. during recovery from diabetic ketoacidosis or during administration of β_2–adrenergic drugs), (c) development of severe weakness in a patient, who is hyperventilating because of metabolic acidosis, (d) the severity of the deficit and the continuing potassium losses, and (e) presence of advanced liver disease, and hepatic encephalopathy.
- Hypomagnesaemia is frequently associated with hypokalaemia. It is important to remember that magnesium is required for potassium entry into the cells. Thus, magnesium administration is frequently necessary for potassium retention in hypokalaemic, critically ill patients and in patients who are refractory to replacement therapy.
- Since hypokalaemia can lead to life-threatening events, one might have to initiate therapy before the investigations can be completed. Full replacement of potassium deficit usually takes a few days. There is lack of proof that treating hypokalaemia (3.0-3.5 mmol/L) really does diminish the cardiac arrhythmias and improves the patient's well being except in a patient who is on digitalis therapy.

GUIDELINES FOR POTASSIUM REPLACEMENT

1. **Check the clinical record of the patient.**

   It is important, from the history and examination findings and the investigative work-up (including ECG) of the patient, to know the urgency of the treatment and the probable cause of hypokalaemia.

2. **Calculate the total amount of potassium to be infused.**

   It is difficult to calculate accurately the degree of hypokalaemia in relation to the extent of total body deficit. A fall in serum potassium from 4 to 3 mmol/L is usually associated with a total body deficit of 100-400 mmol; a much larger deficit is required to lower the plasma potassium from 3 to 2 mmol/L. Therefore, although many rough guidelines exist for relating the deficit of potsssium to the degree of hypokalaemia, these are unreliable in an individual patient.

Moreover, while calculating the total body potassium deficit, one should consider other factors that can independently affect serum potassium. For example, a patient with a serum potassium of 2.5 mmol/L has less total body deficit at a blood pH of 7.5 than at 7.3, because alkalaemia can independently lower the serum potassium by intracellular shift.

3. **Decide the route of potassium replacement. Oral route is safer than IV route.**
    - When considering the quantity of potassium to be administered, the aim should be to get the patient out of danger quickly and to replace the entire potassium deficit more slowly. The main consideration in the initial period is to deliver enough potassium to the cell membrane of the heart so as to avoid a life-threatening arrhythmia. For example, in an adult patient weighing 70 kg, having a serum potassium of 1.5 mmol/L and an abnormal ECG, the aim should be to raise the serum potassium from 1.5 to 3.0 mmol/L in one minute. To do so, one should infuse 4.5 mmol of KCl over one minute under cardiac monitoring. This can be explained as follows: the total blood volume (5 L) circulates each minute (cardiac output is 5 L/min). Because 60% of this blood volume is plasma (3 L), and the target for the serum potassium is 3.0 mmol/L, then (desired K^+ – actual K^+) multiplied by 3L or 1.5 mmol/L × 3L must be given over 1 minute. The infused volume will mix with interstitial fluid before reaching the cell membrane, so there will be a much smaller rise in potassium next to cell membranes. Following this dose, the rate of administration should be slowed down and serum potassium measured in 5 minutes.
    - Except in this extreme situation, in general, oral route is the safest and IV route should be used when GI problems limit the intake or absorption, in the presence of severe degree (< 2.5 mmol/L) of hypokalaemia with either respiratory muscle weakness or cardiac arrhythmias and when there is an anticipated shift of potassium into the intracellular fluid (recovery from diabetic ketoacidosis).

4. **Prepare the drug.**
    - The most common replacement fluid is potassium chloride (KCl), which is available as a concentrated solution (2 mEq/mL), with an osmolality of 4000 mOsm/kg H_2O. It must be diluted before infusion.
    - When correcting hypokalaemia, potassium should not be diluted in glucose-containing solutions because the glucose (via insulin) can lead to an initial lowering of the plasma potassium.

5. **Choose the vein for infusion.**
    Preferably a large central vein should be used for infusion because of the irritant properties of hyperosmotic potassium solutions. However, avoid infusion through central venous catheters with their distal tips in the superior vena cavae or right atrium because delivery of concentrated solution of potassium to the heart can precipitate hyperkalaemic arrhythmias. This is especially important when giving a small bolus dose as described in step 3. On the other hand, concentrations higher than 60mmol/L through peripheral veins may lead to local discomfort, venous spasm, or sclerosis.

6. **Set the infusion rate.**

   When serum potassium level is more than 2 mmol/L and ECG abnormalities are not present, the recommended rate of infusion is 10 mmol/hr of KCl. However, when serum potassium is less than 2 mmol/L or if ECG abnormalities are present or in the presence of muscle weakness/paralysis, up to 40 mmol/hr of KCl in saline may be given. Dose rates as high as 80 mmol/hr have been used safely.

7. **Adopt general measures.**

   - Evaluate and treat the underlying cause. Discontinue offending drugs (diuretics, steroids, β-agonists, laxatives, gentamicin, ampicillin, penicillin, carbenicillin, ticarcillin, etc.).
   - Correct alkalosis, hypomagnesaemia.

8. **After deficits are corrected, start on maintenance potassium therapy.**

   Maintenance therapy is required to cover up the ongoing losses.

References

1. Flakeb G, Villarread D, Chapman D. Is hypokalaemia a cause of ventricular arrhythmias? J Crit Illness 1986; 1:66-74.
2. Freedman BI, Burkhart JM. Hypokalaemia. Crit Care Clin 1991; 7:143-153.
3. Gennari FJ. Hypokalaemia. N Eng J Med 1998; 339(7): 451-458.
4. Kamel KS, et al. Disorders of potassium homeostasis: An approach based on pathophysiology. Am J Kidney Dis 1994; 24:597-613.
5. Rastergar A, Soleimani M. Hypokalaemia and hyperkalaemia. Postgrad Med J 2001; 77:759-764.

Acute Renal Failure

21

Introduction

- Acute renal failure (ARF) is an abrupt (within hours or days) deterioration of renal function because of a decrease in glomerular filtration rate (GFR), or due to a renal tubular injury compromising the kidney's ability to maintain fluid or electrolyte homeostasis. Acute renal failure may or may not be associated with a decrease in urine output. Accumulation of nitrogenous waste products, or failure to maintain water or electrolyte homeostasis in the face of a urine output of less than 400mL in 24-hour period is called oliguric renal failure. When urine output is between 400-1000 mL/24 hr, it is termed non-oliguric renal failure, while a high-output renal failure refers to renal insufficiency despite maintenance of urine output greater than 1000 mL/24 hr.
- Despite efforts devoted to the study of ARF, no consensus definition of ARF exists. Most commonly, investigators define ARF as (a) an increase in serum creatinine of 0.5 mg/dL or greater from baseline, (b) a 50% increase in serum creatinine, (c) a 50% reduction in calculated creatinine clearance, or (d) a decrease in renal function that warrants dialysis. Recently, the following criteria have been proposed to define acute renal failure so that further work on ARF is subject to uniformity.

	Normal	ARI	A/C ARI	ARFS	A/C ARFS	Severe ARFS	Severe A/C ARFS
Creatinine	Normal	>N	Rise>0.5 × N	> × 2 N;	Rise > × 1 N		
BUN	Normal	>N	Rise>0.5 × N	> × 2 N	Rise > × 1 N		
U-O	Normal	<N	<N	<0.5 × N	<0.5 × N		
RRT						Needs RRT	Needs RRT

These criteria need to be preceded by a known cause of ARF developing over a period of 24 hours. The creatinine value and either the BUN or the U-O value must be met.
Abbreviations: ARI, acute renal injury; A/C, acute on chronic; ARFS, acute renal failure syndrome; N, normal range value; 0.5 × N, half of normal value; × 2 N, double normal value; RRT, renal replacement therapy; U-O, urine output (normal > 800 mL/24hr).

- There is enough evidence, to demonstrate the particular vulnerability of the kidney to ischaemia. Such vulnerability involves the renal medulla in particular, and is due to the unique arrangement of the renal vasculature in the medulla and to the countercurrent solute transport between the venous and arterial circulation that surrounds the loop of Henle. Countercurrent solute transport allows the kidney to concentrate urine but, as oxygen is one of the solutes moving from the arterial to the venous circulation in the hairpin loop of vessels surrounding the tubular loop, there is rapid desaturation of arterial blood as it descends into the outer medulla. The consequence of this anatomical and physiological arrangement is, that the medulla lives in an "ischaemic penumbra" at the best of times. Thus, even small decreases in renal blood flow and renal oxygen delivery will trigger medullary ischaemia. Such ischaemia results in ATP utilization and depletion. This, in turn, will liberate increased amounts of adenosine. Being a powerful afferent arteriolar vasoconstrictor, adenosine will decrease the glomerular blood flow, GFR, and urine output. If the ischaemia persists, physical cell injury develops in a continuum that goes from severe dysfunction to cell death. Therefore, to achieve optimal renal resuscitation, restoration of oxygen delivery to the kidney is of paramount importance. As oxygen delivery to the kidney depends on renal blood flow, renal resuscitation should primarily focus on restoring the blood flow.

- Acute renal failure, as commonly seen in the ICU is usually multifactorial. Common causes are hypotension, hypovolaemia, shock, sepsis, post-trauma state, postoperative period and chronic medical problems (liver disease, congestive heart failure, malignancy, post-CPR). These may not represent the classic spectrum of causes as seen by a nephrologist.

- Risk factors for post-traumatic ARF include (a) Hypoperfusion, (b) hypoxia, (c) direct cellular toxicity due to either endogenous nephrotoxins (myoglobin, haemoglobin) released following crush injuries, burns, or major vascular injuries or exogenous nephrotoxins (aminoglycosides, catecholamines, contrast agents, or vancomycin), (d) direct parenchymal injury and or (e) abdominal compartment syndrome. High-risk procedures which increase the risk of postoperative ARF include renal revascularization, aortic cross-clamping, cardiopulmonary bypass, urologic procedures, and transplantation. The risk is intensified in patients with advanced age and pre-existing chronic renal insufficiency [congestive heart failure, diabetic nephropathy, hypertensive nephropathy, liver failure (hepatorenal syndrome) and pregnancy-induced hypertension] as these patients may have a sustained progressive loss of functional nephrons, and may also have less effective compensatory and protective mechanisms.

- While most patients who develop ARF have more than one risk factor, renal ischaemia is the central contributor in at least half of these cases and can result from low renal blood flow or from altered intrarenal haemodynamics. Renal blood flow may be compromised due to (a) Absolute loss of intravascular volume (haemorrhage, gastrointestinal losses, etc), (b) decreased effective intravascular volume (sepsis, peritonitis, rhabdomyolysis, severe soft-tissue injuries, or burns), or (c) diminished cardiac output (congestive heart failure, myocardial ischaemia, dysrhythmia). A variety of medications (non-steroidal anti-inflammatory drugs, angiotensin-converting enzyme inhibitors, radiocontrast media, and amphotericin-B) can alter intrarenal haemodynamics, disrupt renal autoregulation, and produce patchy areas of ischaemia.

- Acute renal failure affects almost every organ system depending on the severity and duration of renal dysfunction. These include: (a) Cardiovascular (pulmonary edema, arrhythmia, hypertension, pericarditis, pericardial effusion, myocardial infarction, pulmonary embolism), (b) metabolic (hyponatraemia, hyperkalaemia, acidosis, hypocalcaemia, hyperphosphataemia, hypermagnesaemia, hyperuricaemia), (c) neurologic (asterixis, neuromuscular irritability, mental status changes, somnolence, coma, seizures), (d) gastrointestinal (nausea, vomiting, gastritis, gastroduodenal ulcers, gastrointestinal bleeding, pancreatitis, malnutrition), (e) haematologic (anaemia, haemorrhagic diathesis), and (f) infections (pneumonia, septicemia, urinary tract infection, wound infection).

- The typical biochemical abnormalities associated with acute renal failure include elevations in serum creatinine and blood urea nitrogen (BUN), hyperkalaemia, hyperphosphataemia, and a wide anion gap metabolic acidosis. Serum creatinine is a function of the amount of creatinine entering the blood (from the breakdown of muscle creatine), its volume of distribution, and its rate of excretion. Since the first two factors are usually constant, changes in serum creatinine concentration generally reflect changes in glomerular filtration rate (GFR). Under steady-state conditions, if the GFR is halved, the serum creatinine doubles. Abrupt cessation of glomerular filtration causes the serum creatinine to rise by 1 to 2 mg/dL/24 hr. Thus, a daily increment of less than 1mg/dL suggests that at least some renal function has been preserved. The blood urea nitrogen (BUN) rises with renal dysfunction, but is also influenced by many extrarenal factors.

- BUN and creatinine levels may not always reflect renal function accurately. For example, BUN may be raised inspite of normal renal function in patients with hypercatabolism, high protein load, gastrointestinal bleed, and haematoma breakdown. BUN may be normal despite a decrease in renal function, when urea synthesis is decreased as in hepatic failure or malnutrition. Similarly, creatinine levels may be raised inspite of normal renal function, because of excessive release of creatinine seen in various conditions e.g. seizures, muscle injury, inflammation, or ischaemia. Normal creatinine levels with decreased renal function may be due to decreased creatinine synthesis (malnutrition and atrophic muscular disorders). Further, serum creatinine is a poor marker of renal function in critically ill non-steady-state patients, particularly in the face of volume expansion. Volume expansion is associated with dilution of the serum creatinine, which may result in serious underestimation of the renal functional deficit.

- Creatinine clearance, which usually parallels GFR closely, can be determined from a 24-hour urine collection (a time-consuming procedure) or from the serum creatinine, using the following equation:

$$\text{Creatinine Clearance} = \frac{[140 - \text{age (years)}] \times \text{weight (kg)}}{\text{Serum Creatinine (mg/dL)} \times 72}$$

The weight used should be either the ideal weight or the actual weight if it is less than the ideal weight. For women, 85% of the value (as calculated from the equation) is taken to correct for their smaller mass. Normal values for creatinine clearance are 95 ± 20 mL/min in women and 120 ± 25 mL/min in men. A serial decline in creatinine clearance is the most reliable indicator of progressive renal dysfunction.

- The primary objective of the management of ARF is prevention, but once ARF has set in, attention must be focused on achieving prompt and complete recovery. In this regard, anything that can be done to minimize the initial injury or prevent secondary complications is desirable. In general, the immediate objectives of management of ARF include, early identification of renal dysfuction, identification and treatment of obstructive or pre-renal failure, and early optimization of intravascular volume and oxygen delivery. Having accomplished this, attention is then directed towards laboratory confirmation of renal parenchymal damage and lessening the initial impact of ischaemic or nephrotoxic injury. The intent has been to reestablish urine flow with the use of diuretics, to restore renal perfusion by treatment with vasodilators, and to preserve tubular epithelial cell integrity by administration of cytoprotective agents (free radical scavengers, xanthine oxidase inhibitors, calcium channel blocking agents, and prostaglandins). Unfortunately, in most cases, the anticipated benefit has not been realized. During the maintenance phase, the objectives of management include elimination of nephrotoxins, correction of associated metabolic abnormalities, institution of renal replacement therapies whenever indicated, provision of adequate nutrition, adjustment of drugs to account for decreased clearance, and control of causative factors. Another major concern during this phase is to prevent secondary renal injury. Potential factors contributing to secondary renal injury are episodes of hypotension/ hypoxia, use of bioincompatible membranes during haemodialysis, and volume depletion and prerenal azotemia associated with the use of diuretics and sodium restriction.

- The observation that patients with nonoliguric ARF generally have a better prognosis than those with oliguric ARF is true only for those in whom nonoliguric ARF occurs spontaneously. There is little evidence that chances of recovery in established ARF are improved either by administration of diuretics or by the pharmacologic conversion from oliguria to nonoliguria. As an example, in a prospective, randomized, placebo-controlled, double-blind study of patients with ARF, it was found that the despite the fact that patients who were given a loop diuretic had a significant rise in urine flow, there were no differences in renal recovery, the need for dialysis or death from those who were not. Although as a group, nonoliguric patients (≥ 50 mL/hr) had a significantly lower mortality than oliguric patients (< 50 mL/hr), this was due to the fact that the nonoliguric patients were less ill and had less severe renal failure at the time of entry into the study.

- Dopamine has been used in critically ill patients who are at risk for developing ARF and in those in whom the renal function is already decreased. While it often increases urine output and sodium excretion, evidence that low doses of dopamine avert the onset or ameliorate the course of ARF in critically ill patients is inconclusive. Thus, until controlled trials are conducted, there seems little justification for the routine administration of dopamine in patients at risk for renal failure in the absence of specific indications.

- In patients with low cardiac output and hypotension (cardiogenic shock or myocardial dysfunction in a patient with septic shock), both, restoration of cardiac output and arterial blood pressure, are required to restore renal perfusion. A number of drugs may be used to achieve these goals. Dopamine (in moderate to high doses), or epinephrine, can be titrated to achieve the given physiological and clinical goals. In a more resistant patient, one may exercise the option of dissociating inotropic from pressure therapy. This can be done by the administration of an infusion of milrinone (typically at a rate of $0.25 - 0.5\ \mu g/kg/min$) to increase the cardiac output, and simultaneous infusion of norepinephrine (typically at a rate of $0.1 - 1.0\mu g/kg/min$).

- Norephinephrine achieves restoration of blood pressure, while maintaining or slightly augmenting the cardiac output, and appears to be the ideal drug in hyperdynamic, hypotensive, oliguric patients with preserved or increased cardiac output (i.e. patients with severe sepsis, or septic shock). High-dose dopamine, in a randomized controlled study, has been shown to be inferior to norepinephrine in this setting. Various studies have shown that administration of epinephrine is also a physiologically sound approach to the hypotensive, hyperdynamic septic patient with renal dysfunction. Even at relatively high doses, epinephrine does not appear to induce any significant degree of renal vasoconstriction and actually results in an increase in renal blood flow through its effects on the arterial blood pressure. Epinephrine may achieve haemodynamic stability in patients unresponsive to other agents, but it compromises regional hepatosplanchnic perfusion and causes profound metabolic alterations, as shown by the development of lactic acidosis. Therefore, its use should be limited.

- The abdominal compartment syndrome (ACS) is often an overlooked cause of oliguria and ARF in critically ill patients. ACS is described when the intra-abdominal pressure is greater than $25\ cmH_2O$ (around 18 mmHg) and it is associated with a rapidly increasing PCO_2, and a decrease in cardiac output and urine output. Intra-abdominal pressure may be increased by haemorrhage, ascites, bowel edema, or intra-abdominal packing. A high intra-abdominal pressure, not only compromises the cardiac output by decreasing the venous return from the inferior vena cava, but it may also exceed the critical closing pressure of renal arterioles (approximately 20 to 30 mmHg), thus inhibiting the flow by increasing intrarenal resistance. Both these processes decrease the renal blood flow and glomerular filtration rate. Volume loading and inotropes can rarely restore renal blood flow in ACS; only prompt decompression of the abdominal cavity is likely to restore renal function to a significant extent.

- When renal function has deteriorated to a critical state, some form of renal replacement therapy (RRT) is required to maintain homeostasis and prevent metabolic and other uraemic complications. Various modes of RRT [peritoneal dialysis, intermittent haemodialysis (IHD), and continuous renal replacement therapy (CRRT)] are available. A recent meta-analysis of continuous versus intermittent renal replacement therapy concluded that there is insufficient evidence to draw conclusions regarding the optimal mode of RRT for ARF in the critically ill. The authors, however, made certain pertinent observations. They noted that mortality, regardless of the modality of RRT, was significantly lower in studies completed after 1992, compared to those before that. They could not demonstrate a beneficial effect on mortality in relation to dialysis dose. They found no overall difference in mortality in patients who received continuous or intermittent RRT, but, after adjustment for study quality and severity of illness, CRRT was associated with an improved survival compared to intermittent renal replacement therapy. The choice of a particular mode of RRT should be decided according to the clinical condition, available resources, and expertise of the intensivist/nephrologist.

- The standard indications for renal replacement therapy include symptomatic uraemia (altered consciousness, neuromuscular excitability, asterixis, uraemic pericarditis, nausea and vomiting), volume overload, acidosis, and hyperkalaemia that prove refractory to medical management.

GUIDELINES FOR DIAGNOSIS AND TREATMENT OF OLIGURIA AND AZOTEMIA

1. **Establish the diagnosis at an early stage.**
   Urine output of less than 0.5 mL/kg/hr for four hours or a rise in serum creatinine of 0.25 mg/dL in one day are early indicators of renal dysfunction.

2. **Wash hands.**
   This reduces the risk of transmission of micro-organisms.

3. **Check Foley's catheter and drainage system.**
   - Check for any kinks or clots in the catheter or drainage tube. The obstruction could also be because of clamps applied inadvertently or forgotten after a planned application.
   - Check whether the Foley's catheter is properly positioned in the bladder. If in doubt, irrigate the catheter with 30-40 mL of sterile water. The return of yellow-pigmented urine on the Foley's effluent correlates with correct positioning.
   - Ensure that the collection bag is at a lower level in relation to the bladder.
   - If obstructive uropathy is still suspected, renal ultrasonography which has a sensitivity of approximately 80% is diagnostic.

4. **Rule out prerenal dysfunction. History, including intake of any drugs, physical examination, intake-output record, status of ECF space (edema/dehydration). Monitor haemodynamic parameters (CVP, PCWP, and/or end diastolic volume index). Laboratory evaluation: (a) Urinalysis, BUN, serum creatinine, UNa to provide clues as to the cause of ARF, (b) complete blood count, electrolyte, calcium, phosphorus, magnesium levels, ECG, and chest roentgenography, to establish patient's baseline status and to provide information about possible complications.**
   - Prerenal azotemia should be suspected in the setting of volume loss, volume redistribution or decrease in effective renal perfusion.
   - On physical examination, signs of volume depletion which should be looked for are: orthostatic hypotension, tachycardia, decreased skin turgor, dry

mucous membrane, and diminished jugular venous pressure.

- Although CVP monitoring may be adequate in some patients, PCWP (pulmonary capillary wedge pressure) monitoring may be considered in high risk patients, including those with advanced cardiopulmonary disease, persistent oliguria resistant to fluid boluses, the elderly critically ill patient, and in septic shock.
- Prerenal azotemia is typically associated with increased urine specific gravity (>1.020), BUN/Cr ratio greater than 20:1, and urinary sodium (UNa) concentration less than 20 mEq/dL. A rapid response to volume repletion is also characteristic.
- A proportionally greater rise in serum urea than in serum creatinine is typical of prerenal acute renal failure. Clearance of urea is reduced as a consequence of impaired GFR. Urea is also reabsorbed from the tubular lumen with sodium and water in response to haemodynamic and hormonal stimuli. In contrast, whereas the clearance of creatinine is also reduced due to impairement of GFR, there is a compensatory secretion of creatinine by the epithelial cells into the tubular lumen.
- Treatment of prerenal ARF focuses on the restoration of euvolaemia, cardiac contractility, and vascular tone, depending on the cause of circulatory collapse. Take blood and urine specimens for investigations before fluid replacement or administration of diuretics or dopamine.

5. **If renal hypoperfusion is suspected, try an empirical fluid challenge (20 mL/kg bolus of normal saline or ringer's lactate).**
    - An increase in urine output combined with improvement in haemodynamic values (decreased tachycardia, increased cardiac filling indices) is diagnostic.
    - Failure to respond to a fluid challenge indicates intrarenal dysfunction, and should prompt a search for evidence of the same.
    - Optimization of preload increases renal blood flow and prevents further tubular epithelial cell injury. Mean arterial pressure is an important determinant of renal perfusion. Recommendation of maintaining the haematocrit more than 30% in any critically ill patient, especially with renal dysfunction, is based on a number of potential benefits. These include increased oxygen carrying capacity, increased preload, augmented cardiac function, improved microcirculation, and minimal edema formation.
    - General haemodynamic management may be done according to the following guidelines:
    (a) – CVP $\geq$ 12 mmHg
        – MAP > 80 mmHg
        – Cardiac index normal or supranormal
    Continue current haemodynamic management
    (b) – CVP $\geq$ 12 mmHg
        – MAP < 80 mmHg
        – Cardiac index normal or supranormal
    Add or increase vasopressor drug
    (c) – CVP < 12 mmHg

      – PAOP < 18 mmHg
      – Cardiac index less than normal
      – MAP < 80 mmHg
Add IV colloids/crystalloids until CVP $\geq$ 12 mmHg and PAOP >18 mmHg
(d) – Cardiac index less than normal
      – PAOP > 18 mmHg
      – MAP < 80 mmHg
Add or increase inotropic drug (s).

(PAOP = Pulmonary artery occlusion pressure)

6. **Use diuretics if oliguria persists. Add furosemide 20-100 mg IV, wait for the response; if no response in 1-2 hours, double the dose, or add a thiazide diuretic (metolazone 2.5-5.0 mg po), or use a continuous diuretic infusion (loading dose 10-20 mg followed by 2.5-10 mg/hr).**
   - Although there is no evidence that converting oliguric ARF to nonoliguric ARF has an effect on renal function or mortality, an attempt to increase urine flow with loop diuretics is still warranted. This avoids fluid overload, treats hyperkalaemia, maintains some level of solute clearance and makes the management easier.
   - In general, diuretic therapy should be reserved for oliguria that persists despite fluid challenge and restoration of stable haemodynamics or when there is an evidence of pigment nephropathy.
   - Continuous furosemide infusion achieves effective diuresis in patients with congestive heart failure at blood concentrations considerably below those achieved by bolus doses.

7. **Continue to monitor the patient at regular intervals.**
   Helps in early detection and management of complications.

8. **Review the medications.**
   Avoid or modify the doses of nephrotoxic drugs such as antibiotics (aminoglycosides, vancomycin etc), non-steroidal antiinflammatory agents, ACE II inhibitors, amphotericin B, radiographic contrast agents etc. Combined use of cephalosporins and aminoglycosides increases the nephrotoxicity of each individual drug.

9. **Treat precipitating factors, if any. Maintain protein and caloric intake.**
   Treat infection aggressively. Decompress the abdominal cavity in case of abdominal compartment syndrome (ACS). A negative nitrogen balance may lead to impaired immune function and an increased risk of morbidity and mortality.

10. **Adopt general supportive measures.**
    General supportive measures include use of aseptic techniques, H_2-receptor antagonists, and antacid therapy (non-magnesium compounds), whenever indicated.

11. **If urine output is more than 0.5 mL/kg/hr, manage as in non-oliguric renal injury.**
    - Consider continuous infusion of a loop diuretic.

- Maintain oxygen delivery and haemodynamic stability.
- Avoid/discontinue nephrotoxic agents.
- Treat underlying illness.
- Add nutritional support.

12. When the urine output does not improve, BUN >100, fluid overload is present or serum potassium is >5.5 mEq/L along with ECG changes or when pH < 7.2, consider adding renal replacement therapy.

- A haemodynamically stable patient (pulse <120/min, MAP > 80mmHg with minimal pressor support) may be considered for intermittent haemodialysis (IHD). Continuous renal replacement therapy (CRRT) may be preferred over IHD for critically ill patients who demonstrate haemodynamic instability or who have systemic inflammatory response syndrome (SIRS) with multiple organ failure. Also, CRRT is associated with a decreased number of hypotensive episodes as compared to intermittent haemodialysis.

References

1. Baldwin L, Henderson A, Hickman P. Effect of postoperative low-dose dopamine on renal function after elective major vascular surgery. Ann Intern Med 1994;120:744-747.
2. Bellomo R, Kellum J, Ronco C. Acute renal failure: time for a consensus. Intensive Care Med 2001;27:1685-1688.
3. Bellomo R, Ronco C. Continuous renal replacement therapy in the intensive care unit. Intensive Care Med 1999;25:781-789.
4. Bellomo R, Ronco C. The use of inotropic and vasopressor agents in patients at risk of renal dysfunction. In: Ronco C, Bellomo R, eds. Critical Care Nephrology. Kluwer Academic Publishers, Netherlands, 1998, pp 1133-1137.
5. Bersten AD, Rutten AJ, Summersides G, et al. Epinephrine infusion in the sheep: systemic and renal hemodynamic effects. Crit Care Med 1994;22:994-1101.
6. Bersten AD, Rutten AJ. Renovascular interaction of epinephrine, dopamine, and intraperitoneal sepsis. Crit Care Med 1995;23:537-544.
7. Brady HR, Brenner BM, Clarkson MR, Lieberthal W. Acute renal failure. In: Brenner BM, ed. The kidney, 6 ed. Philadelphia: Saunders, 2000.
8. Brown CB, Ogg CS, Cameron JS. High-dose furosemide in acute renal failure: a controlled trial. Clin Nephrol 1981;15:90-96.
9. Carcoana OV, Hines RL. Is renal dose dopamine protective or therapeutic? Yes. Crit Care Med 1996;12:677-685.
10. Chertow GM, Sayegh MH, Allgren RL, Lazarus JM. Is the administration of dopamine associated with adverse or favourable outcomes in acute renal failure? Auriculin Anaritide Acute Renal Failure Study Group. Am J Med 1996;101:49-53.
11. Contarovich F, Locatelli A, Fernandez JC, et al. Furosemide in high doses in the treatment of acute renal failure. Postgrad Med J 1971;47(suppl):13-17.
12. Cottee DBF, Saul WP. Is Renal dose dopamine protective or therapeutic? No. Crit Care Med 1996;12:687-695.
13. Heyman SN, Fuchs S, Brezis M. The role of medullary ischemia in acute renal failure. New Horizons 1995;3:597-607.

14. K lienknecht D, Ganeval D, Gouzalez-Dugue LA, Fermanian J. Furosemide in acute oliguric renal failure: A controlled trial. Nephron 1976;17:51-58.

15. Kapadia FN, Bhojani K, Shah B. Special issues in the patient with renal failure. Crit Care Clin 2003;19:233-251.

16. Kellum JA, Angus DC, Johnson JP, et al. Continuous versus intermitted renal replacement therapy: A meta-analysis. Intensive Care Med 2002;28:29-37.

17. Kellum JA, Decker JM. Use of dopamine in acute renal failure: a meta-analysis. Crit Care Med 2001; 29:1526-1531.

18. Kellum JA. Use of diuretics in acute care setting. Kidney Int. 1998;53(suppl 66):567-670.

19. Lawson DH, Gray JMB, Henry DA, Tilstone WJ. Continuous infusion of furosemide in refractory oedema. Br Med J 1978;2:476.

20. Martin C, Papazian L, Perrin G, et al. Norepinephrine or dopamine for the treatment of septic shock. Chest 1993;103:1826-1831.

21. Meldrum D, et al. Prospective characterization and selective management of the abdominal compartment syndrome. Am J Surg 1997;174(6):667.

22. Meyer MM. Renal replacement therapies. Critica! Care Clinics. 2000;16(1):29-58.

23. Moran SM, Myers BD. Course of acute renal failure studied by a model of creatinine kinetics. Kidney Int 1985;27:928-937.

24. Rasmussen H, Ibels L, Acute renal failure: Multivariate analysis of causes and risk factors. Am J Med 1982;78:211.

25. Shilliday IR, Quinn KJ, Allison ME. Loop diuretics in the management of acute renal failure: a prospective, double-blind, placebo-controlled, randomized study. Nephrol Dial Transplant 1997;12:2592-2596.

26. Sladen RN. Oliguria in the ICU. Anesthesiology Clinics of North America. 2000;18(4):739-752.

27. Thadhani R, Pascual M, Bonventre J. Acute renal failure. N Engl J Med 1996;334(22):1448-1460.

28. VanMeyel JJ, Smith P, Russel FG, et al. Diuretic efficiency of furosemide during continuous administration versus bolus injection in healthy volunteers. Clin Pharmacol Ther 1992;51:440-444.

Stress Ulcer Prophylaxis 22

Introduction

Gastric mucosal damage occurs in critically ill patients in the ICU and develops in the setting of severe physiologic stress. Within 24 hours of admission to the ICU, 75% to 100% of critically ill patients demonstrate evidence of stress-related mucosal disease. Major factors responsible for the stress-related mucosal disease are decreased blood flow, mucosal ischaemia, hypoperfusion and reperfusion injury. Three different kinds of stress-related mucosal bleeding may occur in the ICU:

- Occult bleeding is defined as guaiac-positive gastric aspirate or guaiac-positive stool.
- Overt bleeding refers to haematemesis (gross blood or "coffee ground" in the gastric aspirate), haematochezia or malena.
- Clinically important bleeding is overt bleeding complicated by any of the following within 24 hours: a spontaneous decrease in systolic blood pressure of more than 20 mmHg, an increase in heart rate by at least 20 beats/min, decrease in systolic blood pressure of 10 mmHg sitting upright or a decrease in haemoglobin level by more than 2 g/dL.

GUIDELINES FOR INITIATING STRESS ULCER PROPHYLAXIS

1. **Routine preventive therapy is not indicated.**
   Since the risk of clinically important gastrointestinal bleeding is low (0.1%), routine preventive therapy is not indicated.

2. **Prophylaxis therapy is indicated in the following group of patients:**
   (a) Patients having respiratory failure and requiring mechanical ventilation for more than 48 hours.
   (b) Patients having coagulopathy (defined as a platelet count of less than $50,000/mm^3$ or a prolonged prothrombin or partial thromboplastin time).
   The risk of stress-related mucosal disease is increased by nearly 16-fold in those who require mechanical ventilation for more than 48 hours and by nearly 4-fold in those with coagulopathy. Overall, the risk of clinically important bleeding is 3.7% in the presence of risk factors (as mentioned) as compared to 0.1% in their absence.

3. **Consider options available for prophylaxis and their impact on the clinical outcome.**
   The options available include: H_2 receptor antagonists, sucralfate, antacids,

and proton pump inhibitors. Outcome may be considered in terms of clinically important gastrointestinal bleeding, incidence of nosocomial pneumonia, and mortality.

4. **H$_2$RA (ranitidine)/sucralfate.**

    Prevalence of clinically important bleeding is significantly less in patients taking H$_2$RA than in those taking placebo, antacids or sucralfate. However, a number of earlier studies have shown increased risk of nosocomial pneumonia in patients receiving H$_2$RA as compared to those receiving sucralfate.

    A more recent multicenteric, randomized, double blind controlled trial comparing sucralfate and H$_2$RA (ranitidine) confirmed better efficacy of ranitidine in reducing the risk of clinically important bleeding. No significant difference between the two groups (ranitidine vs sucralfate) was noted for ventilator associated pneumonia (VAP) or for mortality (although previous studies have shown an increased risk of VAP with H$_2$RA). Although these data support the benefit of H$_2$RA prophylaxis in reducing the risk of development of stress related mucosal disease, a major drawback to intravenous H$_2$RA is the development of tolerance within 72 hours of administration.

5. **Proton pump inhibitors.**

    There is enough evidence to conclude that acid-suppression prophylaxis for stress ulcer GI bleeding with H$_2$RA significantly reduces the likelihood of clinically important bleeding in the critical care setting. But, evidence regarding the use of proton pump inhibitors for this indication is scarce, although acid suppression with proton pump inhibitors is significantly greater than that achieved with H$_2$RAs.

6. **Role of enteral nutrition.**

    Opinions differ regarding the benefits of continuous nasogastric feeding for the prevention of stress-related mucosal disease. The constant neutralization of gastric acidity by the food (pH of most commercially available enteral nutrition formulations is 6-7) comprises the rationale for this strategy. However, the limited relevant data available do not support this view.

7. **Commonly accepted view.**

    Patients having coagulopathy or requiring mechanical ventilation for less than four days may be given H$_2$RA (ranitidine, 50 mg 8 hourly IV) prophylaxis. Patients having coagulopathy or respiratory failure requiring mechanical ventilation for more than 4 days may preferably be given sucralfate, 1 g 6 hourly through the nasogastric tube.

References

1. Cash BD. Evidence –based medicine as it applies to acid suppression in the hospitalized patient. Crit Care Med 2002;30(suppl):S373-S378.
2. Cook D, Guyatt G, Marshall J, et al. A comparison of sucralfate & ranitidine for the prevention of upper gastrointestinal bleeding in patients requiring mechanical ventilation: Canadian Critical Care Trial Group.

N Eng J Med 1998;338:791-797.

3. Cook D, Heyland D, Griffith L, et al. Risk factors for clinically important upper gastrointestinal bleeding in patients requiring mechanical ventilation. Crit Care Med 1999;27:2812-2817.

4. Cook DJ, Fuller HD, Guyatt GJ, et al. Risk factors for gastrointestinal bleeding in critically ill patients: Canadian Critical Care Trials Group. N Eng J Med 1994;330:377-381.

5. Cook DJ, Reeve BK, Guyatt GH, et al. Stress ulcer prophylaxis in critically ill patients. Resolving discordant meta-analysis. JAMA 1996;275:308-314.

6. Merki HS, Wilder –Smith CH. Do continuous omeprazole & ranitidine retain their effect with prolonged dosing? Gastroenterology 1994;106:60-64.

7. Steinberg KP. Stress-related mucosal decrease in the critically ill patient: Risk factors & strategies to prevent stress-related bleeding in the intensive care unit. Crit Care Med 2002;30(suppl):S362-S364.

An Approach to Acid-base Disorders

23

Introduction

- The partial pressure of a gas is a measure of the concentration of the gas within a medium, e.g. the arterial blood. When a gas mixture is in contact with liquid, the a volume of gas that dissolves depends on the partial pressure of the individual gas forcing the molecules into the liquid and the solubility (the ease with which molecules of the gas can enter the liquid) of the gas. Once equilibrium is reached, the partial pressure of each individual gas within the liquid will be equal to the partial pressure of the same gas in contact with the liquid.

- The relationship of pH to H^+ concentration shows a few important features: (a) pH and H^+ ion concentration are inversely related, (b) normal blood pH of 7.40 (7.36-7.44) corresponds to a normal H^+ ion concentration of 40 (44-36) nmol/L, (c) between the pH range of 7.1 to 7.5, each 0.01 unit change in pH from 7.40 changes the H^+ ion concentration by 1 nmol/L, and (d) 6.8-7.8 is the pH range usually considered compatible with life. This is equivalent to a hydrogen ion concentration of 160-16 nmol/L.

- Acid is defined as any substance that is capable of providing hydrogen ions (H^+) when it is in solution. Base is any substance that accepts hydrogen ions (H^+) when it is in solution; and an alkali is a substance that can donate hydroxide ions (OH^-). Since an alkali can also accept hydrogen ions, it is also a base.

- The body produces a number of acids: hydrochloric acid, lactic acid, ketoacid, pyruvic acid, uric acid, and proteins. The bases produced by the body are: bicarbonate, phosphate, proteins, and ammonia. Proteins may be either acids or bases. This is because they are made up of a long chain of molecules that can either provide or accept hydrogen ions.

- A buffer may be defined as a substance which can absorb or donate hydrogen ions and thereby mitigate, but not entirely prevent, changes in pH. Important buffers are carbonic acid/bicarbonate buffer (H_2CO_3/HCO_3^-), phosphate buffer ($H_2PO_4^-$), proteins buffer (HPr/Pr^-) and haemoglobin.

- The inorganic matrix of bone has vast quantities of sodium, potassium, and calcium that can be exchanged for hydrogen ions, thereby providing a large buffering capacity. Though this takes longer to become effective, it becomes particularly important in chronic acidotic states and when concentration of other extracellular buffers is low.

- Standard bicarbonate refers to the bicarbonate concentration of plasma that has been fully equilibrated with a normal $PaCO_2$ at a standard temperature and pressure and thus reflects only non-respiratory (metabolic) effects. In normal persons, the standard bicarbonate ranges between 21-27 mmol/L. This takes into account only the carbonic acid-bicarbonate system. Consequently, the "standard bicarbonate" underestimates the metabolic changes because it does not measure the activity of the other buffers (for example, plasma proteins) in trying to maintain the pH in the normal range.

- Actual bicarbonate is the concentration of bicarbonate measured in a sample without any corrections as mentioned for standard bicarbonate. Therefore, the actual bicarbonate reflects the contribution of both, the respiratory and metabolic components of the body's acid-base balance, and not the metabolic component alone. The normal value is 21-28 mmol/L.

- Base excess implies a non-respiratory (metabolic) acidosis (negative base excess or base deficit) or a non-respiratory (metabolic) alkalosis (positive base excess). This is calculated by measuring the amount of strong base (or acid) that has to be added to a sample of blood to produce a pH of 7.4, under the specified conditions as stated for "standard bicarbonate". Base excess (negative or positive) takes into account all the buffers in the blood sample and is therefore considered to provide more accurate assessment of the metabolic component of the patient's acid-base status.

- The principle of electroneutrality dictates that total serum cations should be equal to total serum anions. In other words, sodium + potassium + calcium + magnesium = bicarbonate + chloride + phosphate + sulfate + protein + organic acid anions. The value of potassium is small and it is usually omitted. Calcium, and magnesium are considered to be unmeasurable cations (UC), and phosphate, sulfate, proteins, and organic acids are considered to be unmeasurable anions (UA). Thus, sodium + UC = bicarbonate + chloride + UA, or UA -- UC = $Na^+ - (Cl^- + HCO_3^-)$ = serum anion gap (AG). The anion gap, therefore, is the difference between the serum sodium concentration and the sum of measured anions, chloride and bicarbonate. The increase in anion gap could be due to increased UA or decreased UC or both. This method relies on the accuracy of the measurement of sodium, chloride, and bicarbonate. Also the anion gap exists simply because not all electrolytes are routinely measured and more anions are left unmeasured than are cations. In other words, anion gap is an artifact of measurement, and not a physiologic reality.

- The anion gap should be adjusted for hypoalbuminaemia , which tends to reduce it. For every 1g/dL decline in serum albumin level, a 2.5-3.0 mEq/L decrease in AG occurs. Administration of antibiotics, like carbenicillin acting as UA leads to an increase in AG, while polymyxin (being a UC) decreases the AG.

- The common causes of normal anion gap (12 ± 4 mEq/L) metabolic acidosis are pancreatic fistula, saline administration, diarrhoea, carbonic anhydrase inhibitors, renal tubular acidosis, spironolactone, and hyperparathyroidism. Non-anionic gap acidosis usually is the result of administration of large volumes of chloride containing fluid, commonly given in patients with gastrointestinal losses of bicarbonate. The common causes of increased anion gap metabolic acidosis include lactic acidosis (for example in shock, sepsis, hypoxia, seizures, and liver failure), diabetic ketoacidosis, uraemic acidosis, drugs (e.g. iron, isoniazed), and methanol.

- To simplify, when bicarbonate is lost externally through urine or enteric drainage, serum chloride concentration will increase, producing a hyperchloremic normal anion gap acidosis. In contrast, a process such as lactic acidosis, or ketoacidosis increases the anion gap because bicarbonate is consumed in the buffering of hydrogen produced from metabolic acids, with the accumulation of the associated acid anion.

- Metabolic alkalosis is often considered under two general categories: (a) "salt" (NaCl)-responsive, or (b) salt-unresponsive. Salt-responsive metabolic alkalosis may be due to volume depletion, vomiting/diarrhoea, nasogastric suction, diuretics, post hypercapnia, and cationic drugs (e.g. penicillin). The "chloride dose" required to correct a chloride-responsive alkalosis can be approximated as the desired change in chloride concentration times 25% of body weight. Salt-unresponsive or resistant alkalosis (adrenal disorder, corticosteriod administration, and excess alkali administration) is usually accompanied by hypokalaemia.

- Three types of blood gas machine arrangements are possible: (1) A simple blood gas machine, giving information about pH, $PaCO_2$, PaO_2, bicarbonate, and base excess. (2) A blood gas machine and a separate co-oximeter. The co-oximeter can measure haemoglobin (in g/dL), SaO_2, % COHb, and % Met Hb, and arterial oxygen content (CaO_2) can be calculated from these values. (3) A single machine that incorporates blood gas and co-oximetry measurements from a single sample.

- Values for $PaCO_2$, PaO_2 and pH are measured directly. Bicarbonate concentration is usually calculated from pH and $PaCO_2$ using a nomogram derived from the Henderson-Hasselbalch equation. Although the calculated bicarbonate value is as reliable as the pH and $PaCO_2$ values, the calculated percent oxyhaemoglobin saturation value is often inaccurate because of the many unknown variables that cannot be corrected (e.g. 2,3-diphosphoglycerate and binding characteristics of haemoglobin).

- By convention, ABG samples are analyzed at 37°C. Blood gases drawn at temperatures greater than 39°C should probably be corrected for temperature. Because the solubility of oxygen and carbon dioxide increases as blood is cooled to 37°C, the hyperthermic patient is more acidotic and less hypoxaemic than the uncorrected values indicate (or, the measured PaO_2 and $PaCO_2$ will be lower than in the patient). Therefore, for each 1°C that the patient's temperature is greater than 37°C, PaO_2 should be increased by 7.2%, $PaCO_2$ increased by 4.4% and the pH should be decreased by 0.015. It is not necessary to correct the $PaCO_2$ and pH in the hypothermic patient but the PaO_2 at 37°C should be decreased by 7.2% for each degree that the patient's temperature is less than 37°C. Although theoretically this gives a more accurate picture of the patient's status, the current consensus is that for most clinical purposes it is best not to bother with any correction.

GUIDELINES FOR INTERPRETING ACID-BASE STATUS

1. **Decide whether it is an arterial sample or not.**
   - It is best known to the person drawing the sample. If the syringe plunger rises on its own, it is likely to be an arterial sample.
   - Peripheral vein PO_2 is almost always less than 40mmHg. A PO_2 value more than 40mmHg or an oxygen saturation more than 75% is most likely not from a pure venous sample. Sometimes, mixing of venous blood in the sample can lower the PO_2 value. This is more likely with multiple attempts for obtaining the sample or when the sample is drawn from the femoral artery which lies very close to the femoral vein. Remember, an abnormal pH and PCO_2 cannot be used to classify any blood gas data as venous in origin.

2. **Know your patient clinically.**
   The interpretation of ABG should be based on the background of clinical history (e.g. vomiting, diarrhoea, sepsis, diabetes, renal disease or intoxication) and physical examination (e.g. signs of volume depletion, increased or decreased respiratory rate, hypotension).

3. **Consider whether the patient was in steady state, before taking the sample.**
   Before interpreting blood gases, it is important to know whether the patient is in a steady state in terms of oxygenation and ventilation. This becomes important if the blood sample is taken from a patient recently connected to a mechanical ventilator, or changed to a new FiO_2 or the ventimask has inadvertently slipped from the face. It takes only about 3 minutes for people with healthy lungs to achieve a steady state. However, patients with chronic airway obstruction may take upto 20 minutes to reach a steady state. As a general rule, wait for at least 20 minutes before drawing a blood sample after any change in FiO_2. In mechanically-ventilated patients in whom both $PaCO_2$ and PaO_2 may be affected after a change in ventilator settings, wait for at least 30 minutes for the patient to reach a steady state.

4. **Look at the arterial pH.**
   - A normal pH denotes either a normal acid-base status, or a completely compensated acid-base disorder, or a mixed acid-base disorder.
   - A pH < 7.35 denotes acidaemia.
   - A pH > 7.45 denotes alkalaemia.

5. **Look at the $PaCO_2$ and HCO_3^-.**
   In a patient with acidaemia, an increase in $PaCO_2$ level indicates primary respiratory acidosis and a decrease in bicarbonate level indicates, primary metabolic acidosis. In a patient with alkalaemia, a decrease in the $PaCO_2$ level indicates primary respiratory alkalosis and an increase in the level of

bicarbonate suggests primary metabolic alkalosis.

6. **Compare measured pH with expected pH to know if a respiratory disturbance is acute or chronic.**

    In acute conditions, every 10mm Hg change in $PaCO_2$ is associated with an increase or decrease in pH of 0.08 units. In chronic conditions, change in pH is 0.03 units for every 10mmHg change in $PaCO_2$.

7. **Decide whether it is a simple acid-base disorder with compensation, if any or a mixed disorder.**

    - A patient with acidaemia, and elevated $PaCO_2$ levels (primary respiratory acidosis) could have elevated or decreased bicarbonate levels. Elevated levels denote metabolic compensation to the primary respiratory acidosis while decreased bicarbonate levels indicate a superimposed metabolic acidosis as well. To interpret correctly, one should know the expected metabolic compensation for respiratory acidosis: In acute situations, HCO_3^- increases by 1mEq/L for every 10mmHg increase in $PaCO_2$, while in chronic situations the increase in HCO_3^- is 3.5 - 4 mEq/L for every 10mmHg increase in the $PaCO_2$. Therefore, if increase in HCO_3^- concentration is less than expected, it indicates either a complicating metabolic acidosis or that insufficient time has elapsed for the kidneys to compensate. If increase in HCO_3^- concentration is more than expected, it indicates a superimposed metabolic alkalosis. If increase in HCO_3^- concentration is equal to what is expected, it shows a simple disorder i.e acute respiratory acidosis with appropriate metabolic compensation.

      In a patient with acidaemia, decreased HCO_3^- level and negative base excess, (primary metabolic acidosis), look for the $PaCO_2$ level and compare it with the expected $PaCO_2$ level for a given value of HCO_3^-. The expected compensation in metabolic acidosis is:

      Expected $PaCO_2 = (1.5 \times HCO_3^-) + 8(\pm2)$, OR

      Expected $PaCO_2 =$ last 2 digits of pH, OR

      $\Delta PaCO_2 = 1{-}1.3\ (\Delta HCO_3^-)$

      When observed $PaCO_2$ is equal to that expected, it indicates a simple metabolic acidosis with appropriate respiratory compensation. When observed $PaCO_2$ is more than expected, it indicates that the patient has a metabolic acidosis with a respiratory acidosis. When observed $PaCO_2$ is less than expected, the patient has both a metabolic acidosis and respiratory alkalosis.

    - In a patient with alkalaemia and a low $PaCO_2$ (primary respiratory alkalosis), look at the bicarbonate concentration to decide whether appropriate metabolic compensation is occurring or if a concurrent metabolic disorder is present. The expected metabolic compensation in respiratory alkalosis is:

      In acute situations, HCO_3^- falls by 2 mEq/L for each 10 mmHg fall in $PaCO_2$ while in chronic situations, the fall in HCO_3^- concentration is 5 mEq/L for each 10 mmHg fall in the $PaCO_2$.

      Thus, if concentration of HCO_3^- does not decrease by at least 2 mEq/L for every 10 mmHg fall in $PaCO_2$, it suggests either a superimposed metabolic

alkalosis or that insufficient time has been given for compensation.
If concentration of HCO_3^- decreases by more than the expected (5 mEq/L for every 10 mm Hg fall in $PaCO_2$), it suggests an additional component of metabolic acidosis.

If concentration of HCO_3^- decreases according to the expected value, it indicates the presence of simple respiratory alkalosis with appropriate metabolic compensation. *Respiratory alkalosis appears to be unique among the simple acid-base disturbances in its ability to return pH to normal.*

Furthermore, both metabolic acidosis and respiratory alkalosis, are associated with a low $PaCO_2$ – a secondary physiologic compensation in the former and a primary pathologic defect in the latter. If $PaCO_2$ has fallen to compensate for metabolic acidosis, it should bear a predictable relationship to the extent of fall in HCO_3^- concentration. Failure to demonstrate this relationship suggests that a primary respiratory disorder is present. Moreover, a decreased pH goes in favour of metabolic acidosis, while in respiratory alkalosis, pH may be elevated or normal. The clinical history and physical examination are also helpful in interpreting the values.

In a patient with alkalaemia and increased HCO_3^- concentration and positive base excess (primary metabolic alkalosis), look for $PaCO_2$ levels and compare with the expected $PaCO_2$ levels for a given value of HCO_3^- concentration. The expected compensation in metabolic alkalosis is:

Expected $PaCO_2$ = 0.7 × $[HCO_3^-]$ + 20 mmHg., OR
Expected $PaCO_2$ = 0.9 × $[HCO_3^-]$ + 9 mmHg, OR

The last two digits of pH should equal $[HCOO_3^-]$ plus 15 or $PaCO_2$ increases approximately 0.5 to 0.6 mmHg for each 1.0 mEq/L increase in $[HCO_3^-]$.

It has been found that many patients with chronic, stable metabolic alkalosis demonstrate a variable increment in the $PaCO_2$.

As a general rule, one expects some elevation of $PaCO_2$ in metabolic alkalosis. A patient with an elevated HCO_3^- whose $PaCO_2$ is less than normal, clearly shows a concomitant respiratory alkalosis (i.e. $PaCO_2$ is decreasing when it should be increasing). A normal or only slightly increased $PaCO_2$ in patients with substantial HCO_3^- elevation suggests the presence of less than expected compensation or a "relative hyperventilation" (presence of concomitant respiratory alkalosis). A higher than expected $PaCO_2$ indicates a simultaneous presence of respiratory acidosis. It is rare to see a compensatory increase in $PaCO_2 > 60$ mmHg when breathing room air, because at this level of hypercarbia the PaO_2 falls to approximately 60 mmHg and hypoxaemia begins to drive the respiration.

8. **Calculate the anion gap. Make correction for albumin levels.**

    If metabolic acidosis is present, calculate the anion gap.

    - If anion gap is normal, look for a possible cause, based on the history, physical examination and serum potassium levels.
    - If anion gap is greater than 14 mEq/L, look for a possible cause from the list of disease states associated with a large anion gap metabolic acidosis.

9. **Calculate the excess anion gap.**

    The excess anion gap = calculated anion gap minus normal anion gap plus measured HCO_3^-. If the excess anion gap is significantly greater than the normal serum HCO_3^- concentration of 24 mEq/L (i.e. > 30 mEq/L), there is an additional underlying metabolic alkalosis.

If the excess anion gap is significantly lower than the normal serum HCO_3^- (i.e. < 20 mEq/L) there is an additional underlying non gap metabolic acidosis.

10. Combine all the information.

The information collected from clinical history, physical examination, investigations and ABG should be put together to make a diagnosis. Remember, following trends is more important than a single reading of ABG.

References

1. Androgne HJ, Madias NE. Management of life-threatening acid-base disorders. N Engl J Med 1998; 338:26,107.
2. Breen PH. Arterial blood gas and pH analysis. Anesthes Clin North Am 2001; 19(4): 885-906.
3. Brenner M. Pulmonary acid-base assessment. Nurs Clin North Am 1990; 25:761-770.
4. Brewer ED. Disorders of acid base balance. Pediatr Clin North Am 1990; 37:429-447.
5. DuBose TD. Clinical approach to patients with acid-base disorders. Med Clin North Am 1983; 67:799-813.
6. Fencl V, Jabor A, et al. Diagnosis of metabolic acid-base disturbances in critically ill patients. Am J Respir Crit Care Med 2000; 162:2246-2251.
7. Gabow PA, kachny WD, Fennessey PV, et al. Diagnostic importance of an increased serum anion gap. N Eng J Med 1980; 303:854-858.
8. Gluck S. Acid-base. Lancet 1998; 352: 474-479.
9. Hood VL, Tannen RL. Protection of acid-base balance by pH regulation of acid production. N Eng J Med, 1998; 339(12): 819-826.
10. Marini JJ, Wheeler AP. Critical Care Medicine: The Essentials 2 ed. Baltimore: Williams & Wilkins, pp 209-222.
11. Narins RG, Emmett M. Simple and mixed acid-base disorders: A practical approach. Medicine 1980; 59:161-187.
12. Pilon CS, Leathley M, London R, et al. Practice guidelines for arterial blood gas measurment in the intensive care unit decreases numbers and increases appropriateness of tests. Crit Care Med 1997; 25:1308.
13. Preuss HG. Fundamentals of clinical acid base evaluation. Clin Lab Med 1993; 13:103-116.
14. Riley LJ Jr, Ilson BE, Narins RG. Acute metabolic acid-base disorders. Crit Care Clin 1987;5(4):699-724.
15. Salem MM, Mujais SK. Gaps in the anion gap. Arch Intern Med 1992; 152:1625-1629.
16. Schlichtig R, Grogono AW, Severinghans JW. Human $PaCO_2$ and standard base excess compensation for acid-base imbalance. Crit Care Med 1998; 26:1173-1179.
17. Wrenn K. The delta gap: an approach to mixed acid-base disorders. Ann Emerg Med 1990;19: 1310-1313.

Further Reading

1. Driscoll P, Brown T, Gwinnutt C, Wardle T. A simple guide to blood gas analysis. 2nd impresson. London: BMJ publishing group, 2000.
2. Martin L. All you really need to know to interpret arterial blood gases. 2nd ed Philadelphia: Lippincott Williams & Wilkins, 1999.
3. Shapiro BA, Peruzzi WT, Kozelowski-Templin RL. Clinical application of blood gases. 5 ed. Chicago: Mosby-Year Book, 1994.

24

Chest Radiography in ICU

Introduction

- The most commonly ordered imaging procedure in intensive care unit is the portable chest radiograph. Other imaging procedures such as abdominal radiography, ultrasound, computed tomography (CT), magnetic resonance (MR) imaging, and angiography are selectively ordered for specific indications.
- Portable radiographs differ from standard upright chest radiographs in several respects, related to equipment, projection, and the posture of the patient. Portable chest radiographs are inferior in quality to standard upright radiographs. This is principally due to the fact that antiscatter grids are not routinely used in the portable chest radiography of adults.
- In standard erect posteroanterior (PA) radiographs, the patient stands upright, and the X-ray source is 72 inches from the image detector, so that the magnification due to beam divergence is minimal. The central X-ray beam is horizontal, which facilitates detection of air-fluid levels or sub-diaphragmatic free air. Portable (bedside) radiography is generally performed with the patient semi-erect or supine, the distance between X-ray source and the image detector is not fixed, but it is usually considerably less than 72 inches, and the beam is almost never horizontal. Due to an anteroposterior (AP) projection and closer X-ray source, cardiac magnification is increased and because the central X-ray beam is not horizontal, air fluid levels may be difficult to detect (Fig. 24.1 a, b).
- In portable chest radiography, a truly erect position is almost never obtained. So-called erect portable examinations are usually performed with the patient in a semi-erect position. Often, a supine position is used. Patient's position has important effects on distribution of abnormal air and fluid collections, notably pleural effusion and pneumothorax. As a result, the appearance may change dramatically from one examination to the next, if positioning is not consistent.
- Increased severity of pulmonary disease is associated with increased opacity, and often with decreased inflation. Unfortunately, lung opacity varies with the technique and inflation is affected by many factors, including ventilator settings, exposure timings, and voluntary effort. To minimize variations in technique, kilovolts peak (kVp) and distance should be standardized. Exposure should be varied for individual patients by altering the mAs (tube current and exposure time), and a record of previous exposures should be used as a guide for subsequent examinations.

- Underinflation of the lungs is particularly common in portable chest radiographs because of the patient posture, increased upward pressure on the diaphragm in the semi-erect sitting position, and frequently, the patients' inability to fully co-operate.
- When reading radiographs, the effects of mechanical ventilation and gravity should be considered. One should anticipate an apparent decrease in pulmonary opacity with the initiation of assisted ventilation and an apparent worsening of the opacity when the patient is weaned. These changes will be more pronounced when the increased lung density is due to hypoventilation, atelectasis or edema rather than due to pulmonary consolidation.
- In the erect position, gravity results in an increased blood flow to the dependent, lower lobes of the lungs. Thus, the pulmonary vascular diameters are greater in the lower lobes than in the upper lobes. In the supine position, however, gravitational changes result in an equalization of pulmonary blood flow to the upper and lower lobes. Thus, in the supine position, the caliber of the upper and lower lobe vessels is similar.
- Studies have shown that daily interaction with the radiologist results in optimal integration of the clinical history with the radiologic findings and ensures a timely interpretation of the radiographic findings. It is also valuable in determining which diagnostic imaging tests are likely to clarify diagnostic problems, if any.
- It is important to have a systematic approach for interpreting ICU chest X-rays.

This includes: (a) Evaluating the location of all catheters, tubes and support devices, (b) assessing the cardiovascular status of the patient, (c) looking for areas of abnormally increased lung opacification, (d) assessing for pleural fluid, and (e) looking for abnormal air collections.

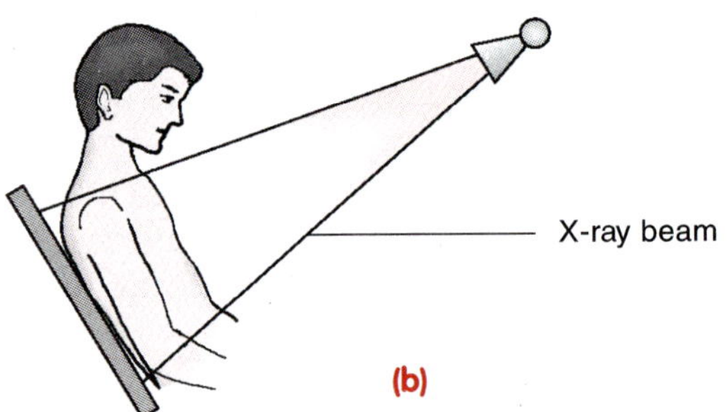

Fig. 24.1 (a, b): (a) Standard erect posteroanterior (PA) chest radiography. The patient is upright, X-ray source is 72 inches from the image detector, and the central X-ray beam is horizontal. **(b)** Portable (bedside) anteroposterior chest radiography. The patient is generally semi-erect, as shown, or supine, X-ray source is usually at a considerably smaller distance (less than 72 inches) from the image detector, and the central X-ray beam is almost never horizontal.

GUIDELINES FOR OBTAINING AND INTERPRETING A CHEST RADIOGRAPH

1. **Fill in the request form.**

   Several studies have documented that in critically ill patients, daily chest radiographs result in a change in patient management in as many as two-third of cases. In patients who are intubated, who are in the ICU for cardiopulmonary disease, and those undergoing diagnostic and therapeutic procedures, utility of daily radiographs is high. In ICU patients with extrapulmonary disease and no cardiopulmonary symptoms, portable radiograph need only be ordered for specific clinical signs and symptoms.

2. **Position the patient correctly.**

   - Optimal position requires cooperation between the radiographic technician and the ICU staff. It is often impossible for a single technician to properly position a semicomatose patient having multiple tubes and catheters. In addition, he needs to be informed about the required position or field of exposure in a given patient. It is the responsibility of the resident/nurse posted, to supervise positioning of the patient and to see that ECG electrodes or ventilator circuit are not superimposed on the chest during exposure.
   - As for radiation exposure of the staff, a lead apron will absorb most of the scattered radiation. Otherwise, standing several feet behind or to the side of the x-ray machine will minimize exposure to scattered radiation.
   - Every attempt should be made to obtain an erect radiograph (unless contraindicated by haemodynamic compromise). In the supine position, the heart and mediastinum are magnified, the upper lobe vessels distend, pleural effusions layer posteriorly, and pneumothorax collects anteriorly and inferiorly.

3. **Look at the position of endotracheal tube (ETT).**

   - A properly positioned ETT tip is 5-7 cm above the carina in the neutral position. The ETT tip descends or ascends approximately 2 cm with flexion or extension respectively of the head and neck from the neutral position. Therefore, the position of ETT should be assessed in relation to the position of the head and neck. In the neutral position, the chin projects over the lower cervical vertebrae (C5 or C6), whereas in flexion the chin is over the upper thoracic vertebrae and in extension, it is above C4. Very often the carina is clearly visible on the X-ray. If it is not very clear, its position is approximately at the level of the T6 vertebral body plus or minus one vertebral body in the vast majority of portable radiographs. Too high ETT may be associated with inadvertent extubation, while too low ETT may cause inadvertent right mainstem bronchus intubation leading to left-sided atelectasis.
   - The ideal ETT is approximately one-half to two-third the width of the trachea. This compromise minimizes laryngeal injury while keeping the airway resistance low. The inflated cuff should fill the tracheal lumen but not

bulge on the tracheal wall or deflect the bevel of the ETT towards the lateral tracheal wall.

4. **Look at the tracheostomy tube.**

    An optimally placed tracheostomy tube should be parallel to the long axis of the trachea, approximately one-half to two-thirds its diameter and ending several cm above the carina. Since the tube is affected little by head or neck movement, a tube closer to the carina is usually tolerated well.

5. **Look at the central venous catheter (Fig. 24.2).**

    - For accurate measurement, the tip of the CVP line should lie within the distal brachiocephalic vein or in the proximal superior vena cava (SVC). On the chest radiograph, the tip should therefore be projected over the first intercostal space to the right of the sternum.
    - One should obtain X-ray chest after every CVP catheter insertion. Up to 6% incidence of pneumothorax has been reported after CVP insertion through the subclavian vein route.

6. **Look at the position of Swan-Ganz catheter.**

    The tip of the catheter should be in the right or left main pulmonary artery within 2 cm of the hilum.

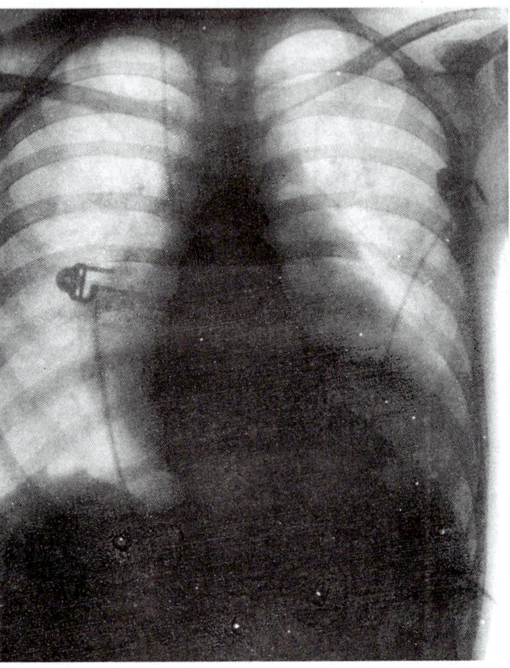

Fig. 24.2 X-ray chest showing CVP catheter inserted through right internal jugular vein.

7. **Confirm the position of intraaortic balloon pump (IABP).**

    The balloon is 26-28 cm long, and the catheter has a rectangular radioopaque tip, which should be positioned just distal to the origin of the left subclavian artery, just below the superior aortic knob contour. Positioning within the arch of aorta predisposes to cerebral embolism. A mid, or distal descending aorta location results in less effective counterpulsation. The balloon may obstruct the celiac, superior mesenteric and renal artery origins and embolization to their vessels has been reported.

8. **Look at the position of cardiac pacemaker (Fig. 24.3 a,b).**

    Right ventricular lead should project over the cardiac apex on PA view and should lie anteriorly on lateral view.

9. **Locate the nasogastric tube.**

    Side port and tip should lie below the left hemidiaphragm.

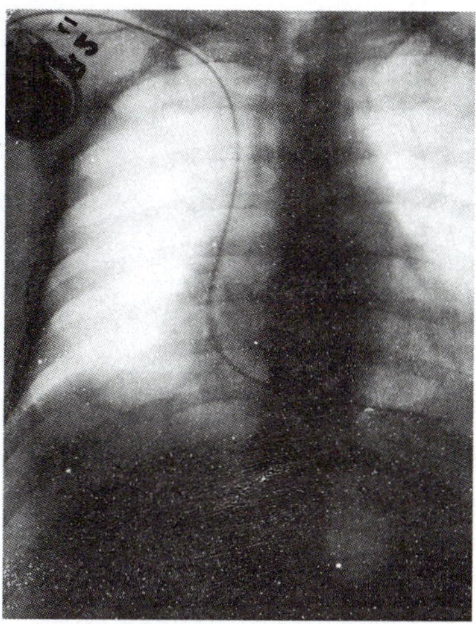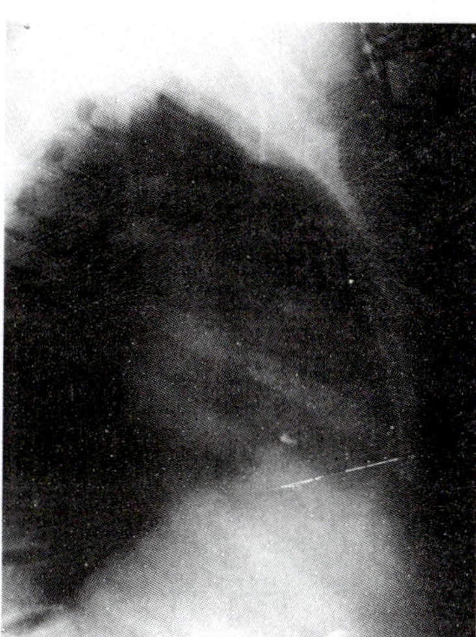

Fig. 24.3a, b X-ray chest AP and lateral view showing pacemaker in situ and the position of pacemaker lead.

10. Confirm the position of the pleural drainage chest tube.

- When inserted for pneumothorax, the tube should be directed anteriorly and superiorly and for pleural effusion, it should be positioned posteriorly and inferiorly. Sonograph and CT guidance may be of additional help in draining loculated effusion or empyema, when a more precise tube positioning is required.
- Tubes that abut on the mediastinal structures may lead to compression or injury of these structures.
- Tubes that are not sufficiently far advanced may have their side holes within the subcutaneous tissues, which results in inefficient drainage and subcutaneous emphysema.
- A tube placed within the lung parenchyma may cause laceration and may lead to bronchopleural fistula formation.

11. Assess the cardiovascular status.

- Assess heart size, vascular pedicle width and pulmonary vascularity.
- On a standard, erect PA chest radiograph, a cardiothoracic ratio greater than 0.5 is considered to be abnormal. Because portable, supine radiographs magnify the cardiac silhouette, it has been suggested that a correction factor of –12.5% be applied to this equation for ICU radiographs.
- Radiographs taken at shallow lung volumes (end-expiration) result in accentuation of the heart size and pulmonary vascularity.

12. Look for areas of abnormally increased lung opacification.

Common causes of opacities in ICU patients are, pulmonary edema, ARDS (Fig. 24.4), pneumonia, aspiration, atelectasis, and pleural effusion.

- An important feature that favours the diagnosis of atelectasis over pneumonia is the presence of volume loss, which may be manifested radiologically by displaced fissures, displaced hila, elevated hemidiaphragm, and shift of the mediastinal structures. Also, atelectasis typically develops and resolves more quickly than pneumonia.

- Complete opacification of an entire hemithorax is either because of complete atelectasis of a lung (due to mucous plug) (Fig. 24.5a,b) or a large pleural effusion, which shifts the mediastinum to the opposite side, in contrast to atelectasis when the shift is towards the side of opacification.
- The radiographic appearance of

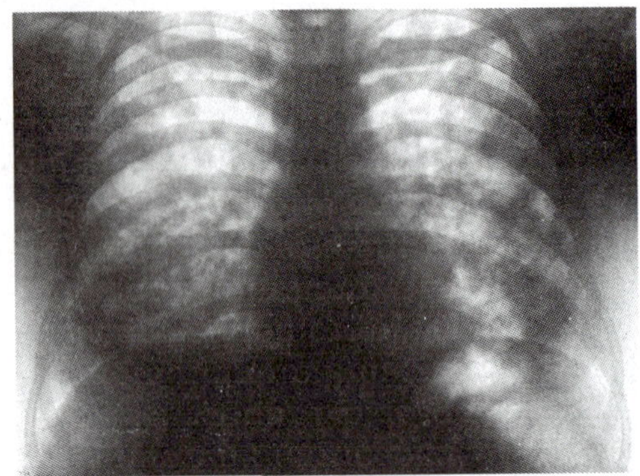

Fig. 24.4 X-ray chest showing multiple, fluffy, soft tissue opacities in both lung fields in a case of ARDS.

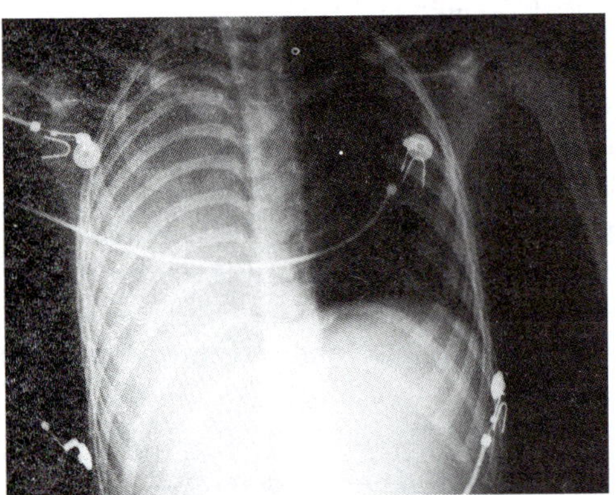

Fig. 24.5(a) X-ray chest AP view showing collapse of right lung with ipsilateral shift of mediastinum, due to obstruction of right main bronchus by mucus plug.

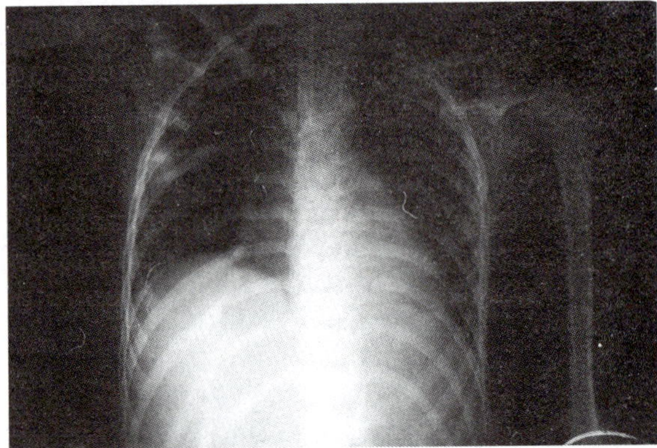

Fig. 24.5(b) X-ray chest showing re-expansion of the lung after bronchoscopic removal of the mucus plug.

aspiration is dependent on the nature and volume of aspirated material and the position of the patient. Aspiration of a small amount of water or blood may not result in any detectable radiographic abnormality, while aspiration of acidic gastric contents results in chemical pneumonitis that resembles pulmonary edema; and that of food or oral pathogens results in aspiration pneumonia. In aspiration, lung opacities are often seen in the dependent portions of the lungs. For example, in a patient who aspirates in the upright position, the basal segments of the lower lobes are usually affected. In the supine position, posterior segments of the upper lobes and the superior segments of the lower lobes are most often affected.

13. Assess pleural fluid.

- The appearance of pleural effusion on an x-ray is dependent on the size of the effusion and the position of the patient. On an erect radiograph, pleural effusion is manifested by blunting of the costophrenic sulcus, which results in a meniscus appearance. It requires approximately 200 mL fluid to produce this picture. On supine radiograph, a unilateral pleural effusion is seen as a diffuse, hazy, opacity throughout the affected hemithorax. A moderate-sized effusion may result in a lateral or apical pleural opacity (apical cap on supine radiograph).

- Loculated pleural fluid collections suggest the presence of an empyema or a haemothorax.

14. Look for any abnormal air collections: Subcutaneous emphysema, Pneumothorax, Pneumomediastinum, Pulmonary interstitial emphysema.

On an erect chest radiograph, a pneumothorax is usually readily identifiable as an apicolateral white line (the visceral pleural line) with an absence of vessels beyond it. In the supine position, air collects preferentially in the anteromedial and subpulmonary portions of the chest. Signs of anteromedial pneumothorax are an unusually sharp outline of the mediastinal vascular structures, heart border, and cardiophrenic sulcus. A subpulmonic pneumothorax is manifested by a hyperlucent appearance of the upper quadrant of the abdomen, a deep costophrenic sulcus, a sharp hemidiaphragm despite lung opacification in the lower lobe, and visualization of the inferior surface of consolidated lung.

A tension pneumothorax will present as mediastinal shift, diaphragmatic inversion, and flattening of the heart border and adjacent vascular structures, such as superior and inferior vena cava.

References

1. Baker SR, Stein HD. Radiologic consultation: its application to an acute care surgical ward. AJR 1986; 147: 637-40.
2. Gibson RN, Hennessy OF, Collier N, Hemingway AP. Major complications of central venous catheterization: a report of five cases and a brief review of the literature. Clin Radiol 1985; 36:205-8.
3. Gooding CA, Kerlan RK, Brasch RC, Brito AC. Medially deployed thoracostomy tubes: cause of aortic obstruction in newborns. AJR 1981; 136:511-4.
4. Goodman LR, Conrardy PA, Laing F, Singer MM. Radiographic evaluation of endotracheal tube position. AJR 1976; 127:433-4.
5. Goodman LR, Curtin JJ. Imaging the mechanically ventilated patient. In; Tobin MJ, ed. Principles and practice of mechanical ventilation. New York: McGraw-Hill, 1994; pp 891-918.
6. Goodman LR. Pulmonary support and monitoring apparatus. In: Goodman LR, Putman CE, eds. Critical care imaging. 3rd ed. Philadelphia: Saunders, 1992; pp 35-59.
7. Jarmolowski CR, Poirier RL. Small bowel infarction complicating intra-aortic balloon counter pulsation via the descending aorta. J Thorac Cardiovasc Surg 1980; 79:735-7.
8. MacMahon H. Pitfalls in Portable Chest Radiology. Respiratory Care. 1999; 44(9): 1018-1032.
9. Milne EN. A physiological approach to reading critical care unit films. J Thorac Imaging 1986; 1:60-90.
10. Trotman-Dickenson B. Radiography in the critical care patient. In: McLoud TC , (ed). Thoracic Radiology: The Requisites. St. Louis: Mosby, 1998: pp 151-172.
11. Zimmerman JE, Goodman LR, Shahvari MBG. Effect of mechanical ventilation and positive end-expiratory pressure (PEEP) on chest radiograph. AJR 1979; 133:811-5.

Introduction

- In the past, loss of spontaneous cardio-pulmonary function was considered to predict permanent non-functioning of the "organism as a whole", and therefore served adequately as a criterion of death. However, the advent of mechanical ventilation and cardiovascular support modalities has presented new challenges for determining the end of life for patients with catastrophic cerebral insults who can be preserved using complex technology. During this era of intensive care, there has been a shift from cardio-pulmonary to brain-oriented definition of death.

- Diagnosis of brain death requires both cessation of function and irreversibility of damage. Cessation of function is determined clinically by showing absence of both cerebral and brain stem function. Irreversibility is determined by: (a) Establishing that the cause of coma is sufficient to account for loss of brain function, (b) excluding the possibility of recovery of brain function, and (c) persistence of the cessation of all brain functions for the period of observation or therapy.

- Cardinal findings in brain death include coma or unresponsiveness, absence of cerebral motor responses to pain in all extremities, absence of brainstem reflexes (pupillary signs, ocular movements, facial sensory and motor responses, and pharyngeal and tracheal reflexes), and apnoea.

GUIDELINES FOR DETERMINATION OF BRAIN DEATH

1. **Wash hands.**
   This reduces the risk of transmission of micro-organisms.

2. **Acquire clinical or neuroimaging evidence of an acute catastrophic cerebral event consistent with the clinical diagnosis of brain death.**
   One of the prerequisites for confirmation of irreversible cessation of brain function.

3. **Ensure that the patient's core temperature is at least 32°C.**
   Hypothermia may alter results of neurological examination by blunting brainstem reflexes.

4. **Exclude conditions that may affect clinical assessment of brain death.**
   These conditions include severe electrolyte or severe acid-base disturbances, acute metabolic or endocrine derangements (e.g. diabetic ketoacidosis,

hyperglycaemic hyperosmolar nonketotic coma and thyroid disturbances), and neuromuscular blockade.

5. **Confirm the absence of drug intoxication or poisoning.**

    In case of possible drug intoxication or poisoning, death should not be declared until the drug or poison is metabolized or until confirmatory testing for cessation of intracranial circulation is considered.

6. **Establish evidence of coma or unresponsiveness.**

    Coma is a cardinal feature of brain death. In brain death, intense stimulation evokes no verbal or voluntary motor responses. Spontaneous voluntary motor activity, shivering, or seizure activity are absent in brain death.

7. **Assess cerebral motor response to pain using noxious stimuli (i.e. supraorbital pressure, nailbed pressure).**

    - Absence of cerebral motor response to pain is a cardinal finding consistent with brain death.
    - If neuromuscular blocking agents have recently been used, examination with a bedside peripheral nerve stimulator is needed. A TOF stimulus should result in four thumb twitches.
    - Motor responses may occur spontaneously during apnoea testing with the occurrence of hypoxia or hypotension and are considered to be of spinal reflex origin. Respiratory acidosis and brisk neck flexion too, may generate spinal cord reflexes. Spinal reflex responses occur more frequently in young adults and include rapid spontaneous flexion and muscle stretch reflexes in the arms and legs, with resulting grasplike, walking-like movements. Spinal reflex movements may occur in the presence of brain death.
    - Involuntary posturing movements (i.e. decorticate or decerebrate) are absent in brain death.

8. **Assess pupillary size and response to light in both the eyes.**

    - Pupillary light reflex is absent in brain death. Round, oval, or irregularly shaped pupils are compatible with brain death. Most pupils are in midposition size (4 to 6 mm) in brain death, although the size may vary from 4 to 9 mm. Dilated pupils are compatible with brain death because intact sympathetic cervical pathways connected with the radially arranged fibres of the dilator muscle may remain intact.
    - Many drugs can influence pupil size, but light response remains intact. In conventional doses, atropine given intravenously has no marked influence on the pupillary response.
    - As nicotinic receptors are absent in the iris, neuromuscular blocking drugs do not noticeably influence the pupil size.
    - Topical ocular instillation of drugs and trauma to the cornea may cause abnormalities in size and can produce non-reactive pupils.
    - Preexisting anatomic abnormalities of the iris or effects of previous surgery should be excluded.

9. Assess oculocephalic (doll's eye) reflexes. Oculocephalic reflexes are elicited by rapidly and vigorously turning the head by 90 degrees laterally to both the sides. Normally, this results in deviation of the eye ball to the side opposite to which the head is turned. Vertical eye movements should be tested with brisk neck flexion.
    - Eyelid opening, and vertical and horizontal eye movements (in response to head movement) are absent in brain death.
    - Cervical spine fracture or instability is a contraindication to performing the oculocephalic reflex.

10. Assess oculovestibular (caloric) reflexes.
    (a) Exclude contraindications.
        - Contraindications to performing this test include perforated tympanic membrane, preexisting meniere's disease, III and VI cranial nerve disorders, or facial trauma involving the auditory canal and petrous bone. Several medications including sedatives, aminoglycosides, tricyclic antidepressants, anticholinergics, antiepileptics, and neuromuscular blocking agents may diminish oculovestibular reflexes. Clotted blood or cerumen may also diminish the response.
    (b) Position the patient. Place the head of the patient in a neutral position with the head end of the bed elevated to 30 degrees.
        - This position brings the lateral semicircular canals to a vertical position, thus allowing maximal stimulation, and also optimizes jugular venous drainage.
    (c) Instill 50 mL of iced water or normal saline into the external auditory canal.
        - The instillation should take between 30 seconds to 3 minutes to allow adequate time for stimulation.
    (d) Observe the patient's eyes for a response for up to 1 minute (Fig. 25.1 a, b).
        - A normal response in the awake patient is nystagmus—a slow component towards the irrigated ear, then a faster component away from the irrigated ear. A normal response in the comatose patient usually results in stimulation of the slow component only.
        - An abnormal (dysconjugate) or absent response to cold water testing in the unconscious patient may indicate brain stem dysfunction and a poor prognosis.
        - In brain death, the deviation of eyes is absent.

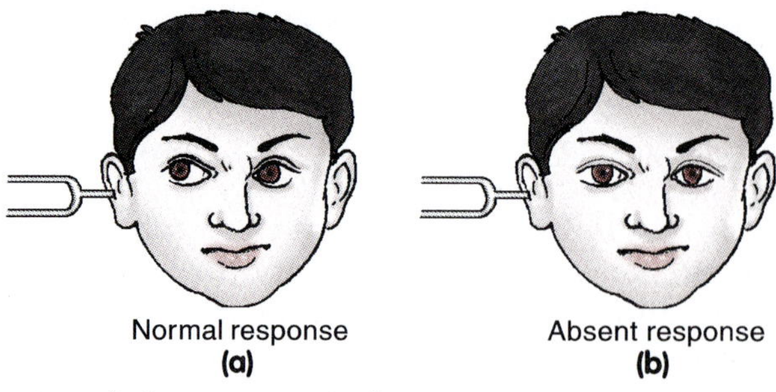

Fig. 25.1 a, b: Cold-water caloric responses in the comatose patient. **(a)** Patient with intact brainstem – slow movement toward the irrigated ear. **(b)** Brainstem not intact – response absent.

(e) Perform the test on the opposite external auditory canal after at least 5 minutes.
- Monitor vital signs both, during and immediately after the test. There could be cardio-respiratory instability.
- Absence of oculovestibular reflexes is a cardinal sign of brain death.

11. Assess corneal reflex (tested with a cotton swab) and jaw reflex.
- Jaw reflex is described as grimacing to pain caused by deep pressure on nail beds, supraorbital ridge, or on the temporomandibular joint.
- Corneal and jaw reflexes are absent in brain death.
- Severe facial trauma may inhibit interpretation of facial brain stem reflexes.

12. Assess pharyngeal and tracheal reflexes. Gag reflexes may be tested by stimulation of the posterior pharynx with a tongue blade. Cough response may be tested by bronchial suctioning.
- Absence of pharyngeal and tracheal reflexes is consistent with brain death.
- In orally intubated patients, gag response may be difficult to interpret.

13. Perform apnoea test.
 (a) Achieve prerequisites necessary for apnoea test.

 (i) Maintain core body temperature more than 36.5°C.
 (ii) Systolic blood pressure ≥ 90 mmHg.
 (iii) Euvolaemia (preferably positive fluid balance in the previous 6 hours).
 (iv) Eucapnia (option: $PaCO_2 \geq 40$ mmHg).
 (v) Normoxaemia (option: arterial PO_2 greater than or equal to 200 mmHg).
 - These may help avoid cardiovascular instability during the test.
 - Connect pulse oximeter probe to the patient.
 - The respiratory neurons are controlled by central chemoreceptors that sense changes in the PCO_2 and pH of the CSF, and these accurately reflect changes in the plasma PCO_2. Advisory guidelines recommend achieving a PCO_2 level of greater than 60 mmHg for maximal stimulation of the brainstem. The target PCO_2 levels for apnoea test may be higher in patients with chronic hypercapnia.
 - Apnoea testing is easy with a starting arterial PCO_2 of 40 mmHg because the target level of 60 mmHg is reached after 6 to 8 minutes of disconnection from the ventilator.
 - The estimated PCO_2 increase is 3 to 6 mmHg per minute and varies with the rate of production.
 - Hypocarbia can be corrected by changing the minute volume by decreasing either the respiratory rate or tidal volume for several minutes. Use of carbon dioxide admixture should be avoided as it may lead to severe hypercarbia and respiratory acidosis.
 (b) Obtain arterial blood gas (ABG).
 (c) Disconnect the ventilator.
 (d) Deliver 100% oxygen at 6 L/min. May place cannula at the level of the carina.
 - Side effects of hypercarbia like cardiac arrhythmias are more likely to occur in the presence of hypoxia.

(e) Observe closely for respiratory movements (defined as abdominal or chest excursions that produce adequate tidal volumes).
- When in doubt, a spirometer can be connected to the patient to confirm that tidal volume is absent.

(f) Obtain ABG after approximately 8 minutes and reconnect the ventilator.

(g) Interpret apnoea test results.

Positive apnoea test:
- Absent respiratory movements.
- Post-test $PaCO_2 \geq 60$ mmHg or 20 mmHg increase in $PaCO_2$ over a baseline of normal $PaCO_2$.
- Supports brain death.

Negative apnoea test:
- Respiratory movements are present regardless of $PaCO_2$ level.
- Does not support brain death.
- May be repeated after some time.

Inconclusive apnoea test:
- No respiratory movements.
- Post-test $PaCO_2 < 60$ mmHg without significant cardiovascular instability.
- May be repeated with 10 minutes of apnoea.

Test resulting in cardio-pulmonary instability:
- Systolic blood pressure falls below 90 mmHg.
- Arterial oxygen saturation falls.
- Presence of cardiac arrhythmias.
- Immediately draw an ABG sample, and reconnect ventilator.
- Left to the discretion of the physician whether a confirmatory test is needed to finalize the clinical diagnosis of brain death.

14. Repeat these tests at intervals of 6 hours for confirming irreversibility of brain function.

   All the above tests are equally essential in declaring brain death.

15. Keep in mind certain clinical observations compatible with the diagnosis of brain death.

   Respiratory acidosis, hypoxia, or brisk neck flexion may generate spinal cord responses. Spontaneous movements of limbs from spinal mechanisms can occasionally occur and are more frequent in young adults. These spinal reflexes include rapid flexion of arms, raising all limbs off the bed, grasping movements, spontaneous jerking of one leg, walking-like movements and movements of the arms upto the point of reaching the endotracheal tube. Further, muscle stretch reflexes are of spinal origin and do not invalidate a diagnosis of brain death.

16. Support clinical findings with confirmatory tests, in cases where results of clinical tests cannot be reliably evaluated.

   Confirmatory tests are not mandatory in all patients for diagnosis of brain death. These include: (i) Cerebral angiography (no intracerebral filling at the level of carotid bifurcation or circle of Willis, external carotid circulation is patent), (ii) electroencephalogram (no electrical activity during a period of at least 30 minutes of recording), (iii) transcranial Doppler ultrasonography (absent diastolic or reverberating flow, or small peaks in early systole, and indicating very high vascular resistance), and (iv) technetium 99m brain scan (no uptake of isotope in brain parenchyma), and (v) somatosensory evoked potentials (N20-P22 response bilaterally absent).

References

1. Black PM. Conceptual and practical issues in the declaration of death by brain criteria. Neurosurg Clin North Am 1991;2;493-501.
2. Brody H, Campbell ML, et al. Withdrawing life-sustaining treatment-recommendations for compassionate clinical management N Eng J Med 1997;336(9):652-657.
3. Guidelines for the determination of death: Report of the Medical Consultants on the Diagnosis of Death to the President's commission for the Study of Ethical Problems in Medicine and Biomedical and Biobehavioral Research. JAMA. 1981;246:2184-2186.
4. Hanley DF. Brain death: an update on the North American view point. Anesth Intens Care. 1995;23:24-25.
5. Lang CJ. Blood pressure and heart rate changes during apnea testing with or without CO_2 insufflation. Intens Care Med. 1997;23:903-907.
6. Lock M. Death in technological time: locating the end of meaningful life. Med Anthropol Q 1996;10:575-600.
7. Minimum technical standards for EEG recording in suspected cerebral death. J Clin Neurophysiol. 1994; 11:10-13.
8. Paolin A, Manuali A, DiPaola F, et al. Reliability in diagnosis of brain death. Intens Care Med 1995; 21:657-662.
9. Payen DM, Lamer C, Pilorget A, et al. Evaluation of pulsed Doppler common carotid blood flow as a noninvasive method for brain death diagnosis: a prospective study. Anesthesiology. 1990;72:222-229.
10. Petty GW, Mohr JP, Pedley TA et al. The role of transcranial Doppler in confirming brain death: sensitivity, specificity, and suggestions for performance and interpretation. Neurology 1990;40:300-303.
11. Shann F. A personal comment: whole brain death versus cortical death. Anesth Intens Care 1995;23:14-15.
12. Taylor RM. Reexamining the definition and criteria of death. Semin Neurol 1997;17:265-270.
13. Wijdicks EFM. Determining brain death in adults. Neurology 1995;45:1003-1011.

Airway Management in Emergency Department/ Ward: Basic Approach

26

Introduction

- The ability to manage an airway appropriately is fundamental to resuscitation. Failure to do so, particularly where that failure could have been anticipated and avoided by the selection of more appropriate technique, is disastrous as failure to maintain a patent airway for more than a few minutes can lead to brain injury or death.
- Emergency airway management, either in the emergency department or in the ward is often a challenging task for many reasons: (i) Patient is comparatively sicker and in respiratory distress, (ii) time is limited, (iii) all the equipment and help may not be timely accessible, and (iv) position of the patient and the operator is awkward. These factors reduce the success rate of endotracheal intubation on one hand and increase the risk of complications on the other. Under these circumstances, it is necessary to employ a systematic approach to improve the success rate of intubation.
- Suggested contents of an emergency intubation bag include: (i) Intravenous catheters (16-22 gauge), (ii) masks of various sizes, (iii) laryngoscope blades: Macintosh and Miller, different sizes, (iv) oral and nasal airways, (v) endotracheal tubes 3-8 mm ID, (vi) Magill forceps, (vii) gum elastic bougie (Fig. 26.1), stylet (Fig. 26.2), (viii) manual ventilation bag with ability to provide adequate oxygen, (ix) syringes (10,5,2 mL), (x) lubricant, (xi) stethoscope, tape and scissors, (xii) suction catheters of different sizes, (xiii) cotton swab, (xiv) nasogastric tube, (xv) various drugs, and (xvi) emergency airway devices in case of failed intubation/ventilation e.g. laryngeal mask (Fig. 26.3); combitube (Fig. 26.4), transtracheal jet ventilation.

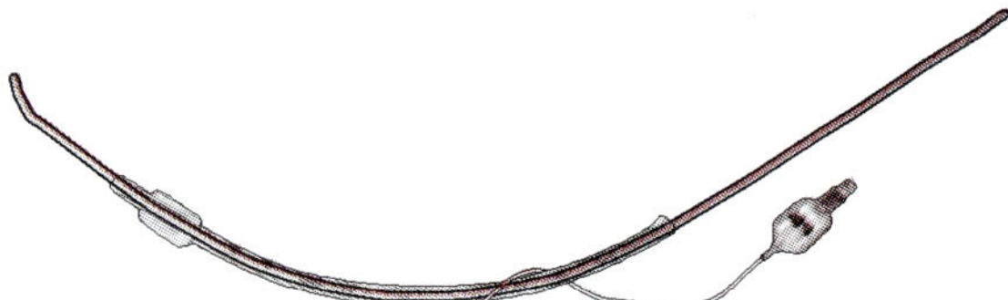

Fig. 26.1: Gum elastic bougie. The gum elastic bougie should be used routinely to minimize the risk of a failed intubation. The bougie has an external diameter of 5 mm and can accommodate tracheal tubes with an inner diameter of ≥ 6 mm. The distal 2.5 cm is angulated at 35°.

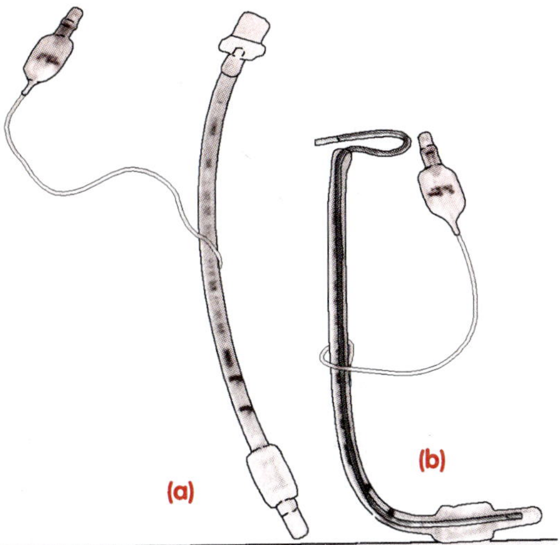

Fig. 26.2: Use of stylet is helpful in difficult-to-intubate "anterior" glottic opening. **(a)**, The endotracheal tube insertion without a stylet, making control of its tip difficult or impossible. **(b)**, The stylet insertion within the endotracheal tube allows control of tube tip and helps it to be directed towards glottic opening. Once at the glottic opening, slowly withdrawing stylet without changing the position of tube further elevates the tip anteriorly and allows the tube to easily advance through the vocal cords.

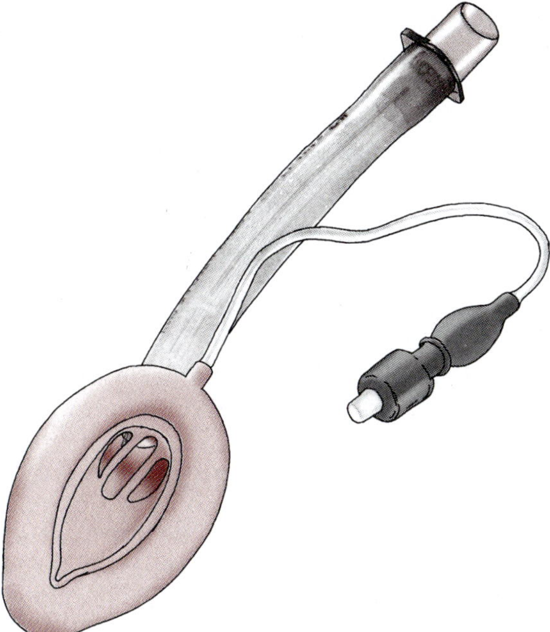

Fig. 26.3: The laryngeal mask airway (LMA) consists of three main components: an airway tube, a mask and an inflation line. The airway tube has a 15-mm standard male adaptor. The mask is in the form of an elliptical cuff and is designed to conform to the contours of the hypopharynx with the lumen facing the laryngeal aperture. The LMA may be a useful alternative when intubation fails.

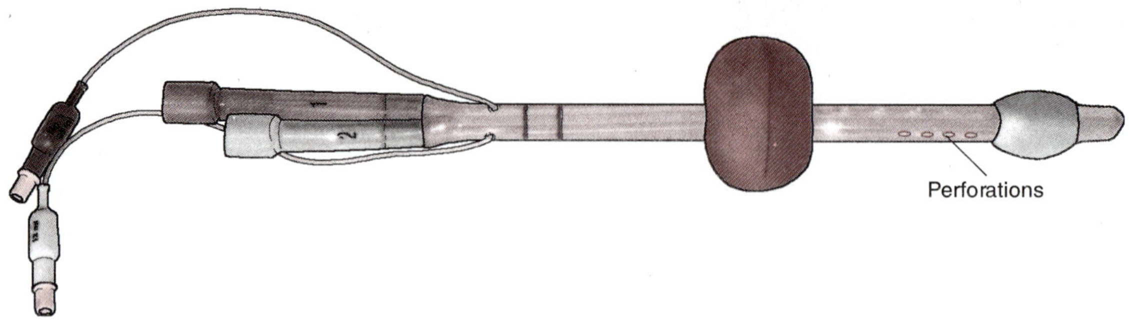

Fig. 26.4: The double lumen combitube has the advantage of blind insertion. The two cuffs are inflated to show their relative positions that allow the combitube to seal the esophagus from the trachea. In the esophageal position, ventilation is via the proximal hypopharyngeal perforations while in the tracheal position, ventilation is via the distal lumen.

- Modified tube changers have a central channel, allowing for passage of oxygen into the pharynx or trachea during an endotracheal tube change. This can be life saving in patients with severe lung disease, in whom hypoxaemia can occur after a few seconds of apnoea.
- Signs indicating a successful endotracheal intubation include a combination of the following: (i) Visual inspection of the tube passing through the cords, (ii) a normal capnographic waveform, (iii) expansion and fall of the chest with ventilation, (iv) moist gas escaping from the tube during expiration, (v) breath sounds heard over both lung fields in the midaxillary line/no breath sounds over epigastrium, (vi) movement of reservoir bag when the patient inspires, (vii) identification of tracheal rings with a flexible fiberoptic scope (viii) maintenance of oxygen saturation, (ix) radiographic evidence.
- American Society of Anesthesiologists (ASA) Task Force defines difficult airway as a clinical situation in which a conventionally trained anaesthesiologist experiences difficulty with face mask ventilation or difficulty with tracheal intubation, or both.
- Difficult mask ventilation may be defined as inability to maintain oxygen saturation greater than 90%, by using 100% oxygen and bag-valve-mask ventilation, in a patient who was capable of doing so before the intervention.
- Difficult laryngoscopy refers to a situation when it is not possible to see any portion of the vocal cords.
- The first response to a failure of bag-and-mask ventilation is better bag-and mask ventilation! Insert nasal airways in both nostrils and an oral airway in the mouth. Optimize airway position by thrusting the mandible forward and holding it there. Use a two-handed mask hold; lift the head to open the airway if the cervical spine is alright. Generate as much positive pressure as possible without inflating the stomach.
- Failed airway is clinically defined as (i) failure to intubate on three attempts by a skilled and experienced operator; This is called "can't intubate, can oxygenate" failure, and (ii) failure to intubate, no matter the number of attempts, along with inability to maintain oxygen saturation at 90% or higher using a bag-and-mask. This is the "can't intubate, can't oxygenate" scenario.

- There are three reasons why intubation may be difficult: poor access (inability to insert laryngoscope into the mouth), poor visualization (of vocal cords or epiglottis), and inability to advance the ETT.

- There are instances when intubation is not possible after a single laryngoscopy. In such cases, few simple techniques such as adjustment of the head position ("sniffing" position) (Fig. 26.5), adjustment of the cricoid pressure, performing the the BURP manoeuvre (displacing the larynx backward against the cervical vertebrae, upward as far as possible, and slightly laterally to the right) (Fig. 26.6), and changing the laryngoscope blade, may be all that is required to facilitate intubation. The gum elastic bougie may be of help where only a small part of the laryngeal aperture can be visualized. It is also useful to consider sedative and paralytic agents to increase the chances of success in selected circumstances.

- In parturients with enlarged breasts, morbidly obese patients, patients with kyphosis and severe barrel-chest deformity, and patients with short necks, insertion of the laryngoscope blade is difficult. To overcome this problem, many solutions have been proposed which include (i) removing the blade from the handle and reconnecting it after it is inserted into the oropharynx, (ii) using a short

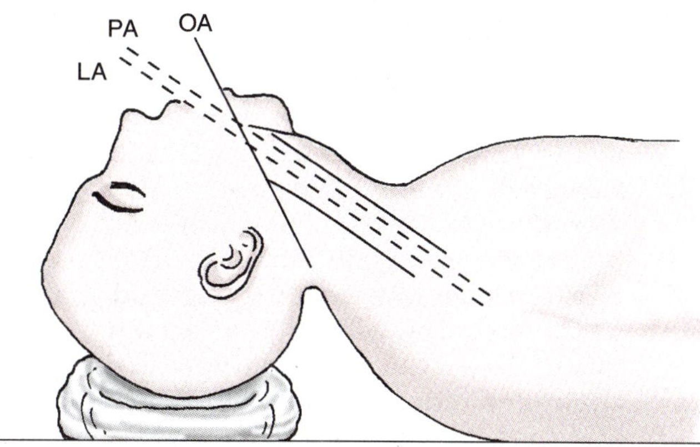

Fig. 26.5: Neck hyperextension in the sniffing position aligns the oral, pharyngeal and laryngeal axes. OA, Oral axis; PA, Pharyngeal axis; LA, Laryngeal axis.

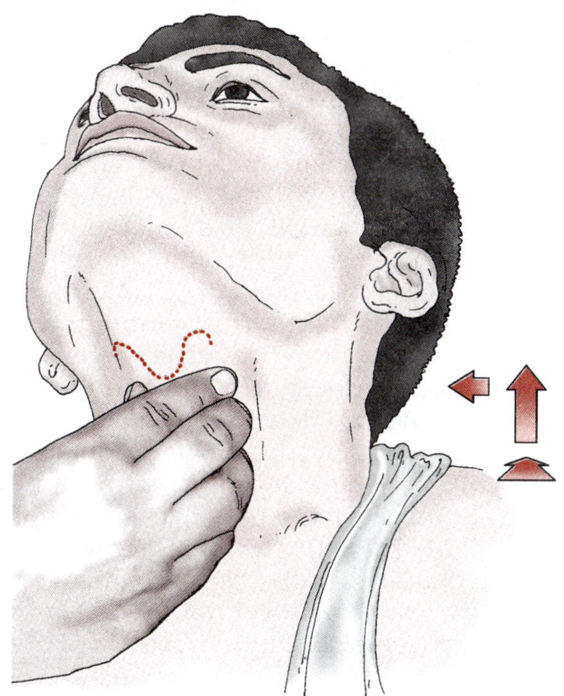

Fig. 26.6: BURP manoeuvre. This is accomplished by displacing the larynx in three specific directions. (i) Backwards against the cervical vertebrae, (ii) upwards, as far superior as possible, and (iii) slightly laterally to the right, on the thyroid cartilage.

laryngoscope handle, (iii) inserting the blade into the corner of the patient's mouth with the handle parallel to the patient's shoulder and then rotating it to the correct position, and (iv) altering the angle, between the blade and the handle (polio laryngoscope blade, Kessel laryngoscope blade, Jellicoe and Harris adaptor, Yentis blade, Dhara and Cheong adaptor).

- In patients in whom a difficult airway is anticipated, LMA may either be used alone as the definitive airway or it may be used as an aid to oral intubation, under general anaesthesia or under topical anaesthesia in an awake patient. However, some authors argue that, in situations where airway difficulty is already recognized, LMA should not be used as a definitive airway as airway protection may be inadequate. In fasted patients and in whom intubation has failed but ventilation with bag-and-mask is possible, LMA can be used alone as the definitive airway or as an aid to oral intubation. When used following a failed intubation in a patient with a potentially full stomach, the risk of aspiration reduces once hypoxia is relieved. However, once the immediate crisis situation is managed, other available options may be considered. Cricoid pressure should be maintained till a definitive airway is achieved. In the emergency situation of "can't intubate, can't ventilate", LMA has been recommended either alone as a definitive airway or as an aid to oral intubation.

- The three non-surgical techniques for emergency airway ventilation in patients with "can't intubate, can't ventilate" situation are transtracheal jet ventilation (TTJV), and ventilation through a laryngeal mask airway (LMA) or a combitube. TTJV requires special equipment and some degree of skill in locating the cricothyroid membrane, especially in obese patients with a short neck. For these reasons, it has been suggested that the LMA and combitube should be tried prior to TTJV. Advantages of LMA include ease of insertion, avoidance of the risk of esophageal and right main bronchus intubation, and the fact that it can be used as an aid to intubation. However it is relatively contraindicated in patients at risk of aspiration and in those with low chest compliance, who require high-pressure ventilation. In patients who are at risk for aspiration, such as obese, obstetric, or emergency patients, the combitube offers an advantage over the LMA in terms of emergent airway control. Once in place, it provides sufficient ventilation and oxygenation as compared with routine endotracheal intubation. In addition, endotracheal intubation can be performed around the combitube without fear of losing the airway, either by direct laryngoscopy or by other manoeuvres (oral or nasal fiberoptic intubation, or lighted stylet). The main disadvantage of the combitube is that it is currently available in only two sizes and, therefore, it cannot be used in patients who are less than 4 feet tall.

- Retrograde intubation may be considered in the following circumstances: (i) Failed attempts at laryngoscopy and/or fiberoptic intubation, (ii) emergency establishment of an airway where visualization of the vocal cords is prevented by blood, secretions, or anatomical derangement, and (iii) electively, in conditions like unstable cervical spine, mandibular fracture, or anatomical anamolies.

- Surgical airway may be indicated, in the initial stage in situations like laryngeal trauma, massive facial injuries, upper airway obstruction, and oropharyngeal distortion. It is also indicated in patients for whom other methods of securing the airway have failed.
- "Call for help" as mentioned below, includes a call for a more experienced anaesthesiologist, additional equipment and/or other personnel (surgeon, technician).
- While the airway is being managed, patients should be monitored (heart rate, blood pressure ECG, and pulse oximetry, if available) continuously.

GUIDELINES FOR MANAGING THE AIRWAY IN AN EMERGENCY

1. Observe the patient.

    At the bedside, first determine whether the patient needs to be intubated immediately without any delay or the condition of the patient can permit a few minutes, in which case, a calm, collected approach with efficient and complete preparation is best. Proceed to step 2.

    Patients requiring immediate intubation without delay include (i) Unresponsive patients, (ii) those having ineffective or no respiration, (iii) those who have already arrested or are near death, (iv) those who are expected to be unresponsive to laryngoscopy. No drugs are necessary in this situation; however oxygen and suction should be readily available. Proper preparation, and positioning of the patient are other prerequisites for a successful intubation. Management includes application of cricoid pressure, mask ventilation, and use of a direct laryngoscopic technique to intubate the trachea with a styletted endotracheal tube. If intubation is successful, proceed with post-intubation management. If it is unsuccessful, assess whether bag and mask ventilation is possible and patient maintain $SpO_2 \geq 90\%$. If ventilation is not possible, it respresents a situation of can't intubate, can't ventilate (failed airway). Proceed to step 12. If it is possible to ventilate and maintain $SpO_2 \geq 90\%$, assess whether the patient is completely relaxed and flaccid. If not, administer a dose of suxamethonium, and make further attempts with optimized 'sniffing' position and manipulation of the larynx (BURP manoeuvre). If successful, proceed with post-intubation management. If intubation is unsuccessful even after three attempts, the situation represents a failed airway. Proceed to step 12.

2. Assemble the necessary intubation equipment and prepare the drugs. Check proper functioning of laryngoscope and select an appropriate size of the endotracheal tube. As a rule, use a malleable stylet to facilitate tube placement in emergency conditions.

3. Assess the patient quickly.
    Nature of the emergency will determine whether assessment should precede the treatment.
    Always assume the patient to have a full stomach.

In case of airway obstruction, attempt head tilt, chin lift or jaw thrust and/or insertion of a nasal or oral airway.

- Take a focused history to assess the cardiorespiratory status and to decide the urgency of endotracheal intubation. Any past history of difficult airway and history of recent ingestion of food should be elicited.
- Assess the airway within a few seconds. If the patient can talk and narrate the history, it indicates an intact airway. Look for any vomitus or blood in the mouth. Suction immediately to prevent aspiration. Listen to sounds: gurgling sound (fluid in the pharynx), snoring sound (soft tissue obstruction), or crowing sound (obstruction at the level of the larynx). Palpate the larynx for any surgical emphysema, or anatomical disruption (may suggest a laryngeal fracture).
- Nasal airway is usually better tolerated in a semiconscious patient because the oral airway has a greater chance of causing gagging and coughing, which may aggravate airway obstruction.

4. Position the patient.
   The sniffing position aligns the oral, pharyngeal and laryngeal axes so that the pathway from the lips to the glottis is nearly a straight line.

   Put the patient in supine "sniffing" position with the occiput elevated using a pillow or folded blankets and the head in extension. If the patient is on a stretcher, bring the stretcher to such a position that there is plenty of room to manoeuvre. In patients with multiple trauma and head or facial injury, the presence of cervical spine injury should always be presumed until excluded. Avoid excessive motion of the spine and stabilize the head and neck in a neutral position. The greatest cervical displacement appears to occur during bag-and-mask ventilation. Administration of anaesthetic agents and neuromuscular blocking agents may be necessary to avoid excessive movement.

5. Check that the suction is available and is functioning properly.
6. Oxygenate the patient.
   Administer 100% oxygen via a tight fitting mask and bag, regardless of the type of oxygen therapy administered prior to the decision to intubate. Most patients requiring intubation in the ward or in the emergency department are in respiratory distress and are hypoxaemic. They do not tolerate even a short period of breathing room air.

7. Establish IV access.
   Start a new IV line if adequacy of the existing line is in question. In cardiac arrest, intubation can precede the establishment of adequate IV access. The endotracheal tube can be used as an alternative route of drug (xylocaine, atropine, epinephrine, isoproteronol, naloxone) administration.

8. Reassess the adequacy of the airway against aspiration and the ability for gas exchange.

   - Observation of the patient's ability to swallow is a valuable sign. If the patient is able to sense secretions in the posterior oral pharynx and is able to swallow them in a co-ordinated way while lying on his back, an adequate level of airway protection is present at the time of examination.

- Even if the airway is patent and protected, if the patient is not able to maintain an adequate gas exchange and $SpO_2 \geq 90\%$ either on air or with an oxygen mask, bag-and-mask assisted ventilation or intubation should be strongly considered.
- Some patients may have adequate gas exchange and the ability to maintain and protect their airway at the time of examination, but are likely to deteriorate with time (e.g. those with head injury, shock, chest trauma, drug overdose with decreasing level of consciousness). In such patients it is advisable to consider early tracheal intubation.

9. **If intubation is indicated, assess the airway.**

Once it has been decided to intubate the patient, the next step is to quickly assess (see Chapter 27) whether the patient's airway is potentially difficult or not. If it is potentially difficult, proceed to step 10. If it is not a potentially difficult airway, proceed with intubation. In most cases, it is preferable to

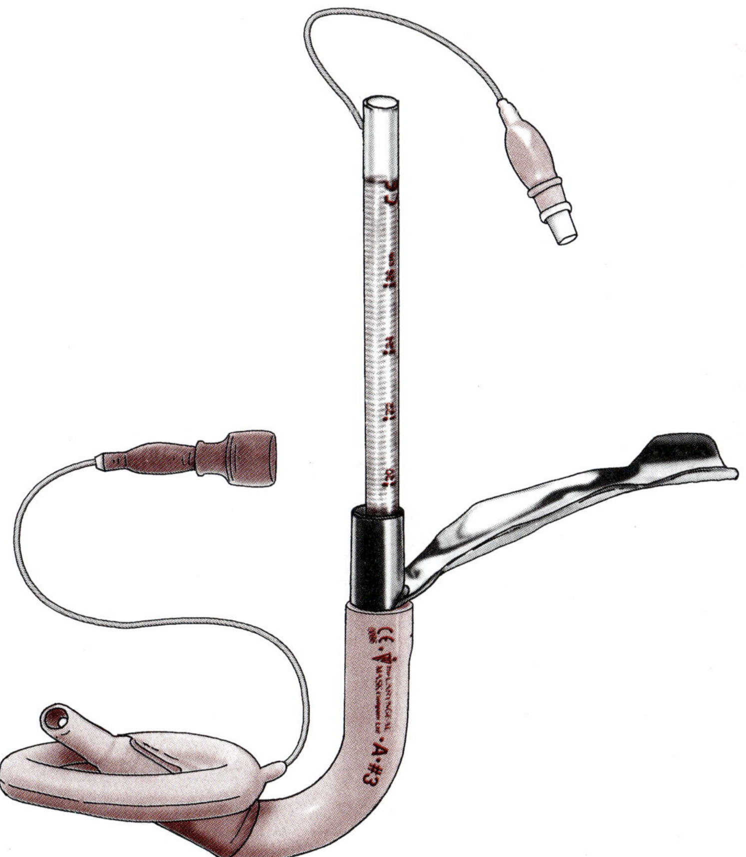

Fig. 26.7: The LMA-Fastrach or intubating laryngeal mask consists of a standard laryngeal mask with epiglottic elevator and a rigid anatomically curved airway. The metal handle facilitates insertion with one hand from various positions without moving the head and neck and without placing the fingers in the mouth. The LMA-Fastrach can be used as a stand alone airway or as a guide for tracheal intubation.

intubate the patient with as little suppression of respiratory drive and airway reflexes as possible and probably in the following sequence: (i) Awake intubation with topical anaesthesia, (ii) sedative agents (e.g. midazolam 0.5 mg, diazepam 1mg) in titrated, judicious doses, only if necessary, (iii) paralysis as a last resort. In extremis, the patient requires much less anaesthesia (or may be no anaesthesia) for intubation, compared to a healthy patient. In most cases, it is possible to intubate with a combination of topical anaesthesia and moderate IV sedation. Exceptions to this general rule, however, do exist. For example, a combative multiple trauma patient may require anaesthesia and paralysis to minimize the chances of excessive motion exacerbating a spinal cord injury. Once the trachea has been intubated, proceed with post-intubation management. If intubation is unsuccessful, proceed as in step 1.

10. **Difficult airway is recognized on assessment.**
    If at any point, $SpO_2 \leq 90\%$, with or without bag and mask ventilation, proceed to step 12 as situation represents failed airway.
    - Ask for help.
    - Reevaluate. If patient is uncooperative but bag and mask ventilation and intubation are predicted to be successful, optimize the sniffing position and BURP manoeuvre, use an alternative laryngoscopy blade (size or type), or a gum elastic bougie if required, and proceed with rapid sequence intubation. Reevaluation as mentioned above includes not only physical assessment but may also include a trial of bag-and-mask ventilation after the use of judicious sedation.
    - When intubation is not likely to be successful, proceed with awake laryngoscopy under topical anaesthesia and judicious sedation. Awake laryngoscopy can be used either to intubate the patient or to assess the ease of intubation. After assessment, awake intubation can proceed either (i) as a blind nasotracheal intubation, or using (ii) direct laryngoscopy, (iii) intubating LMA (FASTRACH) (Fig. 26.7), (iv) fiberoptic bronchoscopy, (v) an illuminating stylet, or (vi) a cricothyrotomy can be performed.

11. **Intubation tried and failed, unrecognized difficulty, patient maintaining saturation, and is possible to ventilate (can't intubate, can oxygenate).**
    (If at any time, $SpO_2 \leq 90\%$ with or without bag and mask ventilation, proceed to step 12 as situation respresents a failed airway (can't intubate, can't ventilate). There is no reason why an alternative option, if available, should not be tried earlier than three attempts.
    - Maintain cricoid pressure.
    - Ask for help.
    - Continue bag-and-mask ventilation to keep $SpO_2 \geq 90\%$.
    - Make an attempt using a bougie (gum elastic, flexible) or intubation stylet/ tube changer. This should be attempted only if a view of the glottis has been obtained and the patient is still oxygenated. Also ensure correct head position, adjust the cricoid pressure, use external manipulation of larynx (BURP manoeuvre), and change the laryngoscopy blades, if options are available.

- If intubation is unsuccessful, consider using an intubating LMA (I-LMA) and/or fiberoptic –assisted intubation (if available).
- If intubation is successful with the above-mentioned measures, proceed with post-intubation management.
- If intubation is still unsuccessful, but $SpO_2 \geq 90\%$, the airway is maintained, and bag-and-mask ventilation is possible, the following options may be considered; blind nasal/oral intubation, use of a light wand, retrograde intubation, and Bullard laryngoscope.
- Once these options have also, failed and $SpO_2 \geq 90\%$, arrange for a definitive airway (cricothyroidotomy or tracheostomy), preferably in the operation theatre.

12. **Patient meets failed airway criteria, and is impossible to ventilate. "Can't intubate, can't ventilate".**
- Maintain cricoid pressure.
- Ask for help.
- Can't intubate and can't ventilate is an emergency situation.
- Use I-LMA (intubating LMA) or combitube as a temporary measure to gain time provided the airway obstruction is not at the level of the glottis (spasm, edema, tumor, abscess, haematoma) or below the level of the glottis. Use of I-LMA or combitube may permit successful tracheal intubation.
- For glottic or subglottic obstruction, use percutaneous transtracheal jet ventilation (TTJV).
- A surgical airway (surgical or percutaneous tracheostomy or cricothyrotomy) is the definite answer in this situation. Cricothyrotomy is a fast and simple procedure that can be performed in less than 1 minute, as it requires very few instruments.

References

1. American Society of Anesthesiologists Task Force on the Difficult Airway: ASA difficult airway to algorithm. Anesthesiology 1993; 78:597-602.
2. Benumof JL Laryngeal mask airway and the American Society of Anesthesiologists' difficult airway algorithm. Anesthesiology 1996; 84:686-694.
3. Benumol JL.. Laryngeal mask airway and difficult intubation. Anesthesiology 1993; 78:995.
4. Bourke DL, Lawrence J, Another way to insert a Macintosh blade. Anesthesiology. 1983; 39:80.
5. Brimacombe J, Berry A, White A. An algorithm for use of the loryngeal mask airway during failed intubation in the patient with a full stomach. Anesth Analg 1993; 77:398-399.
6. Datta S, Briwa J. Modified laryngoscope for endotracheal intubation of obese patients. Anesth Analg 1981; 60:120-121.
7. Finance BT. Emergency airway management. Anesthes Clin North Am 1995; 13(3): 543-564.
8. Hyrford WE. Orotracheal intubation outside the operating room; anatomic considerations and techniques. Respir Care 1999; 44(6): 615-626.
9. Kay NH. Mammomegaly and intubation. Anesthesia 1982;37:221.
10. Kubota y. Mammomegaly and intubation. Anesthesia 1982; 37:779-780.

11. Sakles JC, Laurin EG, Rantapaa AA, Panacek EA. Airway management in the emergency department: a one-year study of 610 tracheal intubations. Ann Emerg Med 1998; 31(3): 325-332.
12. Schwartz DE, Matthay MA, Cohen NH. Death and other complications of emergency airway management in critically ill adults: a prospective investigation of 297 tracheal intubation. Anesthesiology 1995; 82(2): 367-376.
13. Todesco J, Doda C, Tudor Williams R, Williams PJ, Bailey PM. Laryngeal mask airway: Defining the limits. Can J Anaesth .1993;40:816-818.
14. Walls RM. Management of the difficult airway in the trauma patient. Emerg Med Clin North Am 1998; 16(1): 45-61.
15. Wilson WC Application of the ASA difficult airway algorithm. In: Hanowell LH, Waldron RJ, eds. Airway management. Philadelphia: Lippincott-Reven 1996, pp 119-128.

Airway Management: Predicting the Difficult Airway

27

Introduction

- Difficult or failed tracheal intubation is feared by all anaesthetists, intensivists and those involved in emergency care, and there have been many attempts to develop means of predicting it. However, at times even these predictors may fail to predict the difficult airway and therefore, there is a need to always plan an alternative airway management technique, either as a primary approach or as a backup.
- Both, a difficult direct laryngoscopy and blind techniques are more likely to be complicated by tissue trauma, esophageal intubation, cardiovascular and respiratory instability, and aspiration of gastric or pharyngeal contents.
- The body mechanics required for direct laryngoscopy are: adequate mouth opening, mobile soft tissue (tongue and tissue at the floor of mouth), a flexible neck and a normally placed larynx. Most of the predictive tests examine these factors directly or indirectly.
- The temporomandibular joint's (TMJ) integrity as both, a gliding joint and a hinge joint should be individually tested, because each component may be significantly, and independently impaired, thus affecting direct laryngoscopy.
- Length of the mandible is an important predictor. The mandible should be sufficiently large to accommodate a normal sized tongue. A patient with a small mandible will have a tongue that obstructs the view to the larynx during intubation (i.e. the larynx is tucked up under the base of the tongue). Also, a disproportionately large mandible elongates the oral axis (one of the three axes to be aligned during orotracheal intubation), making it more difficult to bring it into alignment with the laryngeal axis.
- Tongue mobility is a function of the mandibular-hyoid distance, since the hyoid bone plays a key role in lingual suspension. This distance also identifies adequate mandibular dimension to permit access to the airway.
- Thyromental distance correlates with the gap between the first and second cervical vertebrae and presumably, the ability to extend the neck at this joint. Tracheal intubation is more difficult in patients whose thyromental distance is less than 6cm.

- The length of the neck and the position of the larynx in the neck are important factors to be considered. The larynx descends in the neck from C_{3-4} level in infancy to C_{5-6} level by 8 or 9 years of age. A larynx that is higher (e.g. in morbid obesity) may be more difficult to visualize than the one that is lower down as it gets tucked under the base of the tongue.

- The Mallampati score of predicting difficulty in airway management involves visualizing oropharyngeal structures in a seated patient with extended neck, having his tongue fully protruded out with the mouth opened widely. A class I score provides a view of the entire posterior oropharynx (soft palate, uvula, fauces, and pillars are visible). In class II, the soft palate, uvula and fauces are visible. In class III, only the soft palate and base of uvula are visible while a class IV view permits no visualization of the posterior oropharynx as the tongue totally obstructs visualization of the uvula. Only the hard palate is visible in class IV.

- Oropharyngeal visualization has been shown to correlate with laryngeal visualization. Class III and IV Mallampati views have been shown to be associated with increasingly poor laryngeal visualization and with higher failure rates of intubation.

- In emergency situations, the formal version of Mallampati is often not possible, but examination of the supine patient with a tongue blade may be useful.

GUIDELINES FOR PREDICTING DIFFICULT AIRWAY IN EMERGENCY DEPARTMENT/WARD

1. **Wash hands, wear gloves.**

   This reduces the risk of transmission of micro-organisms.

2. **Gather past history, if time permits.**

   In an emergency, very often there isn't sufficient time to take a detailed past history. One might have to proceed with step 3 straight away. Relevant information to be gathered includes any history of previous awake intubation, cancellation of surgery following induction of anaesthesia, prolonged (i.e. more than 48 hours) sore throat in the post-operative period, dental damage, or any new factor (facial trauma, cervical spine disease, major dental work) after the last anaesthesia.

3. **Observe the patient for features that may suggest difficulty in intubation/ventilation. Listen for any hoarseness or stridor.**

   Common features include morbid obesity, abnormal facial shape, facial or neck trauma, facial burns, an edentulous mouth with sunken cheeks, prominent upper incisors (reduce visualization and access because they elongate the anteroposterior axis of the mouth, as does a large mandible), narrow facial features and high arched palate (reduced space from side to side in the mouth and large anteroposterior dimension), short bull neck, receding mandible with poorly defined mandibular angles, large breasts, and thyroid goiter.

4. **Evaluate the "3-3-2" rule (three fingers into the mouth, three fingers under the chin, and two fingers at the top of the neck).**

    The first "3" in the rule refers to the ability to place three fingers in the patient's mouth. In other words, the mouth opening should be adequate to permit three fingers to be placed between the upper and lower teeth. The second "3" refers to the space from the mentum to the hyoid bone. Three fingers placed side by side should fit into this space. This indicates adequate mandibular dimension to permit access to the airway. The "2" in the rule requires that two fingers be placed between the thyroid notch and the floor of the mouth (i.e. the hyoid bone). This indicates that the larynx is sufficiently low within the neck to permit access by the oral route.

5. **Perform Mallampati classification, if possible.**

    Class III and IV views are associated with a higher failure rate of intubation.

6. **Assess the ability of the patient to subluxate the mandible.**

    The mandible should move forward by at least 5 mm so that the apical surface of the mandibular teeth rest anterior to the apical surface of the maxillary teeth. If the patient is not able to comprehend the instructions, the patient is asked to bite the upper lip. If the patient is edentulous, then palpation of the mandibular angles may indicate a good mobility when the jaw is protruded.

7. **Evaluate neck mobility.**

    Ask the patient (in the sitting position) to place the chin on the chest and look downwards and then bring the head and neck all the way up to look upwards towards the ceiling behind the head. Neck mobility is reduced in elderly patients and those with systemic arthritis. A trauma patient with suspected cervical spine injury presents a difficult airway because of neck immobilization.

8. **Look for any obstruction in the upper airway.**

    Obstruction may be due to laryngeal tumor, peritonsillar abscess, foreign body, direct airway trauma, and haematoma in the neck.

References

1. Chou HC, Wu TL. Mandibulohyoid distance in difficult laryngoscopy. Br J Anaesth 1993; 71(3): 335-339.
2. Chou HC, Wu TL. Thyromental distance-shouldn't we redefine its role in the prediction of difficult laryngoscopy? (letter). Acta Anaesthesiol Scand 1998; 42(1): 136-137.
3. Frerk CM, Till CB, Bradley AJ. Difficult intubation: thyromental distance and the atlanto-occipital gap. Anaesthesia 1996; 51(8): 738-740.
4. Knill RL. Difficult laryngoscopy made easy with a "BURP". Can J Anaesth 1993; 40(3): 279-282.
5. Mallampati S, Gatt S, Gugino LD, Desai SP, Waraksa B, Freiberger D, Liu PL. A clinical sign to predict difficult tracheal intubation: a prospective study. Can Anaesth Soc J 1985; 32(4): 429-434.
6. Practice guidelines for management of the difficult airway. A report by the American Society of Anesthesiologists Task Force on Management of the Difficult Airway. Anesthesiology 1993; 78(3): 597-602.
7. Randell T. Prediction of difficult intubation. Acta Anesthesiol Scand 1996; 40(8 Pt 2): 1016-1023.
8. Rose DK, Cohen MM. The airway: problems and predictions in 18,500 patients. Can J Anaesth 1994; 41(5 Pt1): 372-383.

9. Tse JC, Rimm EB, Hussain A. Predicting difficult endotracheal intubation in surgical patients scheduled for general anesthesia: a prospective blind study. Anesth Analg 1995; 81(2): 254-258.
10. Walls RM. Management of the difficult airway in the trauma patient. Emerg Med Clin North Am 1998; 16(1): 45-61.
11. Watson CB. Prediction of a difficult Intubation: methods for successful intubation Respir Care 1999; 44(7): 777-796.
12. Wilson ML, Spiegelhalter D, Robertson JA, Lesser P. Predicting difficult intubation. Br J Anaesth 1998; 61(2): 211-216.
13. Yentis SM. Predicting difficult intubation-worthwhile exercise or pointless ritual? Anesthesia 2002; 57:105-109.

Airway Management in Emergency Department/ Ward: Clinical Situations

28

Introduction

- Management of the airway in the ward or in the emergency department is challenging, as patients are generally sicker than those scheduled for elective surgery in the operation theatre. Moreover, timely help and proper equipment may not be as readily available in these situations.
- The approach to intubation in emergency generally depends on the condition of the patient: (a) *Agonal unresponsive patient:* If the patient is unresponsive and exhibits only agonal respiratory effort or cardiac activity, then immediate intubation is indicated. If the jaw is clenched, blind nasotracheal intubation or establishment of a surgical airway may be preferred. If the jaw is not clenched, then orotracheal intubation without medication may be attempted initially and if unsuccessful, should be followed by drug-assisted intubation. In either case, intubation attempt should always be preceeded by optimal oxygenation. (b) *Combative/uncooperative patient:* If the patient is combative or uncooperative, then drug-assisted intubation is indicated. Drug-assisted intubation may involve sedation/hypnosis only (± topical anaesthesia) or sedation/hypnosis and neuromuscular blockade. Blind nasal intubation is relatively contraindicated in a combative or uncooperative patient because of the increased risk of complications like epistaxis, glottic edema and upper airway obstruction. (c) *Cooperative passive patient:* If the patient is not combative and is cooperative, then he may tolerate intubation with minimal amounts of medication together with topicalization of the airway. If the jaw is not clenched, then either direct oral intubation without medication or drug-assisted intubation may be tried, depending on the patient's response to attempts at laryngoscopy. If attempts at oral intubation are unsuccessful because of excessive patient resistance, the patient should undergo drug-assisted intubation.
- Intubation without drugs or adequate airway anaesthesia may result in deleterious patient movements, trauma to the airway, and triggering of airway reflexes. In one prospective nonrandomized study of patients requiring emergency intubation, tracheal intubation without paralysis was associated with a greater number and severity of complications, compared to rapid sequence intubation (RSI). Complications in the nonparalyzed group included

aspiration (15%), airway trauma (28%), and death 3%. None of these complications were observed in the RSI group.

- Preoxygenation is mandatory in all cases before intubation. Preoxygenation is best accomplished with a non-rebreathing mask or with a bag-and-mask apparatus to administer as close to 100% oxygen as possible for 3 to 5 minutes (if there is time). Hyperventilation with eight deep breaths of 100% oxygen can also be used to provide maximal preoxygenation. *Remember, failure to oxygenate kills, not the failure to intubate.*

- Patients presenting in emergency may have a varying combination of the following conditions: Respiratory distress, pre-existing hypoxia, decreased functional residual capacity, haemoglobin concentration, alveolar ventilation and cardiac output (all combining to decrease the capacity for oxygen loading), full stomach, airway trauma, cervical spine instability, bronchospasm, increased intracranial pressure, and compromised cardiac status.

GUIDELINES FOR AIRWAY MANAGEMENT IN DIFFERENT CLINICAL SITUATIONS

1. **Multiple trauma patient.**
   Intubation should be atraumatic and gentle, and should be performed by an experienced person.

   - All blunt trauma patients should be considered to have (i) Unstable cervical spine (until proven otherwise), (ii) full stomach (trauma, pain, apprehension), (iii) unstable haemodynamics (volume depletion, tension pneumothorax, pericardial tamponade). Use benzodiazepines and barbiturates with caution. Ketamine may be preferred.

   - When the patient is apnoeic, has a major facial/nasal trauma, obvious basal skull fracture, or an evidence of increased intracranial pressure, oral rapid sequence intubation, with cervical spine immobilization performed by a second person, is the method of choice for airway management. In the absence of above conditions, awake blind naso-or oro-tracheal intubation under topical anaesthesia may be an appropriate initial choice.

   - In patients with chest injury (pneumothorax, haemothorax, flail chest, pulmonary contusion), preoxygenation may be less effective, and oxygen saturation may fall rapidly after paralysis. Patients with suspected pneumothorax should undergo a tube thoracostomy before rapid sequence intubation if the clinical status permits or else, it should be done immediately after intubation.

2. **Ventilatory failure due to pain and splinting.**

   In a patient with multiple rib fractures or following a thoracotomy, splinting due to pain may result in atelectasis and lead to respiratory failure. Intubation may not be required. Achieving adequate analgesia with an epidural block (thoracic) may result in effective coughing, deep breathing and reexpansion of the atelectatic areas. See Chapter 60.

3. **Head injury with increased intracranial pressure. See Chapter 65.**
   Avoid hypoxia, hypercarbia, hypotension, venous distension, and airway obstruction to minimize secondary brain injury. Preventive measures to minimize increase in intracranial pressure (ICP) during intubation include: (a) Maintain normal oxygen levels, (b) encourage hyperventilation, (c) avoid respiratory depressants, (d) avoid coughing, straining, or vomiting, (e) use prophylactic xylocaine (1-2 mg/kg IV), (f) choose an induction agent that reduces ICP, e.g. thiopental sodium, and (g) use maximal dose of neuromuscular blocking agents. A smooth induction with rapid sequence intubation using Sellick's manoeuvre is preferable to an awake technique.

4. **Respiratory failure due to airway compromise: Tumour, foreign body, trauma, epiglottitis, postoperative state (bleeding following thyroid surgery, carotid endarterectomy, soft tissue swelling following cervical discectomy, edema in massively transfused or burnt patients).**
   - Clinical signs of airway compromise may include change in the quality of the voice, stridor, falling oxygen saturation, chest retraction, etc.
   - In case of bleeding into a closed surgical wound, emergent opening of the wound and relieving pressure on the trachea can be life saving.
   - In massively burnt patients. early intubation avoids potential airway swelling which may occur within a few hours, secondary to release of inflammatory mediators and fluid resuscitation.
   - In other conditions, an awake technique (blind or fiberoptic assisted) under topical anaesthesia and judicious sedation (if at all required) is the preferred technique. When symptoms are modest, but elective intubation is indicated, a combined approach may be used in which an awake technique is used to ensure adequacy of laryngoscopy, then rapid sequence intubation is used for the actual intubation by gentle laryngoscopy.
   - When the patient is uncooperative or time is inadequate, a controlled surgical airway, transtracheal jet ventilation or cricothyroidotomy may be the appropriate choice.

5. **Cardiogenic shock, septic shock.**
   A patient in cardiogenic shock is very sick, has minimum or no cardiac reserve and has a prolonged circulation time (drug effects are delayed). Haemodynamic instability often occurs with intubation Therefore drugs like ketamine which depress cardiovascular performance, should be avoided. An atraumatic, smooth, controlled intubation with Sellicks' manoeuvre is preferred to an awake approach.
   Similar considerations apply in a patient with septic shock with a compromised cardiovascular system.

6. **Acute pulmonary edema.**
   Rapid sequence intubation with Sellick's manoeuvre may be a better choice as compared to awake intubation.
   - A patient with acute pulmonary edema presents certain unique challenges: (a) These patients have little or no functional residual capacity (FRC), so

preoxygenation with 100% oxygen may not be as effective as in patients with normal lungs, (b) Although the cardiovascular system tolerates procedures, medications, and ventilation better in the supine position, patients are often uncooperative and unable to lie flat, (c) high airway resistance and low pulmonary compliance may lead to ineffective bag-and-mask ventilation, (d) frothy secretions may obscure the airway, (e) intubation might precipitate bronchospasm, (f) these patients may be more sensitive to opioids and induction agents, and (g) intubation with its associated reflex responses may further decompensate the cardiovascular system.

- Be ready with vasopressors (e.g. dobutamine, dopamine), pretreatment with fentanyl in a hypertensive or normotensive patient may attenuate some of the stress response, use smaller, titrated doses of benzodiazepines, opioids, or thiopentone. A styletted endotracheal tube increases the chances of successful intubation in the first attempt. Laryngoscopy should be done by an experienced person, and should be smooth and brief. It is best to administer the drugs to the patient in the erect position and then to place him in the supine position for intubation and while fixing the ETT, the tube should be positioned well above the carina.

7. **The comatose patient.**

A comatose patient cannot protect his airway, and is therefore prone for aspiration. The patient might have aspirated prior to arrival and needs intubation to protect the airway. Blind nasal technique may lead to gagging, retching, vomiting and aspiration. Therefore, intubation by direct laryngoscopy technique is preferable.

8. **Bronchial asthma and chronic obstructive pulmonary disease (COPD) (See Chapter 61).**

- Important factors to be considered while managing the airway in a patient of bronchial asthma are: (a) These patients are usually very sick, fatigued, and have reduced functional residual capacity (FRC), and it is therefore very difficult to preoxygenate them optimally, (b) rapid administration of drugs, including ketamine or opioids may lead to loss of respiratory drive, rapid desaturation, and even apnoea, depending on the individual physical reserve, (c) due to transmitted pleural and abdominal pressures, these patients are haemodynamically unstable and exhibit wide swings in blood pressure, (d) most of these patients are volume depleted because of increased work of breathing and decreased oral intake, and (e) it is very difficult to diagnose esophageal intubation because of the difficulty in hearing breath sounds in a patient during a severe asthmatic attack. Considering all these factors, rigid direct laryngoscopic technique using a rapid sequence induction, in a totally paralyzed patient, with optimum intubating conditions, ensuring visualization of cords and successful passing of largest possible sized endotracheal tube (ETT) through vocal cords is preferred over awake intubation techniques which take longer, can exacerbate the hypoxaemia and are unpleasant in an already distressed and fatigued patient. Infuse 1-2 L of N-saline either before intubation or in the early post-intubation period. Ketamine is the ideal induction agent because it is a bronchodilator and also it provides haemodynamic stability. If the patient appears more comfortable sitting upright, drugs are given (pretreatment with xylocaine, ketamine, and succinylcholine) in this position. Once the patient loses consciousness, apply cricoid pressure, place the patient in the supine position, and perform laryngoscopy and oral intubation with a larger diameter ETT to reduce resistance and to facilitate aggressive pulmonary toilette.

- A COPD patient who presents in a moribund condition with ineffective, gasping or agonal respiration, stupor, lack of awareness of his surroundings, inability to respond intelligibly, cyanosis, or impending cardiorespiratory arrest (bradycardia, hypotension), does not need any drugs (sedatives or paralytics) prior to intubation. Ideally, the patient should receive preoxygenation and ventilation with bag-and-mask and 100% oxygen. Rapid orotracheal intubation with Sellicks' manaoeuvre must be done immediately under direct vision.

9. **Primary pulmonary parenchymal problems, i.e. aspiration pneumonitis, respiratory distress syndrome, and sepsis.**

    These patients typically have high minute ventilation and are ideally managed via blind nasal intubation technique under topical anesthesia. If it is unsuccessful, judicious sedation may be added.

References

1. Baraka AS, Taha SK, Aouad MT, El-Khatib MF, Kawkani NI. Preoxygenation: Comparison of maximal breathing and tidal volume breathing techniques. Anesthesiology 1999; 91:612-616.
2. Benumof JL, Dogg R, Benumof R. Critical haemoglobin desaturation will occur before return to an unparalyzed state after 1ml/Kg intravenous succinylcholine. Anesthesiology 1997; 87:979-982.
3. Benumol JL. Management of the difficult airway. Anesthesiology 1991; 75:1087
4. Corbridge TC, Hall JB. Techniques for ventilating patients with obstructive pulmonary disease J Crit Illness 1994; 9:1027-1032.
5. Kardon E. Acute asthma. Emerg Med Clin North Am 1996; 14:93-114.
6. LiJ, Murphy-Lavoie H, Bugas C, Martinez J, Preston C. Complications of emergency intubation with and without paralysis. Am J Emerg Med 1999; 17:141-144.
7. Shatney CH, Brunner RD, Nguyen TQ. The safety of orotracheal intubation in patients with unstable cervical spine fracture or high spinal cord injury. Am J Surg 1995; 170:676.
8. Trupka A, Waydhas C, NastKolb D, etal. Early intubation in severely injured patients. Eur J Emerg Med 1995; 1:1.
9. Walls RM. Airway management. Emerg Med Clin North Am 1993; 11:53-60.
10. Walls RM. Rapid sequence intubation in head trauma. Ann Emerg Med 1993; 22:1008-1013.
11. Walls RM. Airway management in the blunt trauma patient: how important is the cervical spine. Can J Surg 1992; 35:27.

Noninvasive Positive Pressure Ventilation

29

Introduction

- Noninvasive positive pressure ventilation (NIPPV) is defined as any form of ventilatory support applied without the use of an endotracheal airway. As with other forms of assisted ventilation, the ultimate purpose of NIPPV is to enhance alveolar ventilation.
- The goal of NIPPV depends upon the clinical condition for which it is used:
  - (a) During acute decompensation of chronic obstructive pulmonary disease (COPD) or asthma, the goal is to reduce CO_2 by unloading the respiratory muscles and augmenting alveolar ventilation, thereby stabilizing the arterial pH until the underlying problem can be reversed,
  - (b) During acute hypoxaemic respiratory failure, the goal is to ensure an adequate PaO_2 until the underlying problem can be reversed,
  - (c) When applied continuously to patients with chronic ventilatory failure, the goal of NIPPV is to provide sufficient oxygenation and/or CO_2 elimination to sustain life by reversing atelectasis and resting the respiratory muscles,
  - (d) When applied intermittently to patients with obesity hypoventilation syndrome (OHS), the goal is to limit sleep– and position– induced adverse changes in oxygenation and CO_2 elimination and their pathological sequlae by stenting the upper airway, increasing lung volume and augmenting alveolar ventilation, and
  - (e) In acute cardiogenic pulmonary edema (CPE), the goal of NIPPV is to improve oxygenation, reduce work of breathing and increase cardiac output.
- NIPPV has been shown to be effective in reducing the need for endotracheal intubation in several groups of patients with acute respiratory failure. Patients with acute-on-chronic respiratory failure are most likely to benefit from NIPPV in terms of morbidity and mortality. Selected patients with various forms of hypoxaemic respiratory failure may also benefit from NIPPV in terms of intubation rates, duration of hospitalization and complications. NIPPV has been found to be very effective in managing patients with chronic respiratory failure due to restrictive thoracic diseases who can protect their airways.
- One of the major pathophysiological mechanisms of nosocomial pneumonia in mechanically ventilated patients is the aspiration of colonized oropharyngeal secretions. NIPPV reduces the risk of nosocomial pneumonia by maintaining natural glottic barrier.
- Factors vital to the success of NIPPV include: careful selection of patients, properly timed intervention, a comfortable, well-fitting interface, coaching and reassurance of patients, careful monitoring, and a skilled and motivated team.

- Several randomized controlled trials show that use of NIPPV to achieve earlier extubation in difficult-to-wean patients with chronic airflow obstruction can result in reduced periods of endotracheal intubation, reduced complication rates, and improved survival.
- Various studies directly comparing volume-targeted and pressure-targeted ventilators have shown insignificant differences between the two. In general, pressure-limited ventilators are preferred because they are usually more portable, less expensive, have better leak compensating capabilities and lack elaborate alarms that can needlessly awaken patients at night during transient air leaking.

GUIDELINES FOR INITIATING NIPPV

1. **Select the patient.**

    In acute respiratory failure, patient selection may be seen as a two-step process. The first step involves identification of patients needing ventilatory assistance. The criteria include:
    (a) Clinical signs of acute respiratory distress such as moderate to severe dyspnoea, tachypnoea (RR >24/min), use of accessory muscles, and paradoxical abdominal breathing,
    (b) Blood gas abnormalities, e.g. $PaCO_2 > 45$ mm Hg, pH<7.35, or $PaO_2/FiO_2 < 200$.

    The second step involves excluding patients in whom NIPPV is relatively contraindicated. The criteria include:
    (a) Imminent respiratory arrest,
    (b) Haemodynamically unstable (hypotension unresponsive to fluids, ischaemia, arrhythmias) patients,
    (c) Inability to protect airway (impaired cough or swallowing mechanism),
    (d) Excessive secretions,
    (e) Agitated or uncooperative patient, and
    (f) Patients with facial trauma, burns, or surgery or those having anatomical abnormality interfering with mask fit.

2. **Explain the procedure to the patient. Emphasize the importance of his cooperation.**

    Reassure the patient. Very breathless patients may need to start NIPPV sitting up, but in most it is preferable if they are lying back in bed on pillows at an angle of about 45 degrees. This encourages relaxation, puts the diaphragm in an advantageous position (as compared to supine position), and allows the caregiver to assess whether accessory muscle activity has been abolished.

3. **Select the ventilator.**

    The usual critical care ventilator, commonly available in the ICU can be used; however, the main limitation is that it does not compensate for leaks, which are a universal phenomenon with NIPPV. The presently available portable pressure-targeted ventilators, also known as Bi-level ventilators are blower – driven, electrically powered ventilators. In general, these devices can be considered continuous flow ventilators in which flow delivery is based on the set inspiratory and expiratory pressure levels, and the patient demand. Most of these ventilators use a single circuit gas delivery system without a true exhalation valve. Based on current literature, it seems clear that these portable pressure-targeted ventilators compare well with standard ICU ventilators in meeting the ventilatory demands of the patients and function well in the presence of leaks.

4. **Select the interface (Fig. 29.1).**

    The commonly used interfaces are orofacial and nasal masks.

    (a) Facial vs Nasal.

    Orofacial (facial) masks are preferred in acutely distressed patients, in those having large oral leaks while using nasal masks and in patients having mouth breathing. Nasal masks are preferred in chronic respiratory failure and in those patients who feel claustrophobic with facial masks. Fitting a facemask on edentulous patients or on those with denture in place or on bearded patients can be difficult, and a nasal mask may be a better choice. The advantages of nasal masks include less dead space, less risk of aerophagia and aspiration, less claustrophobia, and more patient comfort. In addition, the patient is able to communicate, eat/drink and expectorate better with these masks.

    Presence of sinusitis or any deviation of the turbinates contributing to increased resistance may favour the choice of facial masks.

    (b) Size of the mask.

    Selecting a correct sized mask is critical to avoid large leaks. The facial mask should fit from just above the junction of the nasal bone and cartilage to just below the lower lip. The nasal mask should fit from just above the

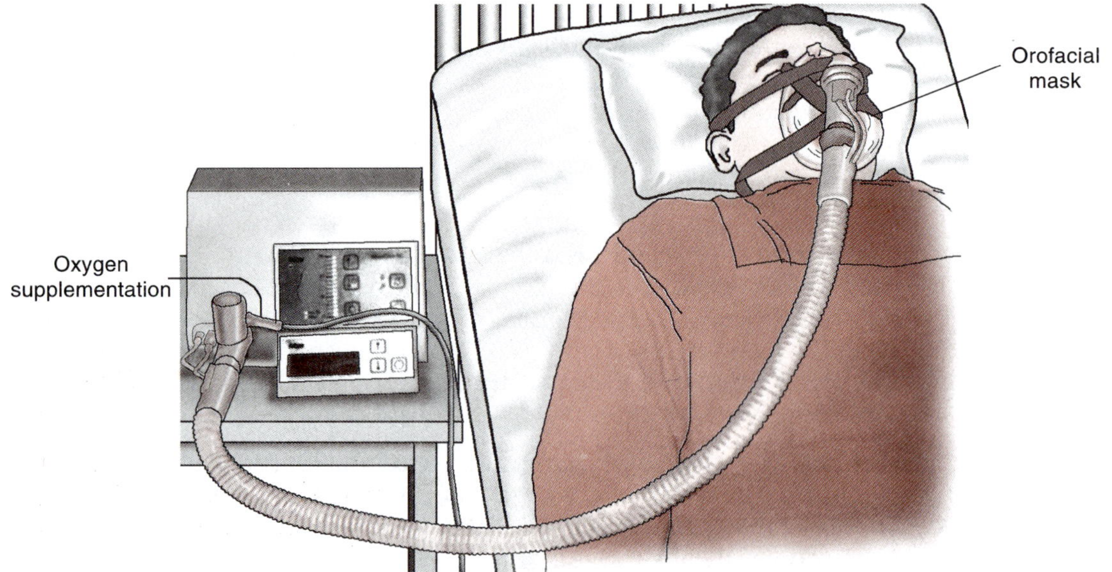

Fig. 29.1: Noninvasive ventilation with orofacial mask.

junction of the nasal bone and cartilage, directly at the sides of both nares, and just below the nose above the upper lip.

(c) Fitting of the mask.

Most masks designed specifically for NIPPV use cloth straps and Velcro to secure the mask. A common mistake is to fit the mask too tightly which decreases patient comfort and compliance and usually does not improve the fit. It should be possible to pass one or two fingers between the straps and the face.

5. **Set the ventilator.**

Common breath types during non-invasive ventilation are:

- Pressure support: patient-triggered, pressure-limited, flow-cycled.
- Pressure assist: patient-triggered, pressure-limited, time-cycled.
- Pressure control: machine-triggered, pressure-limited, time-cycled.
- Volume assist: patient-triggered, flow-limited, volume-cycled.
- Volume control: machine-triggered, flow-limited, volume-cycled.

Start in the spontaneously triggered mode (S/T mode) with a back-up rate. The back up rate is usually set at slightly below the spontaneous breathing rate. Pure control modes have rarely been used in acute respiratory failure, but if they are used, the breathing frequency of the ventilator must be set at higher than the patient's spontaneous breathing frequency to avoid patient's respiratory effort that are not supported by the ventilator. In chronic respiratory failure, timed modes alone may be used if the patient has an unreliable respiratory effort, unstable ventilatory drive or mechanics, apnoeas, or hypoapnoeas, massively overloaded respiratory muscles or when the assist mode fails to augment spontaneous breathing. However, S/T mode combines the advantage of the timed mode and allows augmentation of extra spontaneous efforts that may occur with irregular breathing pattern, which may be seen at the onset of sleep or during rapid eye movement (REM) sleep. The proportion of breaths, which are assisted, and those, which are controlled, will depend upon the backup rate that is set on the ventilator.

6. **Set the pressures.**

Start with low pressures: inspiratory 8-12 cm H_2O; expiratory 3-5 cm H_2O.

7. **Connect the interface to the ventilator tubing.**

8. **Apply the mask.**

To start with, whenever possible, the patient should be allowed to hold the mask in position over his face or nose for a few trial breaths. While this is usually associated with a very poor seal and a large leak around the mask, it allows the patient to get used to the sensation of facial/nasal pressure and increases the chances of success of NIPPV. Once the patient has gained confidence, the mask can be applied over the face and the straps tightened. Avoid excessive strap tension. One should be able to insert one or two fingers between the straps and the face.

9. **Encourage the patient to guide his own therapy.**

The patient can be encouraged to help determine the respiratory rate, length of inspiration, and size of the breath by asking him whether the breaths are of the right length, whether they are deep enough, and coming quickly enough. The patient should be shown how to disconnect the ventilator tubing from the mask himself because this helps promote the feeling that he, rather than the machine, is in control.

10. Increase support as appropriate.

Increase the inspiratory support in steps of 2-3 cm H_2O pressure, according to the patient's tolerance, to obtain an expired tidal volume of 8-10 mL/kg and to meet the goals. The goals of therapy are patient comfort, alleviation of dyspnoea, a respiratory rate less than 25 breaths/min, disappearance of accessory muscle activity (as evaluated by palpation of sternocleidomastoid activity) and good patient-ventilator synchrony. Increase EPAP (expiratory positive airway pressure) in steps to 10 cm H_2O to meet the saturation goal. Supplement oxygen to achieve the desired oxygenation goal. Oxygen may be supplemented either in the circuit beyond the ventilator using a T-piece connection or in the mask. FiO_2 can be calculated by using the following conversion factor: (21% + 3% × oxygen flow in L/min of supplemental oxygen). This conversion factor provides an approximation of the percentage of oxygen delivered. It is influenced by the minute ventilation and the breathing pattern, and may be inaccurate when air leakage occurs around or through the mask.

11. Monitor the patient closely, initially for at least 2-3 hours.

Monitoring should include assessment of patient comfort, level of dyspnoea, respiratory rate, heart rate, blood pressure, oxygen saturation, use of accessory muscles, respiratory paradox, patient-ventilator synchrony, mask leak, discomfort over nose or eyes, and arterial blood gases (30-60 minutes after initiating therapy).

12. Make frequent checks and adjustments to improve patient compliance, as needed.

Reassure the patient, look for mask leaks/strap tension, consider changing the mask (nasal versus facial), check for adequacy of inspiratory and expiratory pressure levels, and consider mild sedation (i.e. midazolam, lorazepam) in a very agitated patient. For short term (< 1-2 days) application, humidification is usually not necessary, unless there is an excessive air leak because normal humidification of the upper airway is left intact. In-line nebulizer therapy may be provided with the nebulizer placed preferably near the mask rather than at the outlet of the ventilator.

13. Avoid enteral feeding for the first 24 hours or so, and monitor for signs of gastric distension.

Gastric insufflation is rarely intolerable. This may be because the lower esophageal sphincter pressure is estimated to be 33 cm H_2O which is well above the peak insufflation pressure commonly used for NIPPV.

14. Consider intubation in those patients who are not responding favourably after initial few hours of therapy.

Criteria indicating failure of NIPPV include: haemodynamic instability, decreased mental status, respiratory rate more than 35/minute, worsening respiratory acidosis, inability to maintain $SpO_2 > 90\%$, inability to tolerate the mask and to manage secretions. NIV failures in upto 40% cases have been reported in a heterogeneous group of patients with acute respiratory failure. Furthermore, successful use of NIPPV in the initial one or two hours has been shown to be a predictor of better outcome.

15. Wean the patient when the condition improves.

Monitor the patient closely for signs of fatigue in the initial two to three hours. Decrease the FiO_2 and inspiratory and expiratory pressures in steps. Therapy may be discontinued when the patient's oxygenation has improved (so that an oxygen saturation of more than 90% is maintained on $\leq$ 2L/min of oxygen) and when the patient's breathing frequency has decreased to < 24 breaths/min. Oxygen supplementation using nasal cannula (to maintain $SpO_2 > 90\%$) should be continued after removing the mask.

16. While monitoring continues, resume NIPPV therapy if indicated.

Resume NIPPV therapy, if the breathing frequency is more than 30 breaths/minute, $SpO_2 < 90\%$ with nasal oxygen of $\leq$ 4L/min, $PaCO_2$ increases by more than 4 mm Hg, dyspnoea worsens, use of accessory muscles increases, or if the patient requests to resume therapy.

References

1. Antonelli M, Conti G, Bufi M, et al. Noninvasive ventilation for treatment of acute respiratory failure in patients undergoing solid organ transplataion. JAMA 2000; 283:235-241.
2. Antonelli M, Conti G, Moro ML, et al. Predictors of failure of noninvasive positive pressure ventilation in patients with acute hypoxemic respiratory failure: a multi-center study. Intensive Care Med 2001; 27:1718-1728.
3. Antonelli M, Conti G, Rocco M, et al. A comparison of non-invasive positive-pressure ventilation and conventional ventilation in patients with acute respiratory failure. N Engl J Med 1998; 339:429-435.
4. Bach JR, Brougher P, et al. Consensus statement: noninvasive positive pressure ventilation. Respiratory Care 1997; 42(4): 365-369.
5. Black JW, Grover BS. A hazard of pressure support ventilation. Chest 1993; 93:333-335.
6. Brochard L. Noninvasive ventilation for acute respiratory failure. JAMA 2002; 288:932-935.
7. Brochard L. Non-invasive ventilation for acute exacerbations of COPD: a new standard of care. Thorax 2000; 55:817-818.
8. Brochard L, Moncebo J, Wysocki M, et al. Noninvasive ventilation for acute exacerbations of chronic obstructive pulmonary disease. N Engl J Med 1995; 333:817-822.
9. Calderini E, Confalonieri M, Puccio PG, et al. Patient-ventilator asynchrony during noninvasive ventilation: the role of expiratory trigger. Intensive Care Med 1999; 25:662-667.
10. Carlucci A, Richard JC, Wysocki M, et al. Noninvasive versus conventional mechanical ventilation. Am J Respir Crit Care Med 2001; 163:874-880.
11. Elliott MW. Non-invasive ventilation in acute exacerbations of chronic obstructive pulmonary disease: a new gold standard? Intensive Care Med 2002; 28:1691-1694.
12. Evans TW. International consensus conferences in Intensive Care Medicine: Non-invasive positive pressure ventilation in acute respiratory failure. Intensive Care Med 2001; 27:166-178.
13. Ferrer M, Bernadich O, Nava S, Torres A. Noninvasive Ventilation after intubation and mechanical ventilation. Eur Respir J 2002; 19:959-965.

14. Hess D. Noninvasive positive pressure ventilation: predictors of success and failure for adult acute care applications. Respiratory Care 1997; 42(4): 424-431.

15. Hilbert G, Gruson D, Vargas F, et al. Noninvasive ventilation in immunosuppressed patients with pulmonary infiltrates, fever, and acute respiratory failure. N Engl J Med 2001; 344:481-487.

16. Hill NS. Complications of noninvasive positive pressure ventilation. Respiratory Care 1997; 42(4): 432-442.

17. Hill NS, Liesching T, Kwok H. Indications for non-invasive ventilation. In: Slutsky AS, Brochard L, (eds). Mechanical Ventilation. Berlin. Springer.

18. Kacmarek RM. NIPPV: patient-ventilator synchrony, the difference between success and failure? Intensive Care Med 1999; 25:645-647.

19. Kacmared RM. Characteristics of pressure-targeted ventilators used for noninvasive positive pressure ventilation. Respiratory Care 1997; 42(4): 380-388.

20. Keenan SP, Kernerman PD, Cook DJ, et al. Effect of noninvasive positive pressure ventilation on mortality in patients admitted with acute respiratory failure: A meta-analysis. Crit Care Med 1997; 25:1685-1692.

21. Keenan SP, Powers C, McCormack DG. Noninvasive positive-pressure ventilation for postextubation respiratory distress. JAMA 2002; 287:3238-3244.

22. Kramer N, Meyer TJ, Mecharg J, Cece RD, Hill NS. Randomized, prospective trial of noninvasive positive pressure ventilation in acute respiratory failure. Am J Respir Crit Care Med 1995; 151:1799-1806.

23. Lightowler JVJ, Elliott MW. Predicting the outcome from NIV for acute exacerbations of COPD. Thorax 2000; 55:815-816.

24. Martin TJ, Hovis JD, Costantino JP, et al. A randomized, prospective evaluation of noninvasive ventilation for acute respiratory failure. Am J Respir Crit Care Med 2000; 161:807-813.

25. Meduri GV, Cook TR Turner RE, et al. Noninvasive positive pressure ventilation in status arthmaticus. Chest 1996; 110:767-774.

26. Mehta S, Jay GD, Woolard RH, et al. Randomized, prospective trial of bilevel versus continuous positive airway pressure in acute pulmonary edema. Crit Care Med 1997; 25:620-628.

27. Moretti M, Cilione C, Tampieri A, et al. Incidence and causes of non-invasive mechanical ventilation failure after initial success. Thorax 2000; 55:819-825.

28. Nava S, Ambrosino N, Clini E, et al. Noninvasive mechanical ventilation in the weaning of patients with respiratory failure due to chronic obstructive pulmonary disease. Ann Intern Med 1998; 128:721-728.

29. Nava S, Carlucci A. Non-invasive pressure support ventilation in acute hypoxemic respiratory failure: common strategy for different pathologies? Intensive Care Med 2002; 28:1205-1207.

30. Nava S, Karakurt S, Rampulla C, et al. Salbutamol delivery during non-invasive mechanical ventilation in patients with chronic obstructive pulmonary disease: a randomized, controlled study. Intensive Care Med 2001; 27:1627-1635.

31. Nourdine K, Combes P, Carton MJ, et al. Does non-invasive ventilation reduce the ICU nosocomial infection risk? A prospective clinical survey. Intensive Care Med 1999; 25:567-573.

32. Pang D, Keenan SP, Cook DJ, et al. The effect of positive pressure airway support on mortality and the need for intubation in cardiogenic pulmonary edema. Chest 1998; 114:1185-1192.

33. Peter JV, Moran JL, Phillip-Hughes J, Warn D. Noninvasive ventilation in acute respiratory failure- A meta-analysis update. Crit Care Med 2002; 30:555-562.

34. Plant PK, Owen JL, Elliott MW. Early use of non-invasive ventilation for acute exacerbations of chronic obstructive pulmonary disease in general respiratory wards: a multicenter randomized controlled trial. Lancet 2000; 355:1931-1935.

35. Rossi A. Noninvasive ventilation has not been shown to be ineffective in stable COPD. Am J Respir Crit Care Med 2000; 161:688-689.

36. Teague WG. Pediatric application of noninvasive ventilation. Respiratory Care 1997; 42(4): 414-423.

GUIDELINES FOR CLINICAL ASSESSMENT OF THE PATIENT BEFORE INITIATION OF MECHANICAL VENTILATION

1. **Clinical parameters.**
    While the patient is being examined, oxygenate the patient with a mask.
    Clinical parameters which should be assessed include: (a) Level of consciousness and the patient's ability to cooperate, (b) use of accessory muscles of respiration, (c) restlessness, anxiety, diaphoresis, posture preferred by the patient, (d) respiratory pattern, (e) presence of cyanosis, (f) altered chest wall movements. Monitor pulse rate, rhythm disturbances if any, blood pressure, and oxygen saturation. Assess for effectiveness of cough reflex and phonation. Examine the chest.

2. **Measure the frequency, tidal volume and minute ventilation (Fig. 30.1).**
    (a) Wash hands and wear gloves, (b) make the patient sit in as upright a posture as is comfortable, (c) remove the oxygen mask and connect the respirometer to the patient through a facemask or a 15 mm adaptor, if already intubated, (d) instruct the patient to breathe normally, (e) measure the exhaled volume while counting the respiratory rate for 1 minute, (f) reoxygenate the patient (apply the oxygen mask), and (g) calculate minute ventilation.

3. **Measure vital capacity.**
    (a) Wash hands and wear gloves, (b) make the patient sit in as upright a posture as is comfortable, (c) remove the oxygen mask and connect the patient to the respirometer through a facemask or a 15 mm adaptor, if already intubated, (d) instruct the patient to inhale as deeply as possible and then slowly exhale as completely as possible, (e) note the volume of air

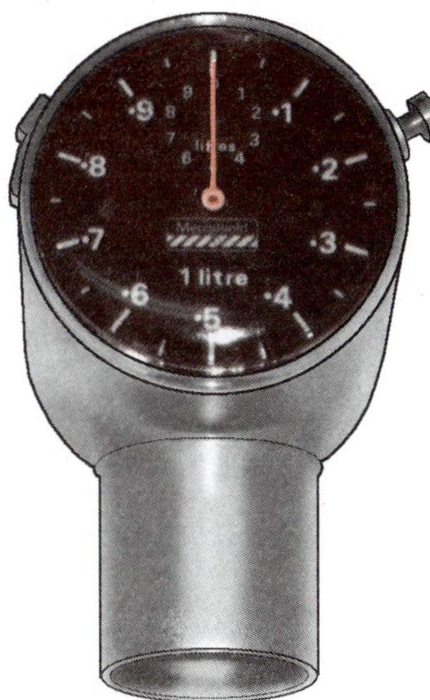

Fig. 30.1: The Wright respirometer.

exhaled, (f) repeat the measurement three times. If necessary, oxygenate the patient between each measurement. Apply the oxygen mask after the final reading, and (h) calculate the average of the three readings.

4. Obtain maximal static inspiratory pressure (PImax).
   See Chapter 43.

5. Obtain peak expiratory flow rate (PEFR) (Fig. 30.2).
   Normal PEFR: 450-700 L/min for men and 300-500 L/min for women.
   Lower values indicate higher than normal resistance to gas flow within the conducting airways, e.g. asthma, COPD, bronchospasm.
   (a) Wash hands and wear gloves, (b) make the patient sit in as upright a posture as is comfortable, (c) remove the oxygen mask and connect the peak expiratory flow meter, (d) instruct the patient to inhale as deeply as possible and then exhale as hard and as fast as possible into the peak flowmeter, (e) note the peak flow, (f) repeat the measurement three times. If necessary, oxygenate the patient between each measurement, (g) calculate the average of three readings, and (h) apply oxygen mask.

6. Reposition the patient.

7. Reposition the oxygen mask. Titrate FiO_2.
8. Remove gloves/wash hands.
   This reduces the risk of transmission of micro-organisms.

9. Record the information.
   Useful for future management of the patient.

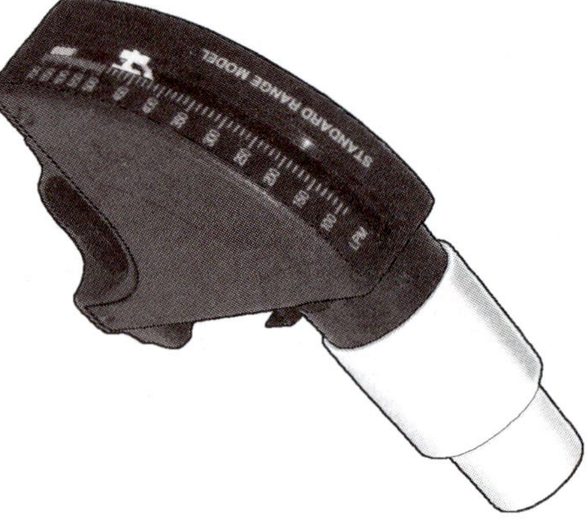

Fig. 30.2: Peak expiratory flow meter.

References

1. Consensus Conference on the Essentials of Mechanical Ventilation. Respir Care 1992; 37:999-1130.
2. Gibson GJ, Pride NB, Davis JN, et al. Pulmonary mechanics in patients with respiratory muscle weakness. Am Rev Respir Dis 1977; 115:389-395.
3. Kacmarek RM, Venegas J. Mechanical ventilatory rates and tidal volumes. Respir Care 1987; 32:466-478.
4. O'Donohue WJ Jr, Baker JP, Bell GM, et al. Respiratory failure in neuromuscular disease. Management in a respiratory intensive care unit. JAMA 1976; 235:733.
5. Pierson DJ. Persistent bronchopleural air leak during mechanical ventilation. Respir Care 1982; 27:408.
6. Powner DJ, Cline CD, Rodman GHJr. Effect of chest tube suction on gas flow through a bronchopleural fistula. Crit Care Med 1995; 13:99-101.
7. Slutsky AS. ACCP consensus conference on Mechanical Ventilation. Chest. 1993; 104:1833-1859.
8. Tobin MJ. Respiratory muscles in disease. Clin Chest Med 1988; 9:263-286.

Initiation of Mechanical Ventilation: Basic Rules   31

Introduction

- Few basic rules may be of help and should be applied before initiating and managing mechanical ventilation.

GUIDELINES FOR INITIATING MECHANICAL VENTILATION: BASIC RULES

1. Wash hands.
   This reduces the risk of transmission of micro-organisms.

2. Assess the patient clinically and decide about the need for respiratory support.
   Examine the patient's condition clinically and monitor the easily accessible parameters, e.g. frequency of breathing, tidal volume, minute volume, vital capacity, maximum inspiratory pressure, peak expiratory flow rate, oxygen saturation, CVP (if CVP catheter is already in place), and ABG (if immediately available). The main indication for ventilatory support is overt or impending respiratory failure. Conditions that can lead to respiratory failure include refractory hypoxaemia, acute hypercapnia, or a combination of both. The clinical symptoms of impending respiratory failure are: tachypnoea (respiratory rate more than 35/min, an important symptom), dyspnoea, paradoxical breathing, agitation, confusion, tachycardia, hypertension, and cyanosis. A PaO_2 of less than 50 mmHg in room air during spontaneous breathing or less than 60 mmHg with an SpO_2 of less than 90% on $FiO_2 \geq 0.5$ and a respiratory rate of more than 35/min are cardinal features of acute respiratory failure.

3. Decide about the degree of respiratory support the patient needs. It may vary from enriching oxygen delivery by facemask, partial ventilatory support, to complete ventilatory support. Nature of mechanical support, i.e. non-invasive versus invasive (i.e. via endotracheal tube) is also a consideration at this stage.
   (a) There is no recommended best overall mode for all types of respiratory failure.
   (b) There is no conclusive evidence to support the superiority of one single ventilatory mode.
   (c) Familiarity and experience with a particular mode is important before selecting the mode.
   Once it has been decided to initiate mechanical ventilation, it is important to know the amount of the work of breathing which will be shared by the ventilator. For example, in respiratory arrest, the ventilator needs to take over the entire

work of breathing. Patients with inadequate ventilatory drive, neuromuscular blockade, heavy sedation, or those in whom ventilatory work places an unacceptable load on the respiratory muscles or heart and those who are already fatigued because of excessive use of respiratory muscles, require a total or near total support of ventilation in the form of assist-control mode or SIMV plus PSV mode with pressure support titrated to an optimum tidal volume (8-10 mL/kg) and a total respiratory rate of less than 25 breaths per minute. Controlling the work of breathing gives the fatigued respiratory muscles time to recover and also reduces the oxygen cost of breathing. When a patient has spontaneous ventilatory activity, and a less severe form of respiratory failure, a partial ventilatory support is indicated. Partial ventilatory support modes allow the patient to perform whatever part of their work of breathing they are capable, with the ventilator performing the remainder of the work. For this, select SIMV plus PSV with the pressure support titrated to achieve an optimal tidal volume (6-8 mL/kg) and a total respiratory rate of less than 30 breaths/min, or PSV alone with the pressure support level optimally titrated to the patient's needs. It is important to remember that PSV should not be used alone in patients with a depressed respiratory drive, as it only augments the existing spontaneous breathing efforts. If there is any doubt, add minimal number of mechanical breaths per minute as a back up rate or use apnoea ventilation parameters. Patients with early cardiogenic pulmonary edema, acute intravascular volume overload, acute those with COPD, hypoxaemia and increased elastic work of breathing associated with flail chest or pulmonary contusion, may benefit from CPAP alone.

4. **Define the ventilatory strategy.**

   The ventilatory strategy is determined by the fact, whether the primary disorder is failure to ventilate (high $PaCO_2$) or failure to oxygenate (low PaO_2). The first problem is best managed by increasing the patient's minute volume to achieve the target $pH/PaCO_2$. Work of breathing should be minimized by keeping mechanical breaths between 10-12 breaths per minute and by optimizing the minute ventilation. The approach to the second problem lies in applying the least PEEP, necessary to recruit collapsed lung units and to achieve a target oxygenation with minimum possible FiO_2.

5. **Keeping in mind the pathophysiology of the disease, and the present condition of the patient, define the goals of ventilation and set the initial ventilatory settings.**
   - Adult respiratory distress syndrome: adopt lung protective strategy, see Chapter 59.
   - Head injury: See Chapter 65.
   - Obstructive airway disease: See Chapters 61 and 62.
   - Neuromuscular disease: These patients usually have healthy lungs and a normal ventilatory drive,. They are at less risk of barotrauma, and need adequate lung inflation and aggressive airway management. Patients are usually more comfortable when ventilated with high flow rates. Whether full or partial ventilatory support is required will depend on the patient's inherent capabilities and the disease process. For example, a patient with C1-C2 lesion (quadriplegia) needs full support.

Initial settings may be: TV 12-15 mL/kg, as the long as airway pressures are low; inspiratory flow rate $\geq$ 60 L/min, constant or descending ramp waveform, and a PEEP of 5–10 cm H_2O, to maintain the FRC.

- Bronchopleural fistula: Ventilatory support should provide adequate inflation of the uninvolved areas of the lung and assure an adequate gas exchange. To facilitate closure of the fistula, use a ventilatory mode and settings that minimize peak and plateau airway pressures necessary to maintain adequate ventilation, use the lowest tidal volume that allows adequate ventilation, consider permissive hypercapnia to minimize inspiratory pressures and volumes, and minimize PEEP. Consider independent lung ventilation or high frequency jet ventilation where large air leaks lead to inadequate lung inflation or failure to adequately oxygenate/ventilate. No single ventilatory mode or approach has been shown to be more effective than the other in treating patients with bronchopleural fistula.

6. Set the ventilator (Fig. 31.1).

Before attaching the ventilator to the patient, attach the ventilator to a test lung, and set various parameters on the ventilator, which are best for

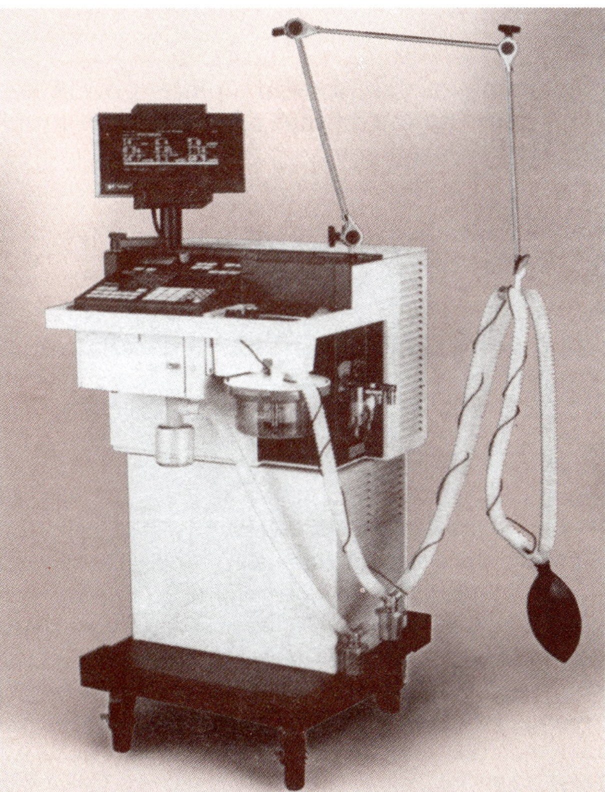

Fig. 31.1: Ventilator with test lung. Parameters already set.

the particular patient at that time. Check the ventilator's performance on the test lung. Reading the manufacturer's operating manual is often helpful before working with any ventilator.

7. **Monitor the ventilator-patient system.**

    Monitoring should initially be continuous and later on, should be caried out at regular intervals.

8. **Be ready to change the settings.**

    Initial ventilatory settings may not be the best for the patient and may require a change depending on the patient's response to ventilation. The response may be apparent within a few minutes.

9. **Never leave the system unattended.**
10. **Give due respect to various alarms.**

    Try to find out the cause for each alarm and manage accordingly (see Chapter 38).

11. **Detect patient/ventilator asynchrony (if any) at an early stage and manage.**
12. **Anticipate your response to problems.**

    Know your next move. When you monitor the patient, ask yourself, "What if...................?"

13. **Anticipate any ventilatory/haemodynamic problem.**

    Haemodynamic problems can arise in a patient because of ventilator-patient interaction (depending on the disease process). Take prophylactic measures, if possible, to avoid such problems.

14. **Keep on monitoring.**

    As the condition of the patient deteriorates or improves, settings will accordingly need to be changed at regular intervals.

15. **Add sedation/neuromuscular paralysis.**

    Make the patient comfortable. Add titrated sedation. Use neuromuscular blocking agents whenever indicated.

References

1. Consensus Conference on the Essentials of Mechanical Ventilation. Respir Care 1992; 37:999-1130.
2. Gibson GJ, Pride NB, Davis JN, et al. Pulmonary mechanics in patients with respiratory muscle weakness. Am Rev Respir Dis 1977; 115:389-95.
3. Kacmarek RM, Venegas J. Mechanical ventilatory rates and tidal volumes. Respir Care 1987; 32:466-478.
4. O'Donohue WJ Jr, Baker JP, Bell GM, et al. Respiratory failure in neuromuscular disease. Management in a respiratory intensive care unit. JAMA 1976; 235:733.
5. Pierson DJ. Persistent bronchopleural air leak during mechanical ventilation. Respir Care, 1982; 27:408.
6. Powner DJ, Cline CD, Rodman GHJr. Effect of chest tube suction on gas flow through a bronchopleural fistula. Crit Care Med 1995; 13:99-101.
7. Slutsky AS. ACCP consensus conference on Mechanical Ventilation Chest 1993; 104:1833-59.
8. Tobin MJ. Respiratory muscles in disease. Clin Chest Med 1988; 9:263-86.

Initiation of Mechanical Ventilation: Setting the Ventilator

32

1. FiO$_2$.

    FiO$_2$ should be set at the minimum level, which maintains haemoglobin saturation at or above 90%. Higher levels of FiO$_2$ are associated with absorption atelectasis and production of free radicals. The risk of oxygen-radicals mediated injury is more in patients on bleomycin or amiodarone. In clinical practice, some guidelines can be made based on the pathophysiology of the disease. (a) Diseases primarily associated with hypoventilation or ventilation/perfusion mismatch respond well to a small increase in FiO$_2$. This includes uncomplicated poisonings, neuromuscular disorders, asthma and chronic bronchitis. High concentrations of oxygen should be avoided in patients with chronic bronchitis, as it may increase dead-space ventilation and result in an increase in PaCO$_2$. Initial FiO$_2$ may be set between 0.24-0.30 to maintain a PaO$_2$ of 55-65 mmHg, and excessive hypercapnia. should be avoided (b) Diseases like pulmonary edema, pneumonia, and atelectasis, where hypoxaemia is primarily because of shunting, require a higher FiO$_2$ as well as recruitment manoeuvres like increased level of PEEP or inverse ratio ventilation to reduce the shunt fraction and maintain oxygenation. It is a common practice to initiate ventilatory support with an FiO$_2$ of 1.0 and to ignore the potential for oxygen toxicity during the first few hours of ventilatory management, and then to titrate the FiO$_2$ to achieve the desired SpO$_2$/PaO$_2$.

2. Inspiratory flow rate.

    - The inspiratory flow rate determines the rate at which the tidal volume is delivered. As an approximation, during volume-cycled ventilation, with constant flow pattern, peak inspiratory flow rate should be at least four times the minute ventilation (e.g. a flow setting of 60 L/min is appropriate for a patient with a minute ventilation of 15 L/min).
    - The flow rate should be increased in patients with respiratory distress (should be set above the patient's peak flow demands, particularly if the minute ventilation requirements are high), in those with airflow obstruction

(to decrease the inspiratory time and prolong the expiratory time, thus reducing the degree of auto-PEEP and dynamic hyperinflation), and in patients where decelerating flow pattern is being used. For a given tidal volume and inspiratory time, the peak flow rate should be approximately 20-25% higher in the decelerating mode than in the constant flow mode. In other words, on changing the flow pattern from constant to decelerating if the peak inspiratory flow is not increased, then for the same tidal volume, the inspiratory time will be longer, thus altering the I:E ratio. Very high peak inspiratory flows cause rapid volume changes, and may increase the shear forces, thereby risking further airway and parenchymal damage. Pressure control and pressure support ventilation can deliver high initial flow rates (flow delivered in decelerating fashion), which may be advantageous in patients with high initial flow demands.

3. **Tidal volume.**

Minute ventilation requirements vary with the metabolic demands and with the proportion of wasted ventilation. An average tidal volume of 8-10 mL/kg has been seen to satisfy minute ventilation requirements and arrest microatelectasis, which leads to a decrease in lung compliance and an increase in intrapulmonary shunting. This is common in any intubated patient in the supine position whether breathing spontaneously or being ventilated mechanically. Lower tidal volumes may be selected in the presence of severe airway obstruction, and in lung injury when limiting plateau pressure between 30 and 35 cm H_2O is more important (even if one has to accept a high $PaCO_2$), in those with only one lung and in hypovolaemic patients. Once the tidal volume has been so selected, the respiratory rate can be adjusted to achieve the desired minute ventilation. Respiratory rate may have to be increased when using small tidal volumes, or in patients with increased dead space or increased carbon dioxide levels (e.g. during laparoscopic surgery). Respiratory rate may have to be decreased in patients with airway obstruction, to give more time for expiration, along with other measures, to decrease the inspiratory time.

4. **I:E ratio.**

Conventionally, ventilatory techniques employ an I:E ratio of < 1:2. The inspiratory time should be kept at 1 to 1.5 seconds or an unacceptably high peak airway pressure may result. Increasing the I:E ratio will increase the mean airway pressure, which may cause air trapping and generate an auto-PEEP.

5. **Inspiratory pause (Fig. 32.1).**

- Inspiratory pause or plateau refers to the option of maintaining the lung volume at end-inspiration for the time set by the operator, by occluding the expiratory port (thus preventing exhalation). It is also referred to as the end-inflation hold time. An inspiratory pause shortens the expiratory phase of the respiratory cycle, thus increasing the I:E ratio.
- The addition of inspiratory pause helps in estimation of the plateau pressure and static compliance, favours the recruitment of previously collapsed or

flooded alveoli, and offers a means of shortening expiration and extending the inspiratory time, and implementing inverse-ratio ventilation in a sedated/paralysed patient during volume-cycled ventilation.

- However, one should remember that though a longer inspiratory pause time results in alveolar recruitment, it may damage relatively normal lung units by keeping them expanded at high volumes and pressures.

6. **Inspiratory waveform.**

   Four types of inspiratory waveforms are available with volume-targeted ventilation:

   (a) *Square waveform* (Fig. 32.2a): Patients who are breathing spontaneously (e.g. assist-control mode or synchronized intermittent mandatory ventilation) are more comfortable when this waveform is used.

   (b) *Sinusoidal waveform:* For all practical purposes, it is very similar to the square waveform.

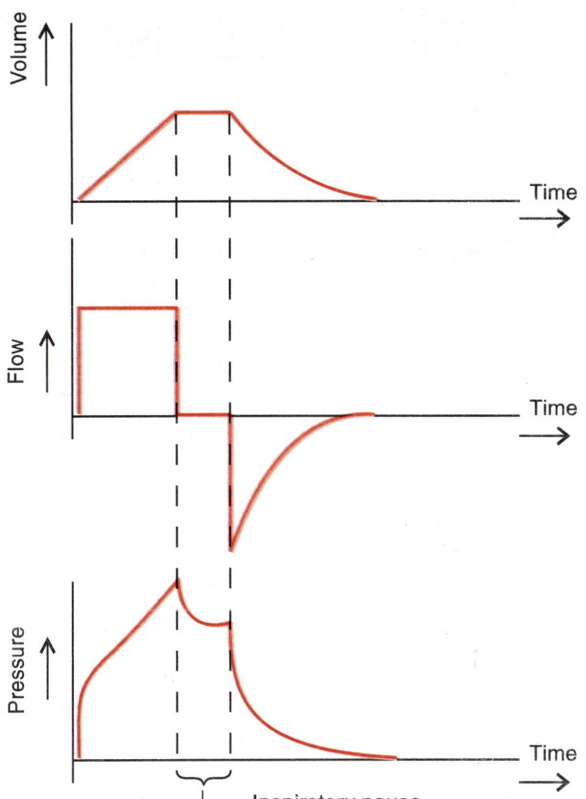

Fig. 32.1: Volume-time, Flow-time and Pressure-time diagrams of volume-oriented ventilation showing inspiratory pause. At the beginning of the pause time, the flow rapidly returns to zero. Lungs are held in inflation after the inspiratory flow has ended. As a result of zero inspiratory flow, there is a drop in the pressure (see pressure-time curve) which is equivalent to the rise in pressure caused by the resistance at the beginning of inspiration.

   (c) *Ascending waveform:* There is no evidence to support the use of this waveform.

   (d) *Decelerating waveform* (Fig. 32.2b): The decelerating waveform is associated with a lower peak airway pressure, higher mean airway pressure and improved gas distribution, resulting in a decrease in the pulmonary shunt and dead space. Therefore, it can be used to improve oxygenation by alveolar recruitment.

   The waveform of inspiratory flow in pressure-targeted modes of ventilation also follows an exponential decelerating pattern. This may help to recruit alveoli with long-time constants, particularly if the inspiratory time is prolonged.

   In patients with normal lungs, diffrent flow waveforms have no significant effect on gas exchange.

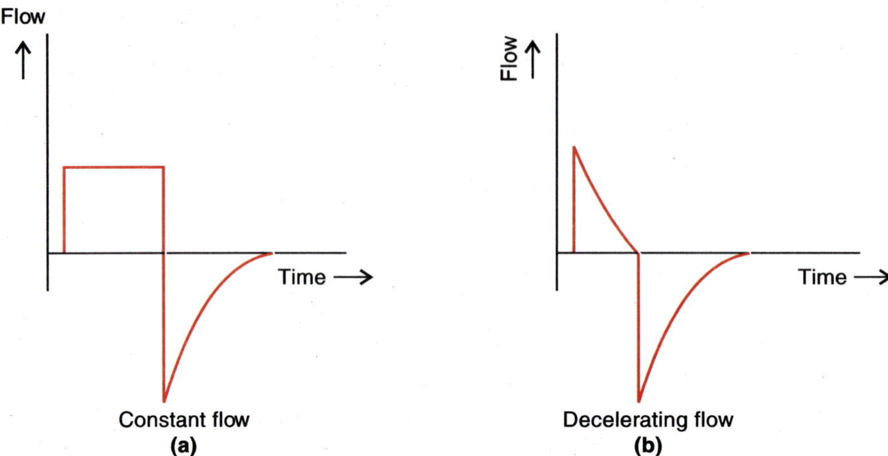

Fig. 32.2 a, b: **(a)** In constant flow, the volume flow rate during inspiration remains constant throughout the flow phase. In other words, volume delivery into the lungs at the beginning of inspiration is the same as that at the end of inspiration. When inspiration starts, the flow rises very quickly to the value set on the ventilator and then remains constant until the set tidal volume has been delivered.
(b) In decelerating flow, the flow is greatest at the beginning of inspiration and decreases with increasing filling of the lungs. The flow decreases to zero at end-inspiration.

For the same tidal volumes and peak inspiratory flow rates, inspiratory time is longer with the decelerating and sinusoidal waveforms, thereby reducing the time for expiration (Fig. 32.3). Therefore, in patients who are obstructed (status asthmaticus), a square waveform is preferred as this increases the peak inspiratory pressure but does not affect alveolar pressure.

7. Respiratory rate.

    Setting of mandatory ventilator gas delivery rate is dependent on the mode of ventilation selected the target $PaCO_2$ level, metabolic rate, the delivered tidal volume, dead space to tidal volume ratio, and the level of spontaneous ventilation.

    (a) *Target $PaCO_2$:* A reduction in respiratory rate with a constant tidal volume, physiological dead space, and CO_2 production leads to a rise in $PaCO_2$ and vice versa. Usually, one aims for a normal $PaCO_2$, except, for example, in a patient with acute COPD where one should aim to maintain the $PaCO_2$ at a level prior to the acute deterioration and in case of acute lung injury, where permissive hypercapnia is being practiced.

    (b) *Metabolic rate:* An increased metabolic rate (e.g. pyrexia) leads to increased oxygen consumption and CO_2 production. Maintaining eucapnia, at the same tidal volume and physiological dead-space, will require an increase in the respiratory rate.

    (c) *Physiological dead space:* In diseases with increased physiological dead space (e.g. COPD), the tidal volume available for gas exchange is reduced, necessitating an increased respiratory rate, to maintain eucapnia.

    (d) *Delivered tidal volume:* A reduction in tidal volume will necessitate an

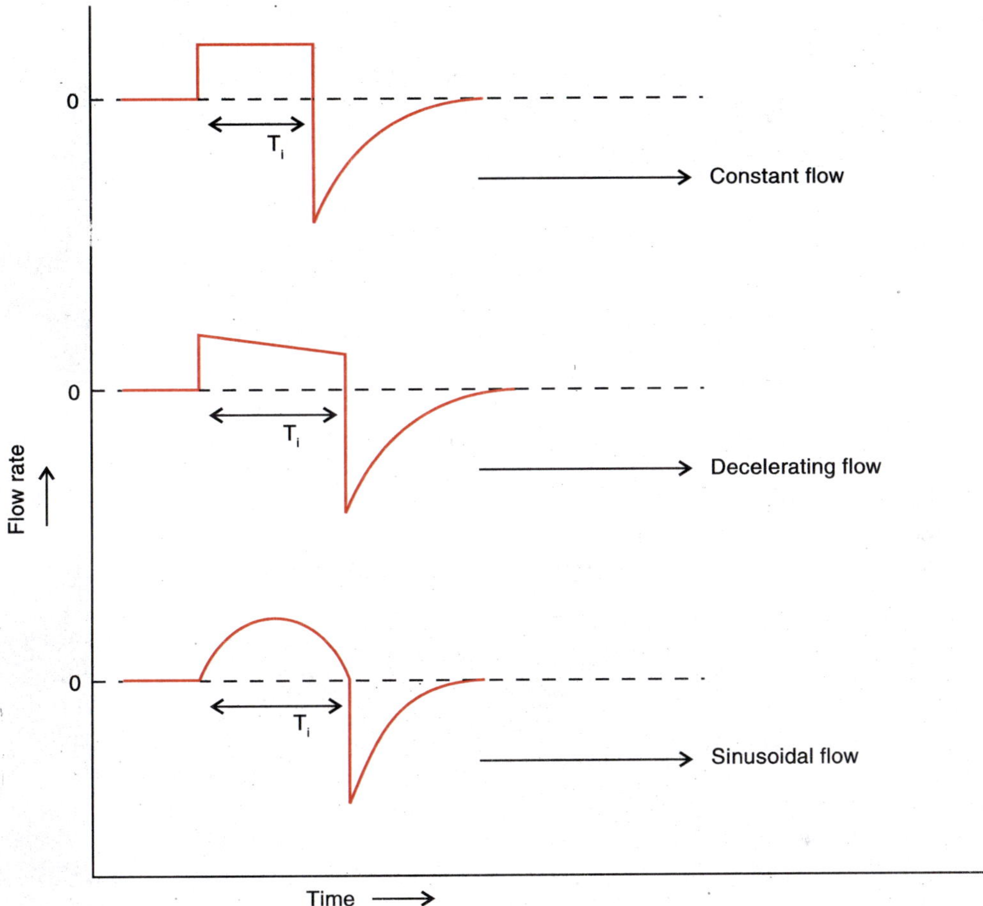

Fig. 32.3: Comparison of different inspiratory flow patterns when using volume-cycled ventilation. Note that the inspiratory time is shortest with a constant flow pattern (at equal peak inspiratory flow rates and delivered volumes).

increase in respiratory rate, assuming that the physiological dead space is unaltered.

Most clinically stable patients require mandatory rates of 8-12/min. In patients with acute COPD, acute asthma (increased airway resistance), or emphysema (increased compliance), a reduction in respiratory rate to 6-8 breaths/min may be required to minimize auto-PEEP.

In patients with acute or chronic restrictive lung disease, mandatory rates exceeding 20/min, may be necessary, depending on the desired minute ventilation and targeted $PaCO_2$.

8. **Sigh.**

Sigh has been used in the past to reduce the risk of atelectasis. For many years the use of sigh during mechanical ventilation was not considered important. However, with the concept of "lung rest" and use of smaller tidal volumes to limit plateau pressure, use of sighs may improve recruitment and oxygenation.

9. **Trigger sensitivity (Fig. 32.4).**

   Patient may trigger the ventilator through changes in either pressure or flow.

   (a) **Pressure triggering.**

   Pressure triggering occurs due to a pressure drop in the system. The pressure at which the ventilator triggers should be set so as to have minimal trigger effort and to avoid auto-triggering. Usually this is 1 – 2 cm H_2O below the PEEP or CPAP level.

   (b) **Flow triggering.**

   Flow triggering occurs due to a change in flow rather than a drop in pressure at the airway. When the flow in the expiratory circuit decreases by the amount of flow sensitivity, the ventilator is triggered. For example, if the base flow is set at 5 L/min and the flow sensitivity is set at 1 L/min, the ventilator triggers when the flow in the expiratory circuit drops to 4 L/min, 1L/min having been inhaled by the patient. Flow triggering is generally more efficient than pressure triggering. Flow sensitivity should be set at 1-3 L/min.

10. **Positive end-expiratory pressure.**

    See Chapter 39.

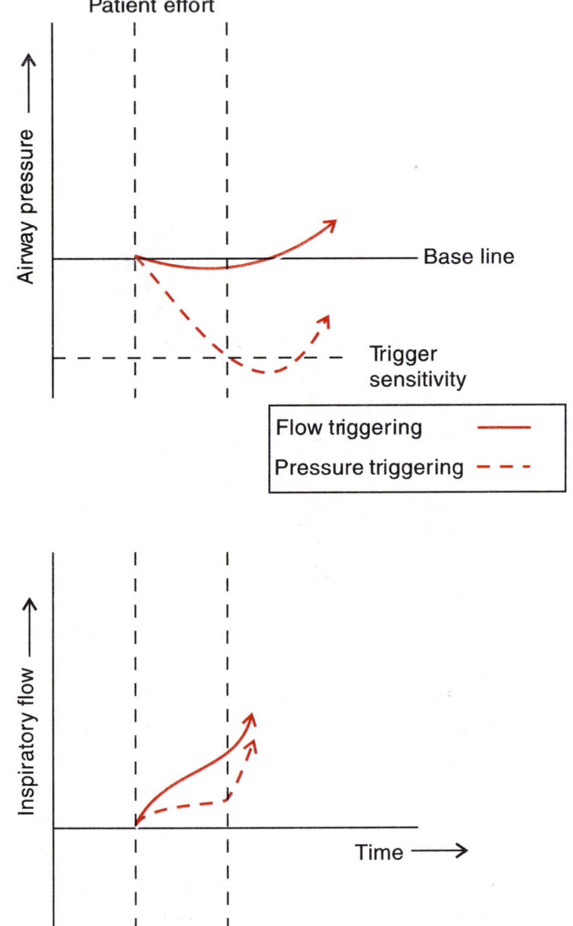

Fig. 32.4: Pressure-time and flow-time diagrams during pressure triggering and flow triggering. In comparison to pressure triggering, flow triggering delivers a low level of constant gas flow (base flow) through the ventilator circuit to meet initial flow requirements and reduces the work required by the patient to initiate a breath. Note that the patient receives no flow during pressure decline with pressure-triggering.

References

1. Acute Respiratory Distress Syndrome Network. Ventilation with lower tidal volumes as compared with traditional tidal volumes for acute lung injury and the acute respiratory distress syndrome. N Engl J Med 2000; 342:1301-1308.
2. Brenson RD, Compbell RS, Davis D, et al. Comparison of pressure and flow triggering systems during continuous positive airway pressure. Chest 1994; 106:540-544.
3. Dreyfuss D, Basset G, Soler P, Saumon G. Intermittent positive-pressure hyperventilation with high inflation pressures produces pulmonary microvascular injury in rats. Am Rev. Respir Dis 1985; 132:880-884.
4. Hess DR, Branson RD. Mechanical ventilation. In: Hess DR, MacIntyre NR, Mishoe SC, et al (eds). Respiratory Care: Principles and Practice. Philadelphia: Saunders: 2002, pp 782-809.
5. Humbmayr RD. Setting the ventilator. In: Tobin MJ (ed). Principles and Practice of Mechanical Ventilation, New York: McGraw-Hill, 1994, pp 191-206.
6. Kacmarek RM, Hess D. Basic Principles of ventilator machinery. In: Tobin MJ (ed). Principles and Practice of Mechanical Ventilation. New York: McGraw-Hill, 1994, pp 65-110.
7. Kacmarek RM, Venegas J. Mechanical Ventilatory rates and tidal volumes. Respiratory Care 1987; 32:466-475.
8. Kolbow T, Moretti MP, Fumagalli R, et al. Severe impairement in lung function induced by high peak airway pressure during mechanical ventilation. Am Rev Respir Dis 1987; 135:312-315.
9. Marcy TW, Marini JJ. Inverse ratio ventilation in ARDS. Rationale and implementation. Chest 1991; 100:494-504.
10. Martz KV, Joiner J, Shepherd RM. Management of the patient-ventilator system. St. Louis: Mosby, 1979.
11. Nelson EJ, Morton EA, Hunter PM. Critical Care Respiratory therapy, Boston: Little, Brawn,1983.
12. Pelosi P, Cadringer P, Bottino N, et al. Sigh in acute respiratory distress syndrome. Am J Respir Crit Care Med 1999; 159:872-880.
13. Sassoon CSH. Mechanical ventilator design and function: the trigger variable. Respir Care 1992; 37:1056-1069.
14. Slutsky AS. ACCP Consensus Conference on Mechanical Ventilation. Chest 1993; 104:1833-1859.
15. Stock MC, Azriel Perel (eds). Handbook of mechanical ventilatory support. Baltimore: Williams & Wilkins, 2 ed., 1997.
16. Vanderwarf C. Mechanical Ventilation. In: Fink JB, Hunt GE (eds). Clinical practice in Respiratory Care. Philadelphia: Lippincott, Williams & Wilkins, 1999, pp 405-435.
17. Wrathall GJ. Respiratory rate, tidal and minute volume, inspiratory time. In: Webb AR, Shapiro MJ, Singer M, Suter PM (eds). Oxford Textbook of Critical Care, 1 ed. Oxford: Oxfort University Press, 1999, pp 1322-1327.

Introduction

- The Synchronized Intermittent Mandatory Ventilation (SIMV) mode consists of two types of ventilatory breaths (Figs. 33.1, 33.2). The first type of ventilatory breath is identical to that in assist-control mode, and provides machine-delivered tidal volumes at a preset respiratory rate. The second type of ventilatory breath allows the patient to breathe spontaneously from the ventilator's demand valve. The volume and rate of these spontaneous breaths depend on the patient's respiratory drive and the mechanical properties of the patient's respiratory system. (This is in contrast to the patient triggered breath in assist-control mode, which is equal to the preset inspiratory tidal volume, as for mandatory breaths). A third type of ventilatory breath may also be seen when the spontaneous breaths between the mandatory breaths are pressure supported (Fig. 33.3).

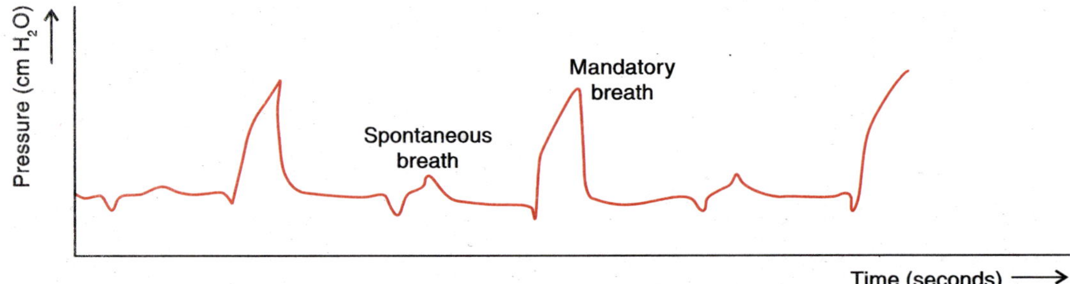

Fig. 33.1: Synchronized intermittent mandatory ventilation illustrating mandatory and spontaneous breaths. The mandatory breaths are volume-controlled.

- Although SIMV was originally developed as a weaning mode, controlled clinical trials show T-piece trials and pressure support ventilation to be superior to SIMV in this respect.
- *Advantages of SIMV* include: (a) Avoidance of respiratory alkalosis, (b) decreased requirement for sedation/muscle relaxation, (c) lower mean airway pressure, (d) better matching of ventilation and perfusion, and (e) prevention of respiratory muscle atrophy.
- *Disadvantages of SIMV* include: (a) Dyssynchrony if set rate is too low, (b) increased work of breathing, (c) respiratory muscle fatigue, and (d) increased risk of CO_2 retention.

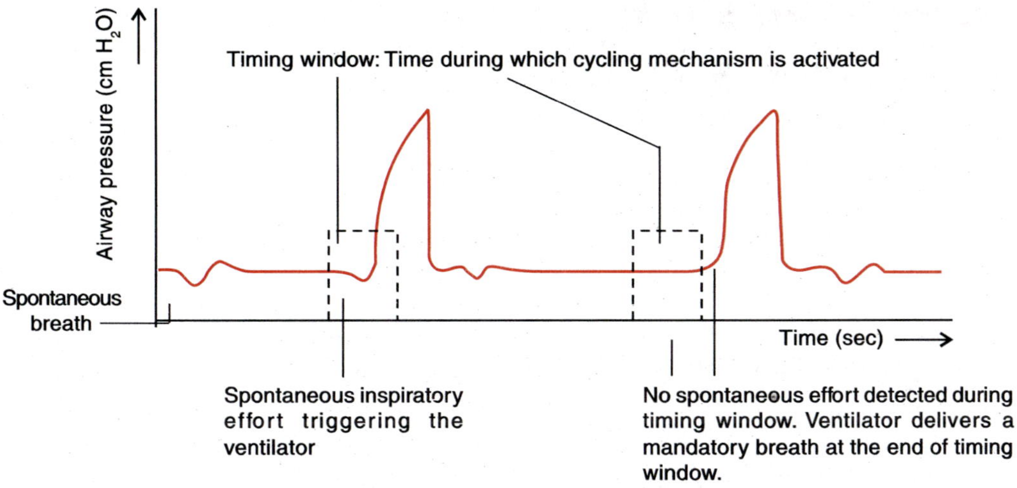

Fig. 33.2: Synchronized intermittent mandatory ventilation. Concept of timing window.

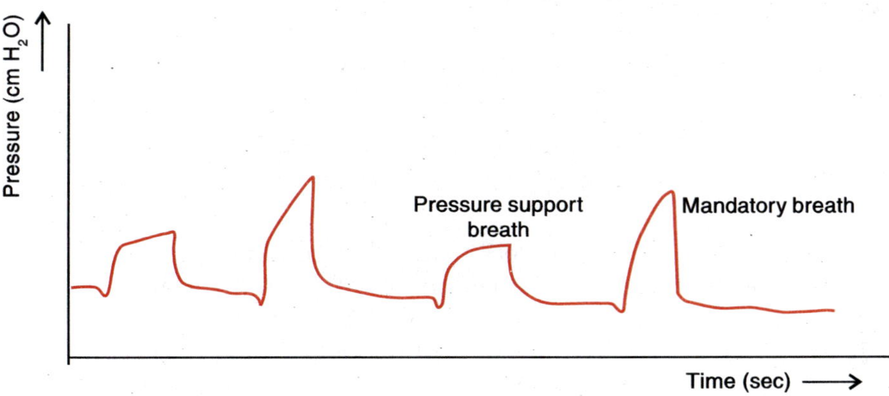

Fig. 33.3: Synchronized intermittent mandatory ventilation with pressure support for spontaneous breaths. The mandatory breaths are volume-controlled.

- With SIMV, electromyogram (EMG) studies reveal that respiratory muscles are stressed equally for both spontaneous and assisted breaths, even at high assist rates, because the respiratory center output cannot adapt when assistance varies from breath to breath. Therefore, when muscle rest is a priority (as in acute COPD), assist-control mode may be preferred over SIMV mode, as it is associated with decreased work of breathing.

GUIDELINES FOR INITIATING SIMV

1. Set PEEP.
   See Chapter 39.

2. **Set machine frequency at 12-14 breaths/min.**

   Define the parameter of the breath provided by the machine (i.e. determine the I:E ratio for the machine breaths).

3. **Set tidal volume at 8-10 mL/kg.**

   See Chapter 32.

4. **Set the peak flow at 60 L/min.**

   A patient requires a peak flow roughly 3-4 times the minute ventilation. However, if patient is breathing spontaneously, then adjustment is required to ensure that the flow matches the patient's efforts. Further, with a decelerating waveform pattern and in patients with airflow obstruction, slightly higher (80-100 L/min) flows should be set.

5. **Set flow trigger sensitivity.**

   Know your ventilator. Flow triggering facility is available in many ventilators.

6. **If flow triggering facility not available, add pressure support (5-6 cmH$_2$O). SIMV with CPAP alone is not indicated.**

   Work of breathing is more with pressure triggered SIMV as compared to that with flow-triggered SIMV. This disadvantage with pressure-triggered SIMV can be offset by adding a pressure support of 5-6 cm H$_2$O.

7. **Use a decelerating flow pattern.**

   See Chapter 32.

8. **Calculate and add pressure support.**

   Pressure support can be added to SIMV to unload inspiratory muscle work during spontaneous breathing cycles for different purposes:

   - The addition of a small amount of PSV (5 cm H$_2$O) to pressure triggered SIMV to overcome the lack of flow triggering in some ventilators.
   - To overcome the endotracheal tube resistance, during spontaneous breaths (6-10cm H$_2$O).
   - To augment tidal volume and unload the elastic work of spontaneous breaths (titrated to get desired tidal volume and minute ventilation). Calculate the amount of pressure support, which may initially be taken as equal to plateau pressure minus PEEP (as on volume controlled breaths).

   Reset the pressure support if required.

9. **Monitor blood gases after 45-60 minutes and then at regular intervals.**

   - If CO$_2$ is elevated: Increase tidal volume if plateau pressure permits (should not exceed 30 cm H$_2$O), or increase the machine breath rate.
   - If CO$_2$ is decreased: decrease tidal volume in steps and/or decrease the machine breath rate.
   - Reduce the mandatory (machine) rate in steps for as long as the arterial pH exceeds 7.35, patient has adequate ventilatory drive and does not show signs of ventilatory muscle fatigue (eg., increase in respiratory rate) (Fig. 33.4 a, b).

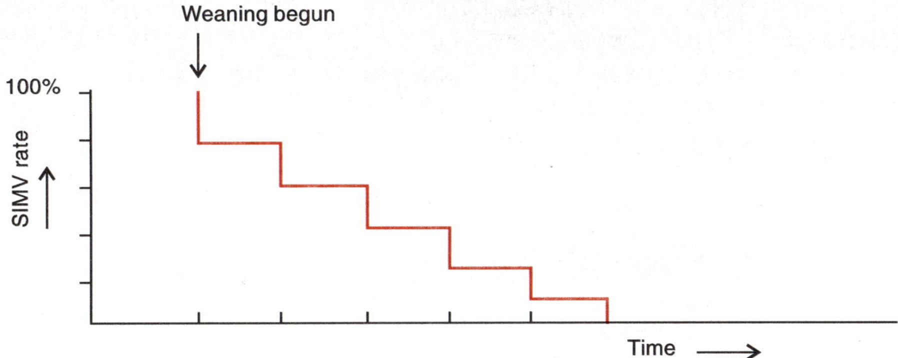

Fig. 33.4(a): Reductions in SIMV rate in steps of 2/min at regular intervals in a stable patient, who is recovering fast.

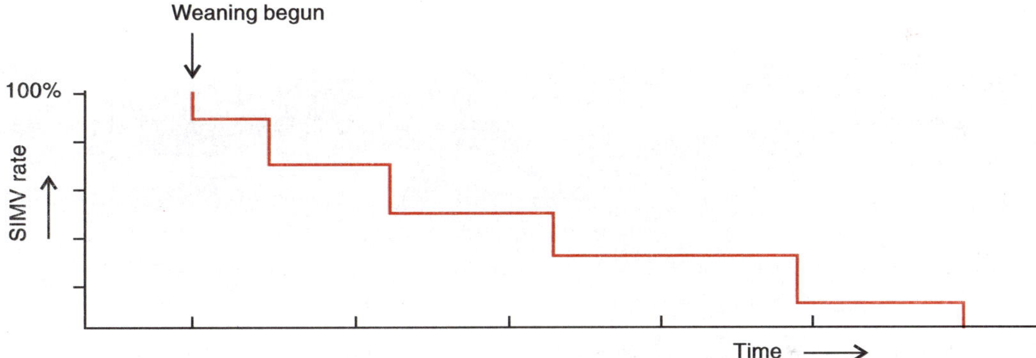

Fig. 33.4(b): Interval between successive reduction in SIMV rate may be increased depending upon the progress of the patient.

10. Switch over to pressure support ventilation.

If patient's lung injury is not advancing, respiratory drive is intact, patient is breathing spontaneously, and mandatory breaths have been reduced to 2-4 breaths/min, switch over to PSV. Recheck if peak flow is adequate.

11. Once on pressure support ventilation, follow guidelines as described for pressure support ventilation.

See Chapter 34.

References

1. Brochard L, Rauss A, Benito S, et al. Comparison of three methods of gradual withdrawal from ventilatory support during weaning from mechanical ventilation. Am J Respir Crit Care Med. 1994; 150:896-903.
2. Downs JB, Klein EF, Desautels D, et al. Intermittent mandatory ventilation: a new approach to weaning patients from mechanical ventilation. Chest 1973; 64:331.

3. Esteban A, Frutos F, Tobin MJ, et al. A comparison of four methods of weaning patients from mechanical ventilation. N Engl J Med 1995; 332:345-350.

4. Imsand C, Feihl F, Perret C, et al. Regulation of inspiratory neuromuscular output during synchronized intermittent mechanical ventilation. Anesthesiology 1994; 80:13-22.

5. Weisman IM, Rinaldo JE, Rogers RM, et al. State of the art: intermittent mandatory ventilation. Am Rev Respir Dis 1983; 127:641.

Introduction

- Pressure support ventilation (PSV) can be defined as a patient initiated, pressure-targeted, patient cycled mode of mechanical ventilation that is generally flow-cycled (Fig. 34.1).

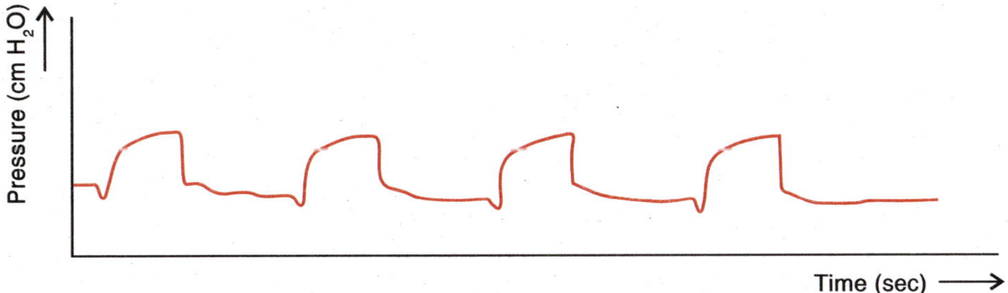

Fig. 34.1: Pressure support ventilation. Every breath is patient triggered, supported to a predetermined airway pressure and is flow cycled.

- The addition of PSV modifies the spontaneous breathing pattern in that, an increase in tidal volume and a decrease in respiratory rate are observed in most patients.
- Monitoring of minute ventilation is not helpful when titrating the level of PSV, as changes in minute volume are not marked during PSV.
- The primary goal of PSV is to support a patient's respiratory effort. Addition of pressure support is associated with changes in breathing pattern, increase in tidal volume, decrease in respiratory rate, decrease in the ratio of dead space volume to tidal volume, increase in alveolar ventilation, decrease in $PaCO_2$ level, and reduction in the work of breathing (which is more or less proportional to the level of pressure given). PSV mode, however, does not reduce the work to trigger a breath.
- The advantages of PSV include: (a) Improvement in patient comfort, (b) helps in better synchrony with ventilator, (c) prevention of respiratory muscle atrophy, (d) overcomes tube resistance, (e) facilitates weaning, and (f) enables evaluation of patient's respiratory status with regard to extubation, i.e. by knowing the pressure needed to obtain a reasonable breathing pattern and gas exchange.
- The disadvantages of PSV are: (a) It requires spontaneous respiratory effort and intact respiratory drive, (b) precipitates fatigue and tachypnea with too low pressure support, (c) activates expiratory muscles with too high pressure

support, (d) development of atelectasis due to smaller tidal volumes in patients with brief inspiratory time and high respiratory impedance, (e) persistent inspiratory pressure assist due to a circuit leak, and (f) episodes of hypoventilation with the use of continuous in–line nebulizers.

- Clinically, PSV can be applied in three different situations:

(a) Low level of pressure support (5-10 cm H_2O) during inspiration, to overcome the resistance component of inspiratory work, imposed by an endotracheal tube during spontaneous breathing. The exact pressure requirement will depend on endotracheal tube diameter and the inspiratory flow characteristics. In ventilators having this facility, consider using automatic tube compensation.

(b) Higher level of pressure support (up to 25-30 cm H_2O) for providing ventilatory support, to obtain desired tidal volume and minute ventilation.

(c) Use of pressure support, via facemask, in non-intubated patients who require transient ventilatory support.

GUIDELINES FOR INITIATING PRESSURE SUPPORT VENTILATION

1. **Set PEEP.**
   See Chapter 39.

2. **Start with pressure support of 18-20 cm H_2O and adjust to a tidal volume of 8-10 mL/Kg or as desired.**
   Start with high-pressure support and gradually lower the level. This will recruit the collapsed lung units. Pressure support is required to decrease the work of breathing during inspiration, which is increased due to loss of lung compliance, increased airway resistance, and other factors increasing work of breathing in an injured lung.

3. **Watch lung compliance and tidal volume.**
   If compliance is reduced or tidal volume is low: increase pressure support. If compliance is increased or tidal volume is more than desired: decrease pressure support.

4. **Look at the pressure waveform.**
   Adjust inspiratory flow (slope) to optimal settings (possible only in those ventilators which have the facility of varying slope).

5. **Watch respiratory rate and accessory muscle activity in the neck, especially sternocleidomastoid muscles.**
   A respiratory rate of less than 25/min may be optimal. Tachypnea indicates either inadequate sedation or an excessive ventilatory muscle load, requiring more pressure support. Bradypnea or episodes of apnea require a decrease in the level of pressure support in the absence of high levels of sedation. Persistent activity in accessory muscles indicates inadequate pressure support; increase the pressure support and titrate with muscle activity (by visual inspection and palpation), the desired tidal volume and optimal respiratory rate.

6. **Wean the patient.**

   Once the primary condition leading to respiratory failure has been managed and the patient is ready to be weaned (see Chapter 42), start decreasing the pressure support by 2-5 cm H_2O/day or more, often as tolerated by the patient (see Chapter 44).

7. **Extubate the patient.**

   If patient is stable at 5-6 cm H_2O pressure support for 10-12 hours, and if patient meets extubation criteria (see Chapter 45), patient may be extubated.

References

1. American Association for Respiratory Care. Consensus statement on essentials of mechanical ventilators. Respir Care 1992; 37:1000-1008.
2. Brochard L, Rauss A, Benito S, et al. Comparison of three methods of gradual withdrawal from ventilatory support during weaning from mechanical ventilation. Am J Respir Crit Care Med 1994; 150:896-903.
3. Esteban A, Frutos F, Tobin MJ, et al. A comparison of four methods of weaning patients from mechanical ventilation. N Engl J Med 1995; 332:345-350.
4. Kacmarek R. The role of pressure support ventilation in reducing work of breathing. Respir Care 1988; 33:99-120.
5. MacIntyre NR, Nishimura N, Usada Y, et al. The Nagoya Conference on system design and patient ventilator interactions during pressure support ventilation. Chest 1970; 97:1463-1466.
6. MacIntyre NR. Respiratory function during pressure support ventilation. Chest 1986; 89:677-683.
7. MacIntyre NR. Weaning from mechanical ventilatory support: Volume assisting intermittent breaths versus pressure assisting every breath. Respir Care 1988; 33:121-125.
8. Meyer TJ, Hill NS. Non-invasive positive pressure ventilation to treat respiratory failure. Ann Intern Med 1994; 120:760-770.
9. Pennock BE, Crenshaw L, Kaplan PD. Non invasive mask ventilation for acute respiratory failure Chest. 1994; 105:441-444.
10. Tobin MJ. Mechanical Ventilation. N Engl J Med 1994; 330:1056-1061.
11. Young KL, Tobin MJ. A prospective study of indexes predicting the outcome of trials of weaning from mechanical ventilation. N Engl J Med 1991; 324:1445-1450.

Pressure-controlled Ventilation

35

Introduction

- Pressure control (PC) only refers to the type of breath delivered, and not the mode of ventilation. Many different modes are pressure controlled. Conventionally the term "PC" refers to an assist-control mode, although SIMV can also be used in pressure control mode on some ventilators.
- In PC, a pressure-limited breath is delivered at a preset inspiratory pressure, rate, and inspiratory time. The tidal volume (TV) is determined by the pressure gradient existing between the airway opening and the alveolus at the onset of inflation, the resistance to airflow, the compliance of the respiratory system, and the time available for inspiration.
- In PC ventilation (PCV), one sets the inspiratory pressure (in contrast to setting peak flow with volume controlled ventilation). The machine constantly adjusts flow so that the inspiratory pressure is maintained during the entire set inspiratory time.
- During PCV, the machine applies approximately square waves of pressure to the airway opening. The flow characteristics during PCV are best studied by observing the flow versus time waveform (Fig. 35.1). Flow will initially enter the lungs rapidly because the ventilator attempts to reach the set airway pressure as quickly as it can (Fig. 35.1, point A). Airways that are open and have the least resistance will receive the greatest amount of gas flow and will reach equilibrium with the preset pressure more quickly than airways with greater resistances. As the open airways fill and the lung pressure reaches equilibrium with the preset pressure, flow will decelerate as the airways with higher resistance continue to fill the gas (Fig. 35.1, point B). The decelerating waveform results in a more laminar flow at the end of inspiration, resulting in a more even distribution of ventilation in patients who have markedly different resistance values from one region of the lung to another. If inspiratory time is adequate (Fig. 35.1, point C), flow into the lungs will continue until the preset pressure reaches equilibrium in all the lung units or it might

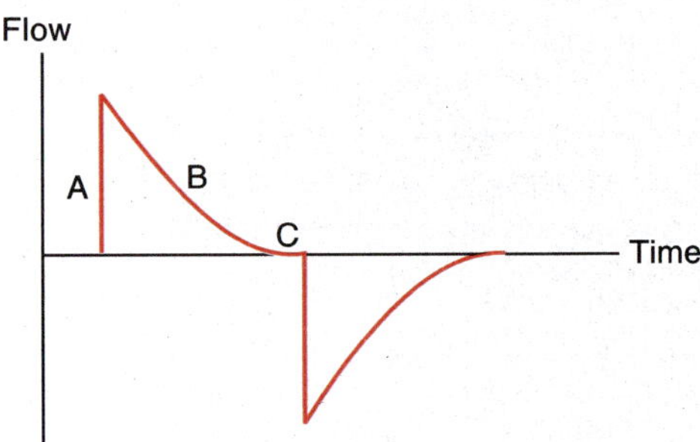

Fig. 35.1: Flow-time diagram during pressure-controlled ventilation.

be terminated by inadequate inspiratory time before touching the baseline in a flow vs time waveform (Fig. 35.2).

- The rapid initial inspiratory flow rate, with decelerating waveform, minimizes the time during which the alveoli are exposed to lower pressure levels that might make them collapse. This rapid initial inspiratory flow is also useful to meet high inspiratory flow demands generated by the patient, thus increasing the probability of patient synchronization and comfort.

- Patient can breath spontaneously on pressure control as long as the inspiratory time has not been unduly prolonged. The trigger mechanism is the same as in volume-controlled ventilation (VCV).

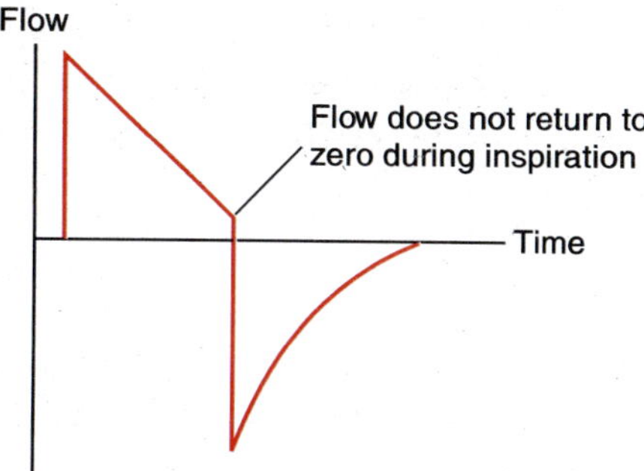

Fig. 35.2: Flow-time diagram during pressure-controlled ventilation in the case of insufficient inspiratory time.

- The advantages of PCV over VCV are: (a) Peak inspiratory pressure (PIP) is limited, (b) inspiratory time is adjustable, (c) a longer inspiratory time often provides better gas distribution and exchange, (d) a decelerating flow pattern allows for rapid flow at the onset of inspiration when the delivered gas is travelling through the larger airways, and a tapering flow as the delivered gas approaches increasingly smaller airways, at the end of inspiration.

- The disadvantages of PCV include: (a) PCV does not guarantee minute ventilation and therefore requires more intensive monitoring, (b) initiation of PCV is slightly more difficult than VCV, (c) it has its greatest application to situations where patient's efforts are suppressed (as with any time cycled mode of ventilation, PCV invites dyssynchrony when patient breathes spontaneously), and (d) when used as the mandatory breath, delivered during SIMV, PCV offers little advantage over conventional flow-controlled, volume cycled SIMV cycles, except the assurance that the peak airway pressure will rise no higher than the nominal value (pressure-support ventilation, a flow-cycled mode would seem a better choice for partial ventilatory assistance).

- While using PCV, the primary problem is that alveolar ventilation varies non-linearly with machine adjustments and, for a given configuration of settings, varies with inflation impedance. To prevent alveolar overdistension and to reduce the transpulmonary pressure gradient, the inspiratory pressure should be set such that the peak inspiratory pressure (applied PEEP plus inspiratory pressure) is less than 35 cmH_2O. Although ventilatory driving pressure and alveolar ventilation can be increased by reducing PEEP at a fixed value of set inspiratory pressure, the resulting decline in mean airway pressure must be offset by extending T_i/T_{TOT} (T_i = inspiratory time, T_{TOT} = total time for a single breath). The latitude to a make such manipulations is limited by the need to maintain some minimum level of end-expiratory alveolar pressure. When restricted to a specific range, pressure modification is, therefore, inherently limited in accomplishing ventilation. Similarly when the lung is stiff, changes in T_i/T_{TOT} also fail to affect total ventilation over the usual clinical range. Over the lower frequency range, increasing frequency tends to improve alveolar, as well as, total ventilation. However, when higher frequencies are used at constant inspiratory pressure and T_i/T_{TOT} (in an attempt to increase minute ventilation), the duration of both inspiration and expiration decreases and auto-PEEP rises. The rise in auto-PEEP decreases the tidal volume, and minute ventilation exponentially approaches an upper limit determined solely by resistance and duty cycle. Also with decreased tidal volume, the wasted fraction of each breath (VD/VT) increases, and it may actually cause $PaCO_2$ to rise rather than fall with increasing frequencies. Because of all these factors, hypercapnia may be an unavoidable consequence of pressure-targeted strategy for managing acute lung injury.

- There is no evidence that pressure control is superior to volume control. One should use the strategy one is comfortable with. Advantages of PCV may be achieved with VCV, by altering flow rates, inspiratory pause, tidal volume, and waveform.

GUIDELINES FOR INITIATING PRESSURE ASSIST-CONTROL MODE

1. Know your ventilator.

   Select a ventilator with PCV software and waveform capability. Flow vs time waveform is of great help for the proper setting of the ventilator parameters.

2. Set PEEP.

   Set PEEP above the lower inflection point of the static pressure/volume curve or between 10 and 15 cm H_2O.

3. Adjust inspiratory pressure to obtain a tidal volume of 6 mL/kg. A convenient starting point may be an inspiratory pressure of 20 cm H_2O.

   Start with high, and gradually lower the inspiratory pressure. This will recruit the collapsed lung units. Also keep in mind that the sum of PEEP and inspiratory pressure should not exceed 35 cm H_2O.

4. Set initial inspiratory time at 0.5 to 0.8 seconds. Adjust the inspiratory time to allow for a full inspiration.

   A better way to set inspiratory time is to analyse flow vs time waveform. Inspiratory time should be long enough for inspiratory flow to reach zero. However, if flow reaches zero and is followed by a long inspiratory pause, it indicates that the inspiratory time is too long. There is no benefit of having such a long inspiratory time: indeed it may lead to significant auto-PEEP with its attendant hemodynamic complications.

5. Set initial rate at 12-14 breaths/min. Adjust the rate to allow the expiratory flow to zero.

   Expiratory time is best adjusted by analyzing flow vs time waveform. Expiratory time should be long enough to complete exhalation so that the expiratory flow touches baseline (atmospheric pressure plus the set PEEP) before the next inspiration starts. If next inspiration starts before exhalation is complete, it will lead to gas trapping and auto-PEEP (Fig. 35.3). In this situation, reduce respiratory rate or inspiratory time so that exhalation is complete and auto-PEEP is minimized.

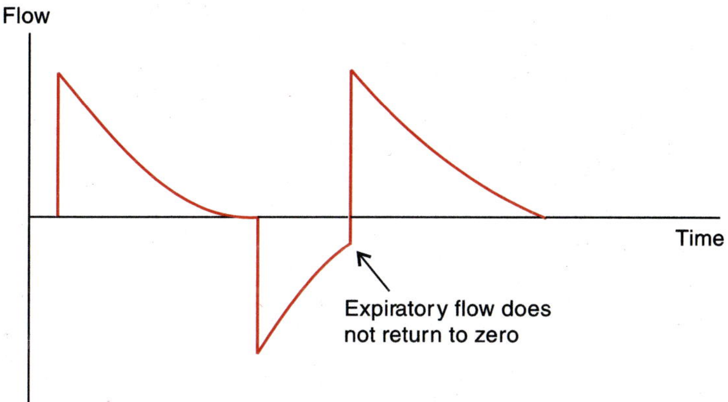

Fig. 35.3: Flow-time diagram during pressure-controlled ventilation in the case of insufficient expiratory time.

6. Set FiO_2 at 1.0.
   Titrate according to PaO_2.

7. Set flow trigger sensitivity.
8. Look at the pressure waveform.
   Adjust inspiratory flow (slope) to optimal settings (possible only in those ventilators which have the facility of varying the slope). Rapid pressurization is needed when flow demands are high; a more gradual pressure build-up is appropriate for quiet breathing.

9. Monitor blood gas after 1 hour.
   If $PaCO_2$ is elevated: increase the respiratory rate, but be careful of auto-PEEP.
   If patient has severe hypoxaemia: Increase the PEEP as necessary, increase the inspiratory time to 1.0–1.5 seconds, sedate and paralyze the patient, and consider prone position or alternative modes like APRV.

10. In case of significant auto-PEEP, reduce tidal volume/respiratory rate.

11. When patient's condition stabilizes, reduce the controlled rate until the patient is on pressure assist (patient only triggers the breath).
12. When respiratory drive is intact, in terms of rate, depth and duration of breath, and there is no tachypnea, switch over to PSV (pressure-support ventilation) and manage further. (See Chapter 34). Reduce the PEEP in steps, considering PaO_2 (see chapter 39).

References

1. Al-Sady N, Benett ED. Decelerating inspiratory flow waveform improves lung mechanics and gas exchange in patients on intermittent positive-pressure ventilation. Intensive Care Med 1985; 11:68-75.

2. Amato MBP, Barbas CSV, medeiros DM, et al. Beneficial effect of the 'open lung approach' with low distending pressure in acute respiratory distress syndrome. Am J Respir Crit Care Med 1995; 152:1835-1846.
3. Manktelow C, Bigatello L, Hess D, et al. Physiological determinants of the response to inhaled nitric oxide in patients with the acute respiratory distress syndrome. Anesthesiology 1997; 87:297.
4. Marini JJ. Pressure –controlled ventilation. In: Tobin MJ (ed). Principles and Practice of Mechanical Ventilation. New York: Mc Graw-Hill, 1994. pp 305-317.
5. Mark PE, Krikorian J. Pressure-controlled ventilation in ARDS: A practical approach. Chest 1997; 112:1102-1106.
6. Tharrat RS, Allen RP, Albertson TE. Pressure controlled inverse ratio ventilation in severe adult respiratory failure. Chest 1988; 94:755-762.

Introduction

- Continuous mechanical ventilation is a supportive measure that maintains cardiopulmonary function until the underlying cause of respiratory failure is resolved. However, the application of positive pressure does alter normal physiology and affects the functions of many body systems. The ventilator part of the patient-ventilator system itself could further add to the problems.
- To simplify monitoring, a terminology called "Patient-Ventilator system checks" has been introduced. A patient-ventilator (PV) system check involves (a) The assessment of the patient's response to mechanical ventilation, (b) evaluation of the current ventilator settings, (c) the presence and functioning of necessary equipment at the bedside, and (d) documentation of findings in the patient's chart. The aim of PV system check is to evaluate the patient's response to his or her current level of mechanical ventilatory support and to assure that the ventilator is functioning properly, ventilator settings are in compliance with the orders, inspired gases are conditioned properly, and that all the necessary equipment is present and functioning properly. It also includes operational verification procedure (OVP), to be done prior to, or at the time the ventilator is first applied to the patient.
- A PV system check should be performed: (a) Prior to obtaining blood samples for analysis of blood gases and pH, (b) prior to obtaining haemodynamic or bedside pulmonary function data, (c) following any change in ventilator settings, (d) as soon as possible following an acute deterioration of the patient's condition, (e) any time ventilator performance is in question. Unstable patients, or those being actively weaned may require check up at 15-30 minute intervals, but more stable patients may be monitored at 4-6 hourly intervals.
- Monitoring ventilator function: The following parameters may be monitored at regular intervals:
  (a) Set-up parameters: (i) Mode, (ii) inspiratory flow rate, (iii) I:E ratio, (iv) FiO_2, (v) tidal volume, (vi) frequency, (vii) minute ventilation, (viii) inspired gas temperature, (ix) trigger sensitivity (pressure, flow), (x) PEEP/CPAP level, and (xi) set the pressure level in case of pressure-support ventilation.
  (b) Patient values: (i) Tidal volume, (ii) respiratory rate, (iii) minute ventilation, (iv) airway pressures (peak, plateau, mean), (v) compliance, (vi) resistance, (vii) waveform/graphics, and (viii) other specific parameters (whenever applicable), e.g. auto-PEEP, occlusion pressure (Fig. 36.1).

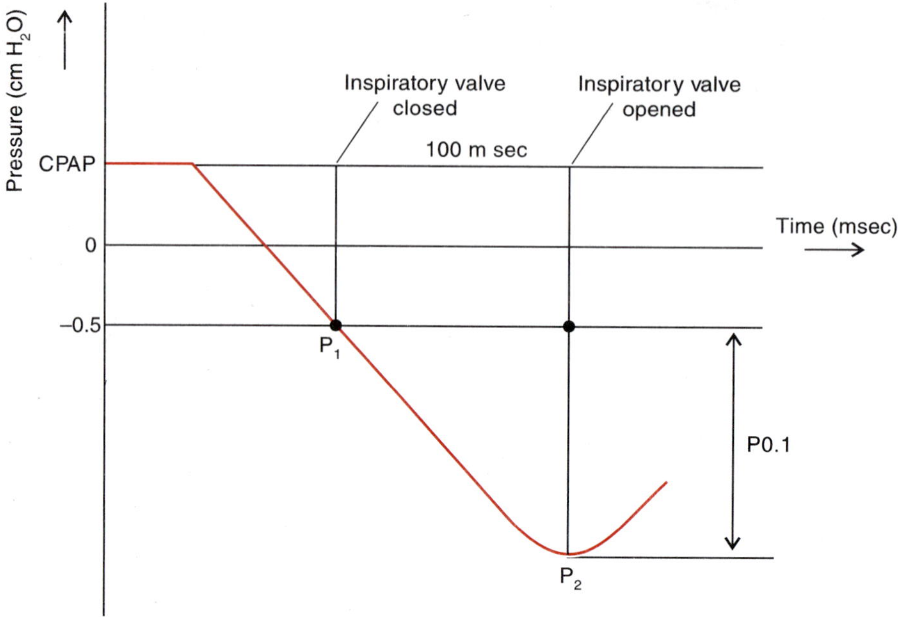

Fig. 36.1: Measurement of occlusion pressure (P0.1): Occlusion pressure is a measure of respiratory effort during spontaneous breathing. The ventilator measures the airway pressure generated by inspiratory effort with the inspiratory valve closed after expiration. A pressure of −0.5 cm H$_2$O (P$_1$) is taken as the beginning of inspiratory effort. The ventilator measures pressure (P$_2$), 100 msec. after inspiratory effort begins. The difference between these two pressures (P$_1$ and P$_2$) denotes the occlusion pressure P0.1. At the end of 100 msec, the inspiratory valve opens and the patient can breathe normally. Normal value is taken as 3-4 cm H$_2$O. High P0.1 values suggests increased respiratory effort which cannot be maintained for long time. P0.1 values over 6 cm H$_2$O, e.g. in patients with COPD, may be an indicator of imminent muscle fatigue.

(c) Check and ensure: (i) Breathing circuit is clear of any condensate, (ii) humidifier container is adequately filled and temperature is properly set, (iii) alarm system is functional and alarms are properly set, and (iv) cylinder pressure is adequate (if ventilator is being run by oxygen cylinder).

GUIDELINES TO MONITOR VENTILATOR FUNCTION

1. **Scan the chart.**

   To obtain information about results of previous P-V system checks.

2. **Wash hands.**

   This reduces the risk of transmission of micro-organisms.

3. **Look at the set-up parameters.**

   Confirm if they are in accordance with the orders given by the intensivist. If not, change them as per the orders.

4. Look for any obvious leaks in patient-ventilator system.
5. Look at the patient values.
   (a) Airway pressures (Fig. 36.2).
      (i) **Peak inspiratory.**
          Peak inspiratory pressure (PIP) is the pressure required to inflate the patient's lungs with a given tidal volume at a given peak inspiratory flow rate, and is determined by compliance (lung-thoracic), airway resistance, and flow pattern. A change in PIP of greater than 8 to 10 cm H_2O or 15% of a previously reported value, should be investigated actively. When a combination of modes is being used (e.g. SIMV plus PSV), the PIP of both mandatory and supported breaths should be measured.
      (ii) **Plateau (Pplat).**
          Plateau airway pressure is defined as the end-inspiratory pressure during a period of at least 0.5 seconds of zero gas flow. During the period of zero gas flow, the airway resistance component of ventilation is eliminated, leaving the elastic recoil component as the force required to maintain inflation. It roughly approximates the average peak alveolar pressure and is a better indicator of risk of barotrauma as compared to the peak pressure. Pplat should be measured on an unassisted breath using a constant inspiratory flow. Patient effort during a Pplat measurement can cause the true pressure to be underestimated. A change in plateau pressure of more than 5 cm H_2O or 15% of the previous value, should be investigated actively. A Pplat greater than 30 cm H_2O above PEEP is associated with ventilator-induced lung injury.
      (iii) **Mean.**
          Mean airway pressure is the average pressure recorded over the entire ventilatory period. It is a useful parameter because it has a direct effect on

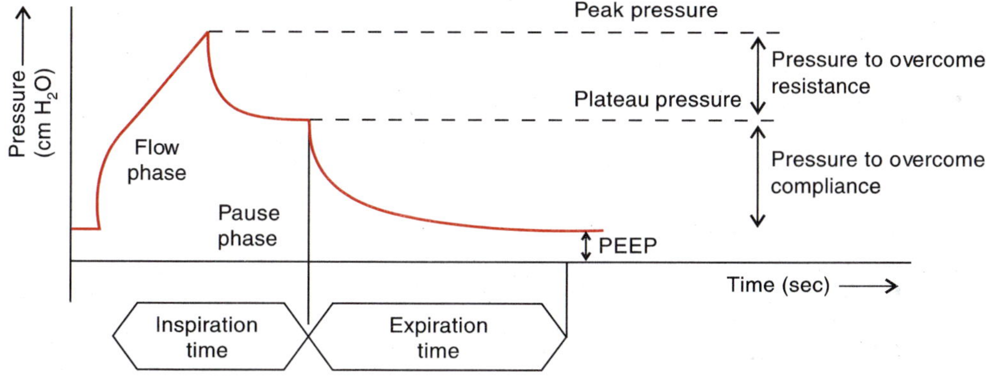

Fig. 36.2: Pressure-time diagram for volume controlled constant flow ventilation. The term "inflation pressure" refers to the pressure required to deliver a tidal volume. Inflation pressure has two components: flow resistive pressure and lung distending pressure. Peak airway pressure represents the maximum pressure applied to the proximal airway to effect flow and volume change. Plateau airway pressure represents the pressure required to distend alveoli (under no-flow conditions).

blood and tissue oxygenation (affects both lung volume and cardiac output). Mean airway pressure is affected by peak airway pressure, PEEP/CPAP levels, inspiratory time (dependent on flow rate and flow pattern), the mandatory breathing rate set on the ventilator, and the mode of ventilation.

(iv) PEEP/CPAP.

Actual PEEP may not be the same as the set-PEEP due to errors in calibration or set-up, or pressure-sensing problems. It is important to maintain a stable PEEP because most ventilators use the set PEEP as a reference value for triggering the ventilator. For example, if PEEP is set at 5 cm H_2O and sensitivity at -1 cm H_2O, the ventilator will trigger only when pressure falls below 4 cm H_2O. If actual PEEP is 3.5 cm H_2O, the ventilator will auto-trigger. If actual PEEP is 6.5 cm H_2O, the patient will need to generate -2.5 cm H_2O to trigger the ventilator on.

(b) Internal PEEP (auto PEEP).

Internal PEEP represents the difference between alveolar pressure and baseline pressure at end-exhalation. The presence of auto PEEP may contribute to haemodynamic instability, barotrauma, increased work of breathing, and miscalculation of dynamic and static compliance. Auto PEEP may be present in as many as 40% of mechanically ventilated patients. Risk factors for the development of auto PEEP include, high minute ventilation (>10 L/minute), small ETT (<7.0 mmID), age (> 60 years), COPD, and intubation and ventilation primarily for respiratory complications (see Chapter 41).

(c) Volume, respiratory rate, minute ventilation.

Each monitored variable may be divided into four distinct types: mandatory, spontaneous, inspiratory, and expiratory. Therefore assess accordingly. Measurement of spontaneous tidal volume is helpful in the assessment of patient's respiratory drive, effort, and ability. It is also used as an end point for titration of pressure support ventilation. Comparison of inspiratory and expiratory tidal volume may be useful in assessing the presence and magnitude of any leak in the patient-ventilator system. Measurement of mandatory tidal volume is complicated by loss of compressible volume in the ventilator circuit. A typical circuit has a compressible volume factor of 2-3 mL/cm H_2O. Thus, at a set TV of 1000 mL and a PIP of 50 cm H_2O, the delivered TV is 850 to 900 mL. This problem is clinically important when small tidal volumes are used in patients with stiff lungs. Different ventilators deal with the issue of compressible volume using a variety of methods, depending on their site of volume measurements. So know your ventilator !!

Spontaneous minute volume may be used to evaluate the patient's respiratory drive, respiratory muscle function, and dead-space ventilation. Weaning is not likely to be successful in patients with spontaneous minute ventilation of more than 10 L/min.

f/TV ratio (breaths/min per L) has been shown to be a good predictor of weaning outcome.

(d) Compliance.

Normal compliance values in patients receiving mechanical ventilation range from 60-80 mL/cm H_2O. Compliance values of less than 25 mL/cmH_2O are

usually not associated with successful weaning attempts or PEEP withdrawal.
(e) Waveforms and graphics (Fig. 36.3-36.6).
The use of waveforms and graphics may aid in rapidly assessing the patient-ventilator interaction and, the appropriateness of ventilator settings. Further, waveforms and graphics allow the intensivist to actually "shape" the patient's breaths while making ventilator manipulations.

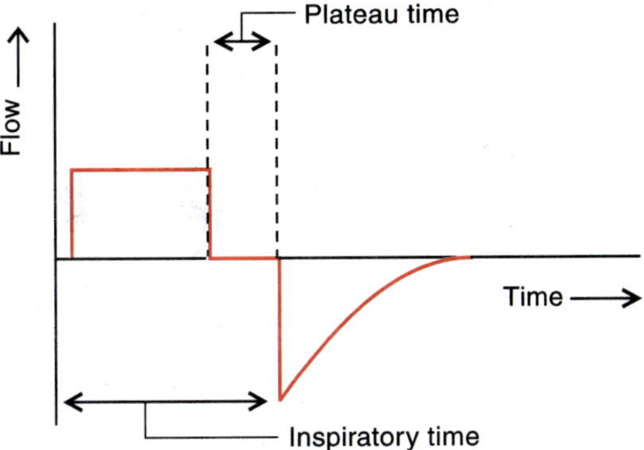

Fig. 36.3: Inspiratory and expiratory flow plotted against time with the ventilator in volume control, constant flow mode. The horizontal baseline represents zero flow. There is an immediate rise to the preset flow at the beginning of inspiration. This is maintained constant until tidal volume has been delivered. At the beginning of the plateau (pause) time, the flow rapidly returns to zero. At the end of the plateau time, the inspiration ends and expiratory flow begins. Flow is then reversed, which shifts the curve abruptly below baseline. The exhalation phase generates a logarithmic curve of gradually decreasing flow. The course of the flow in the expiratory phase gives more complete picture of the overall resistance and compliance of the lung and the system. With decreased compliance, loss of expiratory flow is usually faster, while with obstructive changes, expiratory flow is retarded.

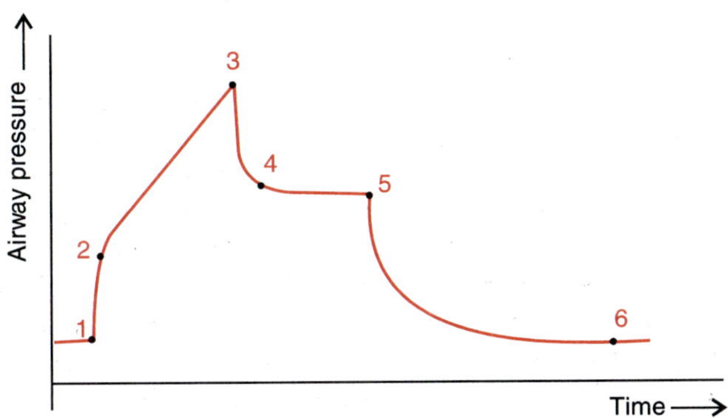

Fig. 36.4: Airway pressure vs time diagram for volume controlled, constant flow ventilation. At the beginning of inspiration the pressure between points 1 and 2 increases dramatically on account of the resistance in the system. After point 2, the pressure increases in a straight line till point 3 (the peak airway pressure). At point 3, the ventilator applies the set tidal volume and no further flow is delivered. Because of no flow, the pressure quickly falls to the plateau pressure (point 4). There may be a slight decrease in pressure between points 4 and 5 due to lung recruitment and leaks in the system. At point 5, expiration begins because of the elastic recoil forces of the thorax and it is a passive process.

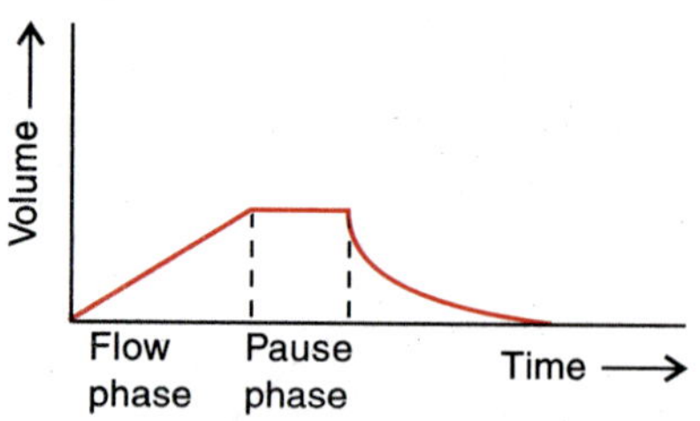

Fig. 36.5: Tidal volume vs time waveform for volume controlled, constant flow ventilation. During the inspiratory flow phase, the volume increases continuously; during the pause phase, it remains constant, and during expiration, the transferred volume decreases as a result of passive exhalation. The baseline represents the zero volume. If the patient does not exhale completely, the curve does not return to baseline.

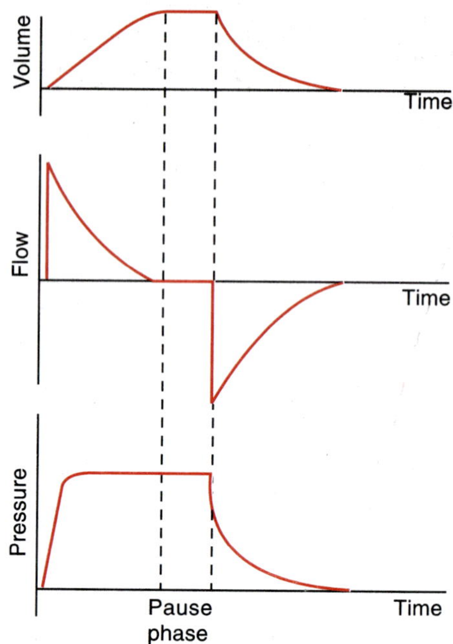

Fig. 36.6: Volume, flow and pressure diagram of pressure-oriented ventilation. The flow falls constantly after having reached an initial high value. Under normal conditions, the flow returns to zero during the course of inspiration. Pressure increases rapidly from the lower pressure level until it reaches the upper pressure level and then remains constant for the set inspiration time. The drop in pressure during the expiratory phase follows the same curve as during volume-controlled ventilation.

6. **Check and ensure the following:**
   - Breathing circuit should be cleared of any condensate with every check. Condensation from the ventilator circuit should be considered an infectious waste and disposed of accordingly.
   - Check humidifier for any leak, set proximal airway temperature, chamber water level, and set alarms. Humidifier should be able to establish a temperature of 30°C to 32°C at the carina with an absolute humidity of 30 mg. Since it is technically difficult to continuously measure humidity levels, the humidity is assessed by the amount and consistency of the patient's sputum. If secretions are thick and tenacious, the amount of delivered humidity should be increased by increasing temperature to a maximum of 37°C.
   - Alarm system should be checked for proper functioning and appropriateness of settings.

7. **Perform ABG analysis.**

   It is important to record ABG here, to know which ventilator settings produced those values (in ABG).

8. **Change ventilator breathing circuits.**

    Breathing circuits should be changed when damaged or dirty. Studies have suggested that the frequency of circuit changes has little impact on the incidence of nosocomial pneumonia and may actually increase the risk of infection (by increased handling probably) and therefore support the use of each ventilator circuit as a "single patient use" item.

9. **Document the measured values.**

    Documentation on the ventilator flow sheet is important for future reference and for legal purposes. Documentation should also include the common bedside interventions like suctioning, repositioning and efforts to wean the patient.

10. **Wash hands.**

    This reduces the risk of transmission of micro-organisms.

References

1. AARC-ARCF Consensus Conference: Consensus Statement on Mechanical Ventilators. Respir Care 1992; 37:1000-1008.
2. American Association for Respiratory Care. Clinical Practice Guideline: patient-ventilator system checks. Respir Care 1992; 37(8): 882-886.
3. Branson RD, Davis K Jr, Campbell RS, et al. Humidification in the intensive care unit; a prospective study of a new protocol utilizing heated humidification and a hygroscopic condenser humidifier. Chest 1993; 104:1800-1805.
4. Branson RD: Flow-triggering systems. Respir Care 1994; 39:138-144.
5. Branson RD. Monitoring ventilator function. Crit Care Clin 1995; 11(1): 127-150.
6. Campbell RS. Managing the patient-ventilator system: System checks and circuit changes. Respir Care 1994; 39:227-236.
7. Hess D, Kacmarek RM. Technical aspects of the patient-ventilator interface. In: Tobin MJ (ed). Principles and practice of mechanical ventilation, New York: McGraw-Hill, 1994, pp 1039-1065.
8. Pierson DJ. What constitutes an order for mechanical ventilation, and who should give the order? Respir Care 1992; 37(9): 1124-1130.
9. Salyer JW, Chatburn RL. Patterns of practice in neonatal and pediatric respiratory care: Respir Care 1990; 35:879-888.
10. Society of Critical Care Medicine, Task Force on Guidelines: Guidelines for standards of care for patients with acute respiratory failure on mechanical ventilatory support. Crit Care Med 1991; 19:275-278.
11. Tobin MJ, Van de Graaff WB. Monitoring of lung mechanics and work of breathing. In: Tobin MJ (ed). Principles and practice of mechanical ventilation. New York: McGraw-Hill, 1994, pp 967-1003.

Introduction

The goal of monitoring the patient is to detect problems and manage them as early as possible. The following parameters should be monitored at regular intervals in a systematic manner and recorded on the monitoring chart. When a new symptom, sign, or a finding appears on routine monitoring, a search for the possible cause should immediately begin. The following parameters should be monitored when a patient is on a ventilator.

GUIDELINES FOR MONITORING THE PATIENTS

Behaviour of the patient

1. Anxiety, fear.
   - Response to new environment/ventilator: Reassure, use sedatives.
   - $\downarrow PaO_2$: Check SpO_2, patient–ventilator system.

2. Restlessness, agitation.
   - $\downarrow PaO_2$: Check SpO_2, patient-ventilator system.
   - Pain: check pain medication.
   - Low PIFR.

3. Confusion, disorientation, decreased responsiveness, no response to stimuli. Use Glasgow coma scale to determine patient's level of alertness.
   - $\downarrow PaO_2$: Check SpO_2, patient-ventilator system.
   - $\downarrow$ Perfusion to brain: Evaluate fluid balance, check blood pressure, examine for any acute event (e.g. stroke).
   - Rising $PaCO_2$: Obtain ABG.
   - Drugs: Check medication record.
   - Inadequate sleep.

4. Twitching/ convulsions/ tetany
   - Decreased serum levels of anticonvulsants in a patient with known convulsive disorder.
   - $\downarrow PaCO_2$ with rising pH.

5. Breathlessness.
   - Anxiety, decreased PaO_2, decreased ventilation, pneumothorax.

Inspection

6. Altered chest wall movements.
   (a) Paradoxical movement.
       Flail chest.
   (b) Inward movement of thorax during inspiration.
       Lower cervical cord transection.
   (c) Asynchronous movement of thorax and abdomen.
       Splinting after abdominal surgery, COPD, diaphragmatic paralysis, respiratory muscle fatigue with impending respiratory failure.
   (d) Unilateral decrease in chest wall expansion.
       Intubation of right mainstem bronchus, splinting secondary to pain, air, blood, or fluid in the pleural cavity, atelectasis, consolidation, obstruction of major bronchus.
7. Asynchrony with the ventilator (distressed patient). Monitor every hour.
   - Anxiety, pain: Reassure, manage pain.
   - Airway obstruction at the level of ETT: Pass a suction catheter to exclude airway obstruction.
   - Migration of tube, either above vocal cords or into the mainstem bronchus.
   - In-line continuous nebulization.
   - Secretions.
   - Fluid accumulation in the ventilator circuit.
   - Inappropriate ventilator settings in terms of flow rate, I:E ratio, FiO_2, trigger sensitivity, total minute ventilation.
   - Leaks in the system (commonly at circuit level or around ETT).
   - Auto-PEEP.
   - Pneumothorax.
   - $\downarrow PaO_2$, $\uparrow PaCO_2$.

   If no obvious cause is found, the first step is disconnection from the ventilator and manual ventilation with 100% oxygen. If patient improves promptly, the ventilator or external circuit is the source of the problem. If patient does not improve, then problem is with the ETT or the patient. Find out the cause and manage accordingly.

Vital Signs

8. Blood pressure. Monitor every 1-4 hours.
   Hypotension: decreased intravascular volume, high external or internal PEEP, cardiac failure and drugs (sedatives and vasodilators). Check drainage system, look for inadvertent discontinuation of inotropes or leak from IV site.
   Hypertension: Anxiety, inadequate sedation, $\uparrow PaCO_2$, other causes of sympathetic stimulation, drugs (vasopressors).
   Disparities between cuff and direct (intra-arterial) pressure measurements of 5-20 mmHg may be considered normal as long as the direct pressure measurement is higher. Disparity may exceed 30 mmHg in the presence of severe vasoconstriction. When cuff pressure is high, check monitoring system for leaks, bubbles, or other causes of damped pressure.

Hypotension is a late sign of decreasing cardiac output. Early signs of a decrease in cardiac output include, tachycardia, cold peripheral extremities, confused or less responsive patient and a fall in the urine output. A normal blood pressure does not guarantee adequate perfusion.

9. Respiratory swing of intra-arterial blood pressure waveform (wherever applicable). During a low flow state, while a prominent Δ down indicates hypovolemia, its total disappearance or lack of a significant Δ down is suggestive of congestive heart failure, reflecting that the inspiratory decrease in venous return has no effect on left ventricular stroke output.

   Δ up is the dominant variable of the arterial pressure waveform in hypervolemia and congestive heart failure. Δ up is of extreme importance during separation from cardiopulmonary bypass. The absence of Δ up segment during separation from cardiopulmonary bypass is a sign of non responsiveness of the left ventricle to increased volume (due most commonly to ischemic left ventricular dysfunction) and is a sign of inadequate or nonfunctioning coronary grafts.

   Respiratory swing of blood pressure is usually not appreciated because the arterial pressure is so high as compared to the magnitude of normal respiratory pressure changes. Also, the pressure scale normally set on the monitor makes changes of 10 mmHg barely visible. The analysis of the morphology of arterial pressure waveform during positive pressure ventilation can provide meaningful information, when the normal cardiovascular consequences of a mechanical breath are fully understood. The main cardiovascular effect of an increase in intrathoracic pressure is the reduction of venous return with relative emptying of the right ventricle. At the same time, filling of the left ventricle is increased because of squeezing of the pulmonary vasculature, leading to an early inspiratory increase in the LV stroke output and systolic blood pressure (Δ up). A few heartbeats after the mechanical breath begins, the decreased right ventricular output reaches the left heart. The LV stroke output declines, diminishing the systolic pressure (Δ down). The Δ down is thus a reflection of the decreased venous return during a mechanical breath. When the baseline preload is low, a further reduction in venous return with each mechanical breath may account for the typical increase in the Δ down value and its correlation with varying degrees of preload value. Baseline for Δ up and Δ down is taken as the systolic pressure during the preinspiratory period or during a short period of apnea. (Δ up is the difference between the maximal systolic pressure and the systolic pressure at apnea, Δ down is the difference between the systolic pressure at apnea and the minimal value of systolic pressure, during the respiratory cycle). The total variation (Δ up plus Δ down) over one respiratory cycle (i.e. the difference between the maximal and minimal values of the systolic pressure) is called systolic pressure variation (SPV). In one study, in which patients were mechanically ventilated following vascular surgery, the mean SPV, Δ up and Δ down were found to be 8.6, 2.7, and 5.9 mmHg respectively. In another study in ICU patients the mean SPV was 9.2 mmHg and correlated significantly with the pulmonary artery occlusion pressure. During active hemorrhage, it was found that the removal of 1000 mL of blood was associated with a systolic pressure variation of 19.6 mmHg, which decreased by about 8.6 mmHg after the first 500 mL volume was replaced. Further volume resuscitation appeared to be adequate when a fluid challenge reduced SPV to 5 mmHg or less, reduced Δ down to 2 mmHg or less, or produced reduction in SPV or Δ down of 2 mmHg or less. However, these guidelines may not be valid in patients with severe lung disease or poor ventricular function. A significant Δ down segment may also appear in the presence of large tidal volumes, low chest wall compliance and nodal rhythm.

10. **Heart rate and rhythm (new arrhythmias, tachycardia, bradycardia). Monitor every 1 hour.**

    Anxiety, inadequate sedation, drugs, $\downarrow PaO_2$, $\downarrow PaCO_2$, $\uparrow PaCO_2$ (check SpO_2, ABG, patient-ventilator system), decreased intravascular volume. Evaluate other haemodynamic parameters for the adequacy of perfusion.

11. **Urinary output. Monitor every 1 hour.**
    - Decreased urine output: inadequate perfusion of kidneys, low intravascular volume, and onset of acute renal failure.
    - Increased urine output: (> 50 mL/hr) in the absence of diuretics or diuretic phase of renal failure: overhydration.
    - Normal urine output: 0.5 to 1.0 mL/kg/hr in adults, 1 mL/kg/hr in children.

12. **Temperature. Monitor every 8 hours.**
    - Fever: overheated humidifier, atelectasis, infection, increased metabolic rate caused by increased inspiratory effort or patient ventilator asynchrony.
    - Geriatric patients have a lower body temperature, and are more easily influenced by enviromental temperature (as in new borns and infants) (as in newborns and infants). In patients over 90 years of age, body temperature of 96°F to 97°F may be normal.
    - Hypothermia: decreased environmental temperature, infection (especially in newborns).
    - Axillary temperature is approximately 0.5°C lower than oral temperature, and rectal temperature (related more closely to core body temperature) is approximately 0.5°C higher than the oral temperature.

13. **Respiratory rate. Monitor every 1-4 hours.**

    Respiratory rate may be influenced by altered ventilator settings, changes in metabolic needs (anxiety, stress, infection, heart failure, pulmonary edema, hypoglycaemia, hypo-or hyper-thermia, sleep), decreased PaO_2, increased $PaCO_2$, drugs (sedatives, narcotics, anesthetic agents), unsuccessful weaning (rapid shallow breathing), increased intracranial pressure.

14. **Weight gain, peripheral edema. Monitor daily.**
    - Heart failure, hypoproteinaemia (low oncotic pressure), venous or lymphatic obstruction, sepsis, shock, trauma etc. (altered capillary permeability).
    - Increasing weight does not necessarily mean an adequate intravascular volume. The patient could be hypovolaemic, because of shifting of fluid to the tissues or to "third space".

15. **Capillary refill time.**

    Normally, after a 5 second compression of the nail bed, the pink colour should return to the blanched area within 3 seconds. If it takes longer, it indicates vasoconstriction or reduced cardiac output with decreased digital perfusion. This may not be reliable when the room temperature is low.

16. Oxygen saturation with pulse oximeter. Monitor continuously.

17. End tidal CO_2.

18. Central venous pressure.
    See Chapter 10.

Physical examination

19. Air leak around ETT. Monitor every 1-2 hours.
    - Deflated/ruptured cuff.
    - ETT lying above vocal cords.

20. Airway secretions. Monitor with every suction.
    - Secretions thick: Inadequate humidity.
    - Secretions copious, thin: Increased humidity, infection, draining of fluid from tubing into trachea (reposition ventilator tubings).
    - Observe the colour of secretions.

21. Breath sounds. Monitor every 1-4 hours.
    - Unilateral decreased breath sounds: blocked ETT, ETT migration into a mainstem bronchus, air, blood, or other fluid in the pleural space, pneumonia.
    - Decreased breath sounds and late inspiratory crackles in the dependent region: atelectasis or any condition of lung that causes a loss of volume (restrictive disorder).
    - Decreased (or absent) breath sounds along with mediastinal shift: tension pneumothorax (suspect in any patient who is difficult to ventilate during CPR or who deteriorates while being ventilated, especially when high peak pressures and PEEP are being used).
    - Presence of wheeze: asthma, congestive heart failure, bronchitis, high flow rate.
    - Inspiratory and expiratory crackles present: bronchitis, respiratory infections and secretions.

22. Subcutaneous emphysema. Monitor every 2-4 hours.
    - Mechanical ventilation of a patient with fresh tracheostomy, laceration of lung or chest wall secondary to trauma or surgery, tension pneumothorax.

23. Air leak via chest tube. Monitor every 1-4 hours.
    - New pneumothorax: Obtain and evaluate X-ray chest and ABG.
    - Broncho-pleural fistula: Change ventilatory settings if required.

24. Skin temperature.
    - Various factors which influence the temperature of skin (especially of feet and hands) are perfusion to the extremity, core temperature of body and environmental temperature. Normally the toe temperature should be at least 2°C warmer than the ambient temperature. A difference of less than

2°C indicates hypoperfusion and a difference of less than 0.5°C indicates a life-threatening situation resulting from reduced perfusion.

- Cold and clammy skin occurs as a result of sympathetic stimulation, and is a compensatory mechanism for a decrease in cardiac output. It may indicate impending shock. A rather practical way to assess a change in temperature is by touching the skin. Back of the hand is moved slowly up the leg starting from the foot and the point or line of temperature change is marked. Though it does not provide an indication of the temperature of the extremity but it gives a fair idea of the change in cardiac output and peripheral perfusion after initiating therapy. If therapy is successful in improving peripheral perfusion, the line of temperature change moves down the leg towards the foot, however, if peripheral perfusion does not improve, the line stays in the same place or advances up the leg and thigh as vasoconstriction increases.

25. Gastric distension. Monitor every 1-4 hours.

Malpositioning of ETT, air swallowing, excessive inspiratory effort by the patient, nutritional intolerance, blocked nasogastric tube.

Laboratory investigations

26. Arterial blood gas (ABG) analysis.

Evaluate with every change in ventilator setting or with any unexplained change in patient's condition.

27. Serum electrolytes.

Daily or twice weekly.

28. Blood urea, serum creatinine.

Twice a week or daily.

29. Liver function tests.

Weekly or twice a week.

30. X-ray chest.

Daily.

31. Cultures from various sites.

As the condition demands. Twice a week or less often.

References

1. Coriat P, Vrillon M, Perel A, et al. A comparison of systolic pressure variations and echocardiographic estimates of end-diastolic left ventricular size in patients after aortic surgery. Anesth Analg 1994; 78:46-53.
2. DelGuercia LRM, Cohn JD. Monitoring: methods and significance, Surg Clin North Am 1976; 56:977.
3. Hudson LD. Monitoring of critically ill patients: conference summary. Respir Care 1985;30:628.
4. Malinowski T. Respiratory monitoring in the intensive care unit. In: Wilkins RL, Krider SJ, Sheldon RL (eds). Clinical Assessment in Respiratory Care. 4ed., St. Louis: Mosby, 2000, pp 281-305.
5. Marik PE. The systolic pressure variation as an indicator of pulmonary capillary wedge pressure in ventilated patients. Anaesth Intensive Care 1993; 21:405-408.

6. Perel A, Pizov R, Cotev S. The systolic pressure variation is a sensitive indicator of hypovolemia in ventilated dogs subjected to graded hemorrhage. Anesthesiology 1987; 67:498-502.

7. Pinsky MR, Vincent JL, Smet JMD. Estimating left ventricular filling pressure during positive end-expiratory pressure in humans. Am Rev Respir Dis 1991; 143:25-31.

8. Pizov R, Ya'ari Y, Perel A. The arterial pressure waveform during acute ventricular failure and synchronized external chest compression. Anesth Analg 1989; 68:150-156.

9. Rooke GA, Scwid HA, Shapira Y. The effect of graded hemorrhage and intravascular volume replacement on systolic pressure variations in humans during mechanical and spontaneous ventilation. Anesth Analg 1995; 80:925-932.

10. Shoemaker WC. Routine clinical monitoring in acute illness. In: Shoemaker WC, Velmachos GC, Demetriades D (eds). Procedures and monitoring for critically ill. New Delhi: Harcourt (India), 2002; pp 155-166.

11. Tobin MJ. Respiratory monitoring in the intensive care unit. Am Rev Respir Dis 1988;138:1625.

Introduction

When routine monitoring of the ventilator discloses a problem or a potential problem, a search for the cause should begin. The following guidelines offer some common causes/situations to initially look for in case of a particular problem. However, there will be situations when one may not be able to discover the cause of a problem. That is the time when one needs to consult the senior faculty member or a technical person to look into the internal function of the ventilator.

GUIDELINES FOR ANALYSING THE CLUES

Clues and possible common causes

1. Decreased minute or tidal volume alarm.
   - Patient not connected to the ventilator.
   - Leaks – around ETT, around humidifier, through the chest tube and in the breathing circuit.
   - Malfunctioning flow sensor.
   - Altered settings.
   - Decreased patient triggered respiratory rate.
   - Airway secretions.
   - Decreased lung compliance.
   - Dynamic hyperinflation.

2. Increased minute or tidal volume alarm.
   - Increased patient –triggered respiratory rate.
   - Malfunctioning flow sensor.
   - Altered settings (e.g. decreased trigger sensitivity).
   - Patient getting nebulized with an external nebulizer.
   - Increased lung compliance.
   - Hypoxia.

3. Sudden increase in peak inspiratory pressure.
   - Artificial airway: Secretions, kinking or malpositioning of ETT, mucosal plugging, cuff herniation.
   - Ventilator circuit: Water/condensate in tubing, kinked circuit tubing, high inspiratory flow rate.
   - Patient factors: Bronchospasm, pneumothorax, abdominal distension,

diaphragmatic and intercostal muscles disco-ordination, active expiration, restlessness, pain, change in position from supine to lateral or prone.

4. Sudden decrease in peak inspiratory pressure.
   - Low gas inlet pressure, discontinuation of source gases.
   - Leaks in the system.
   - Clearing of secretions.
   - Relief of bronchospasm.

5. Increase in plateau pressure.
   - Auto-PEEP, severe hyperinflation.
   - Stiffness of lungs (e.g. pneumonia or congestive heart failure).

6. Increased peak-plateau pressure difference (Fig. 38.1, 38.2).
   - Bronchospasm.
   - Narrowing/kinking of ETT.

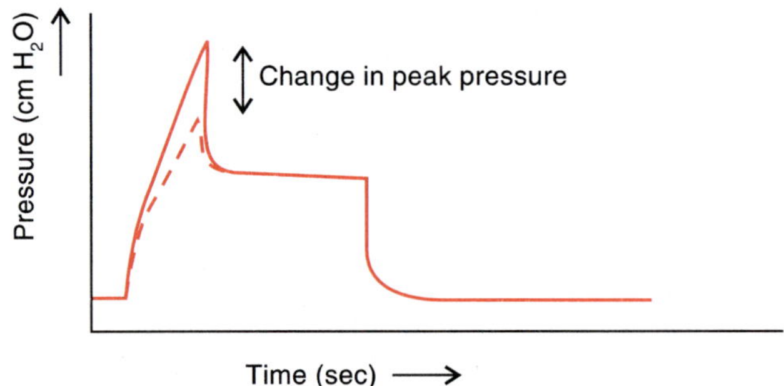

Fig. 38.1: Pressure-time diagram for volume controlled, constant flow ventilation: When the inspiratory airway resistance changes, the peak pressure changes in the same direction and the plateau pressure remains the same.

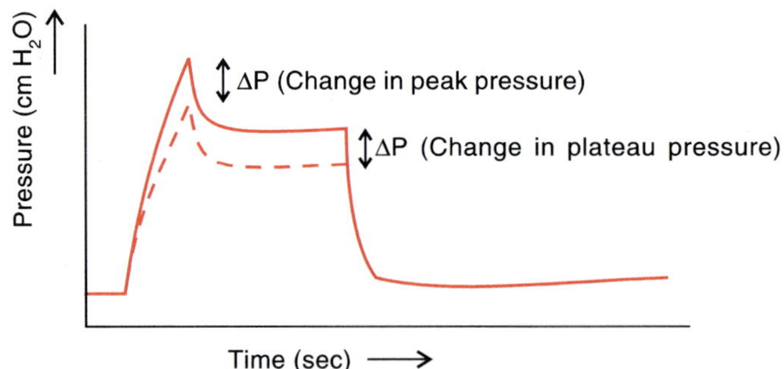

Fig. 38.2: Pressure-time diagram for volume controlled, constant flow ventilation: With changes in compliance, the peak and plateau pressures change by the same amount of the pressure difference ΔP.
increasing compliance → both pressures fall
decreasing compliance → both pressures rise

- Airway edema.
- Mucosal plugging.

7. Change in respiratory rate.
    - Altered settings.
    - Hypoxia.
    - Change in metabolic demand.
    - Drugs (sedatives, narcotics).
    - Exhaustion during weaning trial.

8. Change in oxygen concentration.
    - Oxygen sensor malfunction.
    - Pipeline failure/empty cylinder.

9. Altered I:E ratio.
    - Altered inspiratory flow rate.
    - Leaks in the system.
    - Airway secretions (pressure limited ventilation).

References

1. AARC consensus group. Essentials of mechanical ventilation. Respir Care 1992; 37:1001-1009.
2. Branson RD. Monitoring ventilator function. Critical Care Clin 1995; 11(1): 127-149.
3. Durbin CG. Monitoring gas exchange: Clinical effectiveness and cost considerations. Respir Care 1994; 39(2): 123-137.
4. MacIntyre NR. Ventilator monitors, displays, and alarms. In: MacIntyre NR, Branson RD (eds). Mechanical Ventilation. Philadelphia: Saunders, 2000, pp 131-145.
5. MacIntyre NR, Day SD. Essentials for ventilator-alarm systems. Respir Care 1992; 37:1108-1112.
6. Martz KV, Joiner J, Shepherd RM. Management of the patient-ventilator system. St, Louis: Mosby, 1979.
7. Nelson EJ, Morton EA, Hunter PM. Critical Care Respiratory Therapy. Bosten: Little, Brown 1983.
8. Pilbeam SP. Introduction to ventilators. In: Cairo JM, Pilbeam SP (eds). Respiratory Care Equipment, 6ed. St Louis: Mosby, 1999, pp 272-339.
9. Reily DJ, Lanken PN. Ventilator alarm situations. In: Lanken PN (ed). The intensive Care Unit Manual. Philadelphia: Saunders, 2001, pp 553-561.

Application and Weaning of Positive End-expiratory Pressure (PEEP)

Introduction

- Functional residual capacity (FRC) is markedly decreased (20-40% of predicted value) in patients with acute respiratory failure due to cardiogenic or non-cardiogenic pulmonary edema. The decrease in FRC results from a reduction in the number of ventilatory alveoli, consequent to terminal airspace flooding and collapse. The collapsed airways are: (a) A source of ventilation / perfusion mismatch leading to hypoxaemia, and, (b) are tremendously difficult to reinflate, leading to increased work of breathing and oxygen consumption.
These changes are accompanied by a lower compliance and a more flat pressure-volume (P-V) curve compared to that in normal subjects. The main effect of application of PEEP on the respiratory system of the patients with acute respiratory failure is to increase the abnormally low FRC, as a result of recruiting previously flooded and collapsed alveoli. It also causes a redistribution of extravasated lung water from the alveoli to the compliant interstitial regions. Furthermore, it keeps terminal airspaces open especially during expiration, when these airspaces tend to collapse due to the weight of the flooded airspaces.
- At low levels of PEEP, mechanical tidal ventilation is preferentially distributed to the non-dependent regions of the lung. With increasing PEEP, more tidal volume is shifted to the dependent regions in the supine patient.
- PEEP reduces the severity of ventilation-induced lung injury by keeping the alveoli open and avoiding the shear stress and parenchymal injury because of repetitive alveolar opening (during inspiration) and collapse (during expiration).
- The optimal level of PEEP is that which puts the majority of lung units on the favourable part of the pressure-volume curve (remember, each lung unit has a different P-V curve) and achieves the best balance between the beneficial and the potentially harmful effects of PEEP. The beneficial effects of PEEP include: (a) Alveolar recruitment, (b) vascular derecruitment, (c) improvement of PaO_2, (d) protection against ventilator- induced lung injury, and (e) reduction of inspiratory workload. Adverse effects of PEEP include: (a) Overdistension of more compliant alveoli (barotrauma and increased dead space), (b) depression of cardiac output (decreased delivery of oxygen), and (c) reduction of inspiratory muscle force.
- The major aims of PEEP in an acute respiratory failure are to improve oxygenation in acute hypoxaemic failure, and to unload inspiratory muscles

and minimize inspiratory work in cases of acute exacerbation of chronic obstructive pulmonary disease (COPD).

- Differing concepts have been used to define optimal PEEP over the last three decades. Some of these are as follows:

  (a) In 1975, it was pointed out that changes in the delivery of oxygen should be used as the reference standard for the evaluation of PEEP. The level of PEEP corresponding to the highest oxygen delivery was labelled as optimal PEEP. These conclusions were subsequently challenged.

  (b) Later, the concept of Super–PEEP was described. It was reasoned that PEEP should be increased until intrapulmonary shunt decreases below 15% of the cardiac output and intravenous fluid therapy and vasopressors be administered to maintain cardiac output. This strategy required very high levels of PEEP (up to 43-57 cm H_2O) and did not gain popularity.

  (c) Pulmonary mechanical indicators of the optimal alveolar inflation point determine PEEP. This refers to the inflation pressure at which lung compliance no longer increases or remains constant but instead begins to decrease, indicating that the pressure increases are no longer opening collapsed alveoli but are merely inflating or over inflating alveoli that are already open. A number of methods have been described to determine this lung compliance inflection point.

  (i) While measuring lung compliance (VT/Pplat) at increasing levels of PEEP with a constant VT, inspiratory flow, and respiratory rate, optimal PEEP is that PEEP level at which compliance begins to decrease. Intrinsic PEEP, if present, should be subtracted from Pplat for calculation of compliance.

  (ii) On constructing a static pressure-volume curve by slow progressive inflation of the lungs using a large-volume syringe, optimal PEEP corresponds to the pressure just above the lower inflection point on the inspiratory limb of P-V curve (Fig. 39.1). However, such an inflection

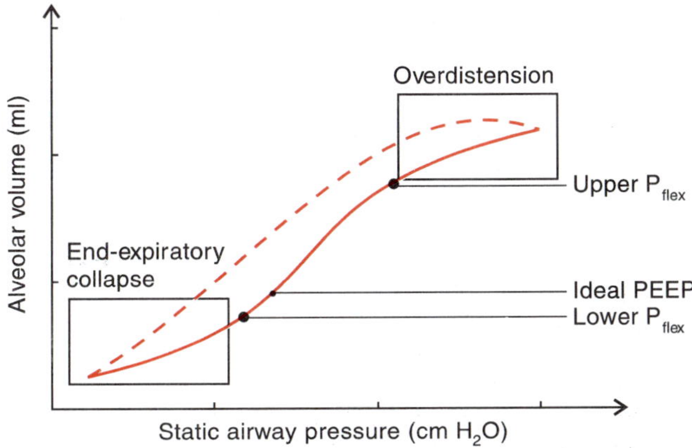

Fig. 39.1: Static pressure-volume curve demonstrating an upper and a lower inflection point (upper P$_{flex}$ and lower P$_{flex}$) in patients with ARDS. The solid line is the inflation limb and the dotted line the deflation limb. The upper box indicates the alveolar volume and pressure at which alveolar distension may contribute to lung injury. The lower box indicates the alveolar volume and pressure at which end-expiratory alveolar collapse occurs. PEEP should be set above the lower inflection point to prevent repeated alveolar collapse and opening during the ventilatory cycle.

point is usually present only in patients with pulmonary edema and in the early stages of ARDS, so the method has a limited sphere of application. The inflection point may also be due to the presence of intrinsic PEEP.

(iii) A simple, more practical method for day-to-day use has been described. This method recognizes that at constant VT, inspiratory flow and respiratory rate, inspiratory resistance changes very little with increase in PEEP, and peak airway pressure (PIP) will be higher than plateau airway pressure (Pplat) by a constant amount, when PEEP is increased. Thus, when PEEP is gradually increased, increase in PIP, which is similar to or lesser than the increase in PEEP, suggests constant or increasing compliance (suggesting alveolar recruitment), whereas a PIP increment larger than the PEEP increment, suggests decreasing compliance. Optimal PEEP is the level of PEEP less than that which induces an increment in PIP that is greater than the PEEP increment.

- The most appropriate method of determining PEEP level during a lung protective ventilatory strategy has not been established. In one of the studies, three approaches for determining PEEP level after a recruitment manoeuvre were compared. These were: (i) 2 cm H_2O above the lower inflection point on the inflation pressure-volume curve, (ii) at the point of maximum curvature on the deflation pressure-volume curve, and (iii) at the PEEP level that maintained target arterial oxygen partial pressure at a fraction of inspired oxygen of 0.5. It was found that although generating higher plateau pressure, PEEP 2 cm H_2O above the lower inflection point resulted in the best gas exchange; PEEP set 2 cm H_2O above the lower inflection point and the PEEP set at the point of maximum curvature, resulted in less lung injury as evaluated by histologic and inflammatory mediator insult when compared to PEEP setting based on maintaining target arterial oxygen partial pressure. PEEP based solely on oxygenation response (group iii), despite a lower plateau pressure, resulted in progressive deterioration in gas exchange, marked inflammatory mediator response, and lung injury.

GUIDELINES FOR APPLICATION OF PEEP

1. **Patient having PaO_2 > 60 mm Hg with FiO_2 < 0.5.**

    No more than a normal physiological PEEP (3-5 cm H_2O) is required (Remember, intubation bypasses the larynx). The major goal of PEEP therapy is to maintain a PaO_2 of more than 60-70 mm Hg at FiO_2 < 0.5. It is already being met.

2. **Inquire if the patient is adapted to a low PaO_2.**

    In a patient who is chronically hypoxaemic, and adapted to low a PaO_2, e.g. COPD, no increase in PEEP is required, unless PEEP is added to counterbalance intrinsic PEEP to decrease the work of breathing.

3. **Determine if minute ventilation is adequate with optimal respiratory rate. Review I:E ratio.**

Decreased minute volume can be the cause of a decreased PaO_2 and increased $PaCO_2$.

4. **Evaluate cardiac status.**

   Fluctuations in blood pressure and unexplained tachycardia could indicate hypovolaemia or cardiac dysfunction. Addition of PEEP may aggravate the problem. These should be corrected, whenever possible, before increasing PEEP.

5. **Set FiO_2 at 1.0. Record baseline blood pressure, peak airway pressure (PIP), plateau airway pressure (Pplat), compliance (C), resistance (R), ABG, PaO_2/FiO_2, and SpO_2.**

   Since the patient is already sick, it is necessary to establish baseline values, as PEEP may have adverse effects.

6. **Keep tidal volume, inspiratory flow and respiratory rate constant.**

   It is presumed that with these parameters being kept constant, change in resistance will be very little and changes in PIP will be proportionately higher by a constant amount, as PEEP is increased.

7. **Add PEEP in steps of 3-5 cm H_2O, wait for 5-10 minutes.**

   While adding PEEP, keep a watch on various parameters.

8. **Measure blood pressure, PIP, Pplat, C, R, cardiac rhythm, and SpO_2 at regular intervals, and for 5-10 minutes after each step.**
   - PIP increase should either be equal to or smaller than the increase in PEEP, suggesting constant or increasing compliance (alveolar recruitment).
   - Increase in PEEP may also cause a decreased cardiac output resulting in decreased blood pressure and oxygen saturation.

9. **PIP increases more than the PEEP increment.**

   This suggests a decreasing compliance (over inflation), or bronchoconstriction (increased airway resistance), secretions, or kinked endotracheal tube. Compare resistance with baseline value, look for rhonchi/wheeze and take corrective measures.

10. **Reduce the PEEP by 2-3 cm H_2O.**

    Optimal PEEP is the level of PEEP less than that which induces an increase in PIP that is greater than the PEEP increment.

11. **Obtain an ABG after 20 minutes.**

    Look for any improvement in PaO_2 and PaO_2/FiO_2 ratio as compared to baseline values.

12. **Reduce FiO_2 in steps until PaO_2 is 60-65 mm Hg and SpO_2>90%.**

    The aim is to maintain a desired PaO_2 and SpO_2 at a minimum safe FiO_2. Perform recruitment-manoeuvre and set the PEEP and FiO_2 to the identified level.

13. **Retreat and resume the original level of PEEP.**
    - If at any time between point 7 to 11, SpO_2 drops or the patient exhibits signs of exhausion (e.g. increase in respiratory rate, increased use of accessory muscles, tachycardia, arrhythmias, or alterations in blood pressure), resume the original level of PEEP.

- Repeat the steps, after the patient is stable and other causes of deterioration have been managed.

14. Wean PEEP therapy.

- Once the pulmonary pathology has resolved and there is adequate gas exchange at an $FiO_2 < 0.5$, wean PEEP therapy slowly and in steps, as described later.

A more conservative approach of applying PEEP is to titrate it with SpO_2. Perform a recruitment manoeuvre (RM) and set the PEEP at 20 cm H_2O. Reduce the FiO_2 to the lowest level maintaining the SpO_2 between 90 and 95%. Following this, decrease the PEEP by 2-3 cm H_2O every 20-30 minutes until the patient desaturates. The PEEP level before desaturation is the PEEP level that prevents the majority of derecruitment. Once this is identified, the RM is repeated, and the PEEP and FiO_2 are reset to the identified level.

GUIDELINES FOR WEANING PEEP

1. Perform clinical assessment.
   Obtain baseline ABG.
   - Patient should be haemodynamically stable. Underying pathology should have settled.
   - $PaO_2 \geq 80$ mm Hg with $FiO_2 \leq 0.4$.
   - No change in PEEP level during the past 12 hours.

2. Reduce PEEP by 5 cm H_2O (reduce by 2.5 cm H_2O if oxygenation is borderline).

3. Obtain ABG after 5 minutes and return PEEP to the previous level while awaiting ABG report.
   - If the patient's PaO_2 falls by less than 20% of that at the previous PEEP level, then the patient is ready to tolerate the lower PEEP level. Repeat the assessment for further decrease in PEEP in the same manner, after 12 hours.
   - If the reduction in PaO_2 is more than 20%, continue with previous PEEP. Wait, re-evaluate and try again (steps 2 and 3) after 6-12 hours.

4. When patient is stable at 4-5 cm H_2O PEEP only, consider T-piece trial (if other criteria are also being met).
   - When T-piece trial is successful, consider criteria for extubation.
   - If reducing PEEP to zero (i.e. on T-piece trial) results in worsening of condition, leave the patient at 5 cm H_2O until fit for extubation. Extubate and apply 5 cm H_2O of CPAP by mask.

References

1. Amato MBP, Barbas CSV, Medeiros DM, et al. Effect of a protective-ventilation strategy on mortality in the acute respiratory distress syndrome. N Engl J Med 1998; 338:347-354.

2. Benito S, Lemaire F. Pulmonary pressure–volume relationship in acute respiratory distress syndrome in adults: role of positive end expiratory pressure. J Crit Care 1990; 5:27-34.

3. Gattinoni L, Pesenti A, Avalli L, et al. Pressure-volume curve of total respiratory system in acute respiratory failure. Am Rev Respir Dis 1987; 136: 730-6.

4. Gattinoni L, Mascheroni D, Torresin A, et al. Morphological response to positive end expiratory pressure in acute respiratory failure: computerized tomography study. Intensive Care Med 1986; 12: 137-42.

5. Hudson LD, Weaver LJ, Haish CE, et al. Positive end-expiratory pressure: reduction and withdrawal. Respir Care 1988; 33:613-617.

6. Lu Q, Rouby JJ. Measurement of pressure-volume curves in patients on mechanical ventilation: methods and significance. Crit Care 2000; 4:91-100.

7. Marcy T, Marini J. Inverse ratio ventilation in ARDS: rationale and implementation. Chest 1991; 100: 494.

8. Neff MJ, Steinberg KP. Acute respiratory distress syndrome. In: Hess DR, MacIntyre NR, Mishoe SC, et al (eds). Respiratory Care: Principles and practice. Philadelphia: Saunders, pp 1022-1034.

9. Rossi A, Renieri MV. Positive end-expiratory pressure. In: Tobin MJ(ed) Principles and Practice of Mechanical Ventilation, New York: McGraw-Hill, 1994, pp 259-303.

10. Slusky AS. Consensus conference on mechanical ventilation. Intensive Care Med 1994; Part1, 20:64-79; Part II, 20:150-162.

11. Smith TC, Marini JJ. Impact of PEEP on lung mechanics and work of breathing in severe airflow obstruction. J Appl Physiol 1988; 65:1488-1499.

12. Steinberg KP, Pierson DJ, Clinical approach to the patient with acute oxygenation failure. In: Pierson DJ, Kacmarek RM. Foundation of respiratory care. New York: Churchill Livingstone, 1992, pp 721-739.

13. Suter P, Fairley H, Insenberg M. Optimum end-expiratory airway pressure in patients with acute pulmonary failure. N Engl J Med 1975; 292: 2984-89.

14. Takeuchi M, Goddon S, Dolhnikoff M, et al. Set positive end-expiratory pressure during protective ventilation affects lung injury. Anesthesiology 2002; 97:682-692.

15. Tobin MJ, Lodato RF. PEEP, Auto-PEEP, and waterfalls. Chest 1989; 96:449-451.

16. Tuxen DV. Permissive hypercapnia. In: Tobin MJ (ed). Principles and Practice of mechanical ventilation, New York: McGraw-Hill, 1994, pp 371-392.

Recruitment Manoeuvres 40

Introduction

- Recruitment manoeuvres (RMs) are used to establish initial alveolar patency that then can be maintained at a lower tidal pressure and positive end expiratory pressure (PEEP) levels, than would otherwise be required. They are based on the principle that acutely injured lung units can be held open at pressures well below those needed to open them.
- Alveoli or small airways require much higher pressures to reinflate them once collapsed than to maintain inflation, especially in surfactant –depleted lungs, as expected from Laplace's law. Laplace's law states that the pressure generated within a spherical bubble by surface tension forces is equal to 4 t/r, where t is the surface tension and r the radius of the sphere. The air-liquid interface in the small airway, proximal to a collapsed alveolus, has a very small radius of curvature, so a high pressure is required (the opening pressure) to advance this interface and inflate the alveolus, especially in surfactant-depleted lungs. Once the alveolus is inflated to a normal or high volume, the radius of curvature is much larger, and so the pressure required to overcome surface tension forces is much less.
- A number of strategies have been reported as recruitment manoeuvres (RMs). These include increasing the PEEP setting on the ventilator, using sustained inflation, use of frequent sighs on the ventilator, high frequency oscillation, use of ventilator modes that encourage spontaneous breathing, and prone positioning.
- The success of RMs depends on whether the pathophysiology of ARDS is primarily atelectasis, consolidation, or edema. If the underlying pathology is atelectasis, then one might expect a large benefit from RMs. ARDS due to extrapulmonary causes (sepsis, trauma etc) can be recruited more easily than pulmonary ARDS. In pulmonary ARDS (e.g. associated with pneumonia), not only are RMs less effective, but may even be harmful because they may cause over-distension injury to the unaffected lung. In patients with brain injury, RMs marginally improve arterial oxygenation and may adversely affect cerebral haemodynamics.
- Contraindications to performing RMs include haemodynamic instability, barotrauma, localized atelectasis (e.g. unilateral lung disease), and bullous lung disease.
- Although performing RMs in the course of ARDS/ALI, regardless of the etiology, is recommended, many questions still remain to be answered: (a) The specific

group of patients in which RMs show maximum benefit, (b) how frequently should RMs be performed, (c) which technique or a combination of techniques is best, (d) how to monitor the effect of recruitment, (e) are these RMs effective in terms of terminal outcome, and (f) do they actually prevent lung injury and promote repair.

GUIDELINES FOR RECRUITMENT MANOEUVRES

1. **Perform RM whenever the lung is derecruited or the ventilator disconnected.**
    In ARDS/ALI, ventilator disconnection can rapidly lead to derecruitment and severe hypoxaemia. RM should also be performed whenever there is sustained (>5 minutes) decrease in SpO_2. These patients should preferably be managed with closed suction catheters and aerosol therapy adaptors to avoid ventilator disconnection.

2. **Expect a different response to different recruitment pressures in an individual patient.**
    The successful response is more likely in early ARDS (within 1-2 days) and in those without impairment in chest wall mechanics. As ARDS progresses, the lungs become more and more fibrotic, leading to reduced efficacy of RMs in improving PaO_2 and an increased risk of barotrauma.

3. **Monitor the patient before initiating and while performing a recruitment manoeuvre.**
    Monitor arterial pressure, heart rate and rhythm, and oxygen saturation.

4. **Use sedation.**
    Sedation ensures passive inflation during the recruitment phase.

5. **Ensure haemodynamic stability.**
    Application of high-sustained airway pressure can give rise to haemodynamic compromise and development of barotrauma.

6. **Set the FiO_2 to 1.0.**
    This ensures oxygenation.

7. **Wait for 10-15 minutes.**

8. **Use 30 cm H_2O CPAP for 30-40 seconds (or 10 cm H_2O above the plateau pressure level in a given patient).**
    Lungs may have recruitable alveoli, which may not be recruited with normal tidal ventilation and normal inspiratory time. This is because of the viscosity of the fluid lining the collapsed lung, the high surface tension of these units, and parenchymal tethering. Collapsed lung units, whether healthy or injured, require both-high airway pressure and longer time to recruit. Therefore, when applied, two conditions must be met for a successful RM: (a) The pressure applied must be in excess of the plateau pressure, and (b) the pressure must be sustained in order to inflate lung units with long time constants.

9. **If the response is inadequate and there is no haemodynamic instability, wait for 10-15 minutes, repeat the manoeuvre with 35 cm H_2O CPAP for 30-40 seconds.**

Successful RM should result in improved oxygenation, reduced end-tidal CO_2 and improved compliance. A highly successful series of RMs should result in a PaO_2/FiO_2 ratio >300.

10. If the response is still inadequate, but tolerance is good, wait for 15 minutes, and repeat the manoeuvre with 40 cm H_2O CPAP for 30-40 seconds.

11. If unresponsive, wait for 15 minutes, and then repeat the RM with 20 cm H_2O pressure control with 30 cm H_2O PEEP, 1:E ratio of 1:1, rate 10/min for 2 minutes. Some pulmonary units have high opening pressures.

12. If still unresponsive, wait for 15-20 minutes, and then repeat the RM with 20 cm H_2O pressure control with 40 cm H_2O PEEP, I:E ratio of 1:1, rate 10/min for 2 minutes.

13. If still patient does not respond, consider other measures for recruitment, e.g. prone position.

    Prone position sustains a high recruiting force in the dorsal regions, which are compressed in the supine position by a higher local pleural pressure and by the weight of the heart and mediastinal contents. Arterial oxygenation improves in 50% to 70% of ARDS patients in the prone position.

14. Reset the ventilator.

    After performing a recruitment manoeuvre, put the patient back on the ventilator with previous settings, which were being used prior to performing the manoeuvre.

15. Monitor the patient.

    Monitor the patient carefully for the expected response to a successful recruitment manoeuvre.

16. Repeat the RM.

    Even when successful, the benefits of each RM tend to fade over time. Derecruitment could be because of reabsorption atelectasis caused by low ventilation/perfusion ratios or lack of adequate PEEP level to maintain the patency of alveoli, opened by a recruitment manoeuvre.

References

1. Albert RK, Hubmayr RD. The prone position eliminates compression of the lungs by the heart. Am J Respir Crit Care 2000; 161:1660-1665.
2. Barbas CSV. Lung recruitment manoeuvres in acute respiratory distress syndrome and facilitating resolution. Crit Care Med 2003;31(suppl): S265-S271.
3. Barbas CSV, Silva E, Garrido A, et al. Recruitment manoeuvres with different pressure control levels in ARDS patients. AM J Respir Crit Care 2001; 163:A163.
4. Bein T, et al. Lung recruitment manoeuvre in patients with cerebral injury effect of intracranial pressure and cerebral metabolism. Intensive Care Med 2002; 28:554-558.
5. Crotti S, mascheroni D, Caironi P, et al. Recruitment and derecruitment during acute respiratory failure. A clinical study. Am J Respir Crit Care Med 2001; 164:131-140.

6. Foti G, Cereda M, Sparacino ME, et al. Effects of periodic lung recruitment manoeuvres on gas exchange and respiratory mechanics in mechanically ventilated acute respiratory distress syndrome (ARDS) patients. Intensive Care Med 2000; 26:501-507.

7. Grasso S, Mascia L, Del Turco M, et al. Effects of recruiting manoeuvres in patients with acute respiratory distress syndrome ventilated with protective ventilatory strategy. Anesthesiology 2002; 96; 795-802.

8. Hess DR, Bigatello LM. Lung Recruitment: the role of recruitment manoeuvres. Respir Care 2002; 47:303-318.

9. Mickling KG. The pressure-volume curve is greatly modified by recruitment: a mathematical model of ARDS lungs. Am J Respir Crit Care Med 1998; 154:194-202.

10. Hubmayr RD. Perspective on lung injury and recruitment. A skeptical look at the opening and collapse story. Am J Respir Crit Care Med 2002; 156:1647-1653.

11. Lachmann B. Open up the lung and keep the lung open. Intensive Care Med 1992; 18:319-321.

12. Lapinsky SE, et al. Safety and efficacy of a sustained inflation for alveolar recruitment in adults with respiratory failure. Intensive Care Med 1999; 25:1297-1301.

13. Marini JJ. Efficacy of lung recruiting manoeuvres: It's all relative. Crit Care Med 2003; 31(2): 641-642.

14. Marini JJ. Recruitment manoeuvres to achieve an "open lung" –whether and how? Crit Care Med 2001; 29:16471648.

15. Medoff BD Harris RS, KesselmanH et al. Use of recruitment manoeuvres and high positive end-expiratory pressure in a patient with acute respiratory distress syndrome. Crit Care Med 2000; 28:1210-1216.

16. Patroniti N, Foti G, Cortinovis B, et al. Sigh improves gas exchange and lung volume in patients with acute respiratory distress syndrome undergoing pressure support ventilation. Anesthesiology 2002; 96:788-794.

17. Pelosi P, Cadringher P, Bottino N et al. Sigh in acute respiratory distress syndrome. Am J Respir Crit Care Med 1999; 159:872-880.

18. Pelosi P, Goldner M, McKibben A, et al. Recruitment and derecruitment during acute respiratory failure: An experimental study. Am J Respir Crit Care 2002; 164:122-130.

19. Rimiensberger PC, Pache JC, McKerlie C, et al. Lung recruitment and lung volume maintenance: a strategy for improving oxygenation and preventing lung injury during both conventional mechanical ventilation and high frequency oscillation. Intensive Care Medicine 2000; 26:745-755.

20. Suter PM. Does the advent of (new) low tidal volumes bring the (old) sigh back to the intensive care unit. Anesthesiology 2002; 96:783-784.

21. Takeuchi M, Goddon S, Dolknikoff M, et al. Set positive end-expiratory pressure during protective ventilation affects lung Injury. Anesthesiology 2002; 97:682-692.

22. Villagra A, et al. Recruitment manoeuvres during lung protective ventilation in acute respiratory distress syndrome. Am J Respir Crit Care Med 2002; 165:165-170.

Dynamic Hyperinflation and Auto-PEEP 41

Introduction

- Dynamic hyperinflation (DH) is defined as the failure of lung volume to return to passive FRC (volume at which elastic recoil equals external PEEP), prior to onset of the next inspiration. Whenever this happens, alveolar pressure remains higher than the external PEEP throughout expiration, and unless airways completely collapse, expiratory flow continues till the onset of next inspiration.
- Auto-PEEP is the difference between the alveolar pressure and the external airway pressure at end expiration. Whenever the expiratory flow continues until the end of expiration, a difference in the pressures (i.e. auto-PEEP) will always exist. In the passive patient, this can result only from dynamic hyperinflation (DH) (Fig. 41.1), since alveolar pressure in this case reflects only passive elastic recoil, and a gradient in the pressures means that lung volume did not return to passive FRC.

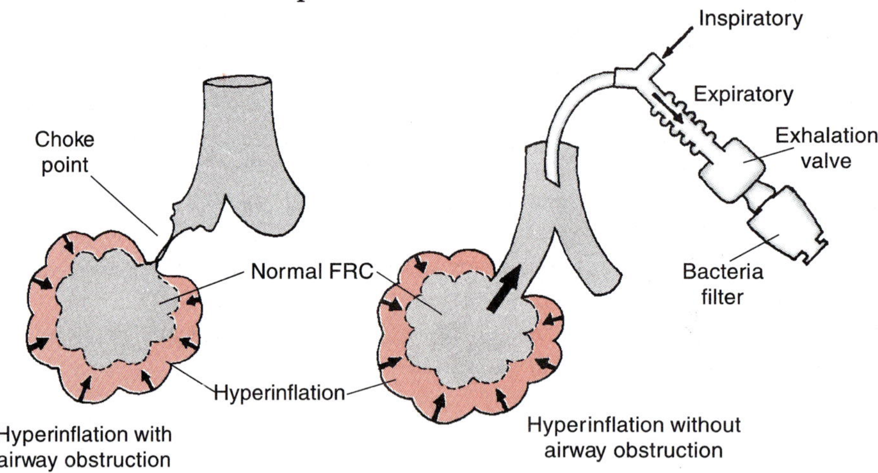

Fig. 41.1: Auto-PEEP with hyperinflation.

- Since auto-PEEP reflects only alveolar pressure, and not transalveolar pressure (the difference between alveolar and pleural pressure), it is possible to have auto-PEEP without hyperinflation (Fig. 41.2). This occurs in patients with active expiratory muscles (e.g. in the presence of high respiratory drive and/or high expiratory resistance), when the pressure generated by expiratory muscles affects alveolar pressure. Auto-PEEP can therefore exist, even though the volume is at, or even below, passive FRC. Therefore, presence of auto-PEEP in the active patient does not necessarily signify the presence, or magnitude of DH. Also, the physiologic consequences and management of auto-PEEP differ, depending on whether the auto-PEEP is due to DH or due to expiratory activity.

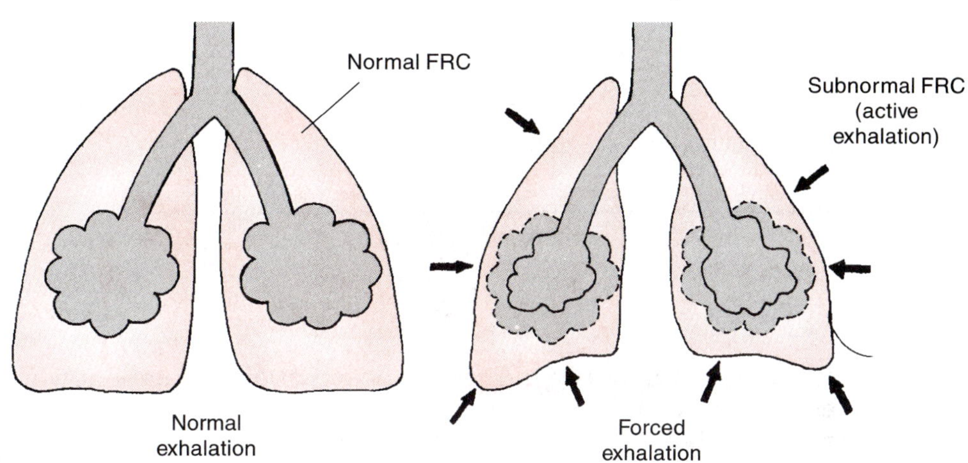

Fig. 41.2: Auto-PEEP without hyperinflation.

- Various factors important for the development of DH include, compliance of the respiratory system, volume from which exhalation begins, and the expiratory time. Expiratory time may be prolonged when expiratory flow is retarded, like patients with obstructive lung diseases, reduced elastic recoil of the lung, narrow ET tube, kinking or water clogging of exhalation tube or poor exhalation valve. DH at end-expiration may arise in patients with airflow limitation as a result of dynamic airway collapse (air trapping). It can also arise in patients without dynamic airway collapse if there is inadequate time available for expiration for the pressure in the alveoli to come to equilibrium. This frequently occurs when respiratory frequency and/or tidal volume are relatively high and expiratory time is relatively short, for the resistance and compliance (i.e. time constant) properties of the respiratory system.
- Auto-PEEP and DH have been described in many conditions, e.g. COPD, asthma, ARDS and can occur in any situation, whenever minute ventilation is high.
- The consequences of DH and auto-PEEP are related to the associated changes in lung volume and pleural pressure: (a) Hyperinflation places the lungs on the flatter portion of their P-V curve; so higher pressure is needed to inhale tidal volume. This is equivalent to a situation wherein one tries to inhale tidal volume after taking a deep breath, (b) hyperinflation also flattens the diaphragm; flattened diaphragm has to generate a greater tension to achieve a given change in thoracic pressure (Laplace Law), (c) it interferes with triggering in the assisted mechanical ventilation or pressure support modes; the patient has to generate enough pressure to offset auto-PEEP plus trigger sensitivity before triggering occurs, (d) because of factors (a), (b), and (c), the work of breathing is increased and there is delay in triggering a breath. It is one of the factors (Fig. 41.3) that

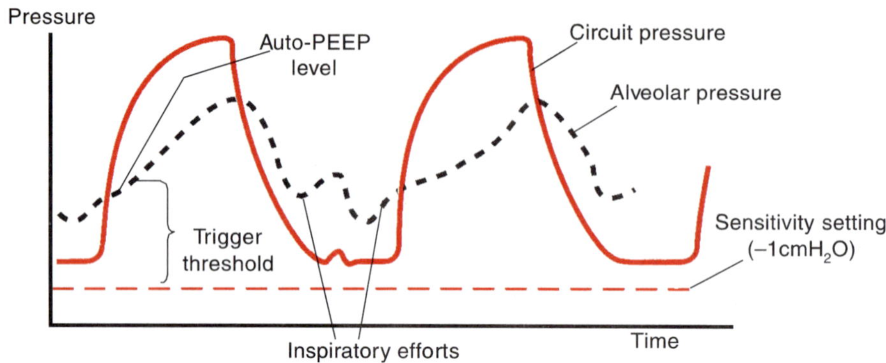

Fig. 41.3: Auto-PEEP elevates the triggering threshold

may account for the not so infrequent observation of a patient who is unable to trigger a ventilator despite obvious respiratory efforts, (e) when thoracic compliance is being measured, failure to take the level of auto-PEEP into account may lead to very substantial underestimation of thoracic compliance, and (f) auto-PEEP (in the passively ventilated patient), increases mean intrapleural pressure, pulmonary artery wedge pressure, pulmonary vascular resistance, and right ventricular afterload, and decreases venous return (preload). Unless the presence of auto-PEEP is recognized, elevated wedge pressure, decreased cardiac output and hypotension may be viewed as an evidence of cardiogenic shock. This is more relevant either during intubation or immediately post-intubation, if there is excessive manual ventilation. It can also give rise to electromechanical dissociation (undetectable blood pressure despite a coordinated ECG).

- Auto-PEEP in the absence of DH (i.e. end-expiratory lung volume at or below passive FRC) does not place the lungs on the flatter portion of P-V curve, has little effect on triggering, does not increase the work of inspiratory muscles, and does not result in underestimation of true compliance.
- Measures to prevent or reverse auto-PEEP include: (a) Prolonging expiratory time (increased peak inspiratory flow rate, use of non-distensible ventilator tubing that decreases the total tidal volume delivered, which in turn, can be delivered during a shorter period), (b) minimizing expiratory airflow obstruction (use a larger diameter ETT, treat bronchospasm aggressively, and suction frequently to remove secretions), and (c) employing appropriate ventilatory strategies (use lower tidal volumes, use PEEP to decrease the inspiratory force necessary to trigger the ventilator, thereby decreasing the work of breathing).
- Applied external PEEP does not increase end-expiratory lung volume. For a given expiratory resistance, the main determinant of the rate of lung emptying and therefore, of end-expiratory lung volume (EELV) in patients with dynamic airway compression, is the difference between alveolar pressure and the critical pressure that narrows the airways and limits airflow. Because the critical pressure is higher than the central airway pressure, adding pressure

downstream does not increase alveolar pressure or volume, until the critical pressure is exceeded.

- In patients receiving mechanical ventilation, auto-PEEP is often called occult PEEP because, unlike externally applied PEEP, it is not registered on the ventilator pressure manometer because the latter is open to the atmosphere. If, however, the expiratory port of the ventilator circuit is occluded immediately before the onset of the next breath, the pressure in the lungs and ventilator circuit will be equilibrated and the level of auto-PEEP will be displayed on the ventilator manometer (Fig 41.a and b).

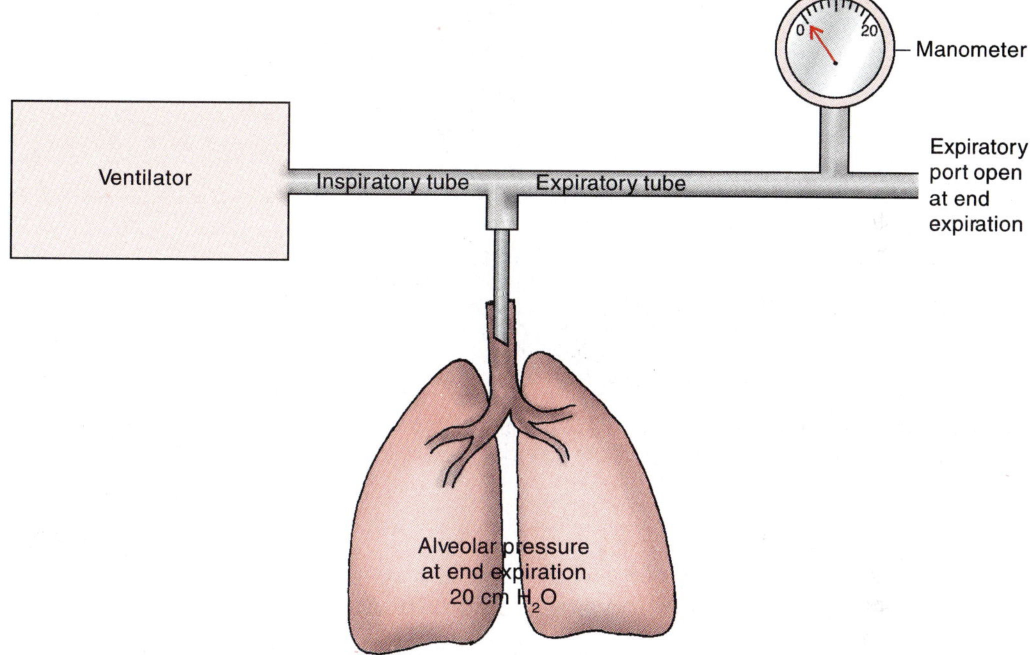

Fig. 41.4(a): Ventilator circuit and manometer at end-expiration without end-expiratory occlusion. Manometer has equilibrated with atmospheric pressure due to its close proximity to the expiratory port of the ventilator. Manometer registers 0 cm H$_2$O even though alveolar pressure is 20 cm H$_2$O.

GUIDELINES FOR MEASUREMENT OF AUTO-PEEP

1. Have a high index of suspicion for those patients likely to be having auto-PEEP.
   Suspect auto-PEEP if any of the following is noted:
   - Minute volume requirement greater than 10 L/min.
   - The patient has: bronchospasm, COPD, rapid respiratory rate (i.e. >25/min), or prolonged inspiratory time (i.e. >1sec).
   - Presence of dyssynchrony between patient and ventilator.
   - Presence of severe hypotension in a patient of status asthmaticus or severe bronchospasm due to other causes. Auto-PEEP is present because of vigorous bagging immediately after intubation, or high respiratory rates set on ventilator.

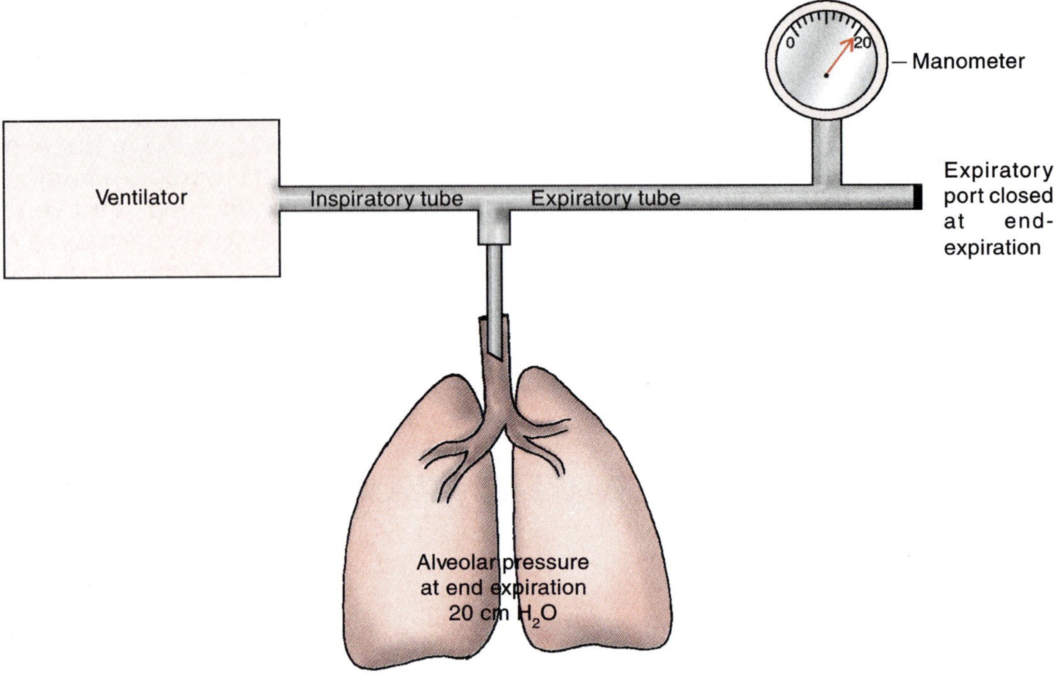

Fig. 41.4(b): Ventilator circuit and manometer at end-expiration with end-expiratory occlusion. Expiratory port has been occluded at end-expiration and it permits equilibration of the alveolar compartment with the tubing circuit and manometer. Manometer registers 20 cm H$_2$O as auto-PEEP.

2. Observe patient-ventilator system.

Auto-PEEP can be detected in several ways:
- On physical examination, if exhalation persists till the onset of the next breath.
- Identification of a delay between the onset of inspiratory effort and a drop in airway pressure at the start of machine-delivered flow.
- Patient unable to trigger machine-assisted breaths or pressure support, thereby decreasing the overall minute ventilation.
- Ventilator-patient dyssynchrony: because the ventilator is unable to sense the patient's inspiratory efforts, controlled breaths also are not synchronous with the patient's respiratory pattern.
- In the paralyzed or heavily sedated patient, reduction of Pplat after a prolonged exhalation is indicative of auto-PEEP.
- On flow-time graph, expiratory flow persists until interrupted by the next breath (Fig 41.5).
- Add external PEEP and monitor the peak inspiratory airway pressure. The addition of external PEEP normally increases peak inspiratory airway pressure. Failure to produce this is an evidence of auto-PEEP.

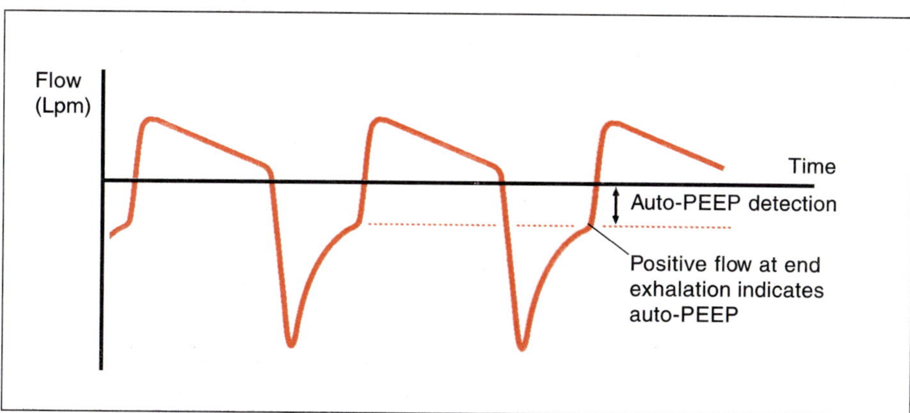

Fig. 41.5: Flow waveforms showing auto-PEEP

3. Determine if the ventilator has a specific auto-PEEP or end-exhalation hold command. If no such command is available, proceed to step 5.

   Newer generation ventilators are often so equipped.

4. Push the end-exhalation hold command at the end of exhalation, or activate auto-PEEP command.

   Observe carefully to make sure that the auto-PEEP level reaches a sustained steady value, either on the manometer or with airway pressure graphics. If the patient actively fights the manoeuvre, the value may be inaccurate. If insufficient end-expiratory hold time is used, there may not be full equilibrium of the manometer with the alveolar space, and auto-PEEP will be underestimated. This requires either little or no respiratory effort on the part of the patient, or patient should be paralyzed.

5. If the ventilator does not have a specific auto-PEEP or end-exhalation hold command, identify the expiratory port of the ventilator.

   As a generic concept, all ventilators have an expiratory port that can be occluded at an appropriate time.

6. Turn the ventilator rate to one or two breaths per minute. Following the last breath, occlude the expiratory port of the ventilator with a gloved hand at the end of expiration, just before the initiation of the subsequent mechanical breath. Occlusion should be complete.
   - Patient should not trigger a breath in between.
   - Occlusion too early in exhalation will over-estimate auto-PEEP.
   - If the machine rate is not temporarily reduced, the auto-PEEP occlusion manoeuvre will be interrupted by a machine cycle breath.
   - Maintain the occlusion for a sufficient period to permit equilibration of alveolar pressure with the patient's tubing. It may take many seconds. If the occlusion is of insufficient duration, auto-PEEP will be underestimated.

7. Note the pressure on the manometer, when the needle finally rests. Immediately release the expiratory port.

8. **Return the ventilator rate to the previous value, or set new values.**

   Make final adjustments in the ventilatory parameters, if required, based on the value of auto-PEEP.

References

1. Brochard L. Intrinsic (or auto) PEEP during controlled mechanical ventilation. Intensive Care Med 2002; 28:1376-1378.
2. Brochard L. Intrinsic (or auto) positive end-expiratory pressure during spontaneous or assisted ventilation. Intensive Care Med 2002; 28: 1552-1554.
3. Leatherman JW, Ravenscraft SA. Low measured auto-positive end-expiratory pressure during mechanical ventilation of patients with severe asthma: Hidden auto-positive end-expiratory pressure. Crit Care Med 1996; 24:541-546.
4. Lessard MR, Lofaso F, Brochard L. Expiratory muscle activity increases intrinsic positive end-expiratory pressure independently of dynamic hyperinflation in mechanically ventilated patients. AM J Respir Crit Care Med 1995; 151:562-569.
5. Lodato RF, Tobin MJ. Estimation of auto-PEEP. Chest 1991; 99:520-522.
6. Ninane V, Yernault JC, De Troyer A. Intrinsic PEEP in patients with chronic obstructive pulmonary disease. Am Rev Respir Dis 1993; 148:1037-1042.
7. Pepe PE, Marini JJ. Occult positive end-expiratory pressure in mechanically ventilated patients with airflow obstruction. Am Rev Respir Dis 1982; 126:166-170.
8. Ranieri VM, Eissa NT, Corbeil C, Chasse M, et al. Effects of positive end expiratory pressure on alveolar recruitment and gas exchange in patients with the adult respiratory distress syndrome. Am Rev Respir Dis 1991;144:544-551.
9. Renieri VM, Guiliani R, Cinnella G, et al. Physiologic effects of positive end-expiratory pressure in patients with chronic obstructive pulmonary disease during acute ventilatory failure and controlled mechanical ventilation. Am Rev Respir Dis 1993, 147:5-13.
10. Tobin MJ, Lodato RF. PEEP, auto-PEEP, and waterfalls. Chest 1989; 96:449-451.
11. Tobin MJ, Van de Graaff WB. Monitoring of lung mechanics and work of breathing. In: Tobin MJ (ed). Principles and Practice of mechanical ventilation, New York: McGraw-Hill, 1994, pp 967-1003.
12. Tuxen DV. Detrimental effects of positive end-expiratory pressure during controlled mechanical ventilation of patients with severe airflow obstruction. Am Rev Respir Dis 1989; 146:16-21.
13. Tuxen DV, Lane S. The effects of ventilatory pattern on by perinflation, airway pressures, and circulation in mechanical ventilation of patients with severe air-flow obstruction. Am Rev Respir Dis 1987; 136:872-879.

Introduction

- Over 90% critically ill patients require mechanical ventilation and during this period, 40% of the time is spent in the process of weaning from it. Prolonged mechanical ventilation is associated with increased morbidity and mortality, prolonged stay in the ICU, and increased resource consumption.
- For the majority of mechanically ventilated patients (70-80%), weaning can be accomplished quickly and easily. There is, however, a smaller group of ventilated patients (20-30%), whose progress is generally manifested by peaks and valleys, and who remain ventilator dependent for prolonged periods of time. Short-term mechanical ventilation ($\leq$ 2 days) is generally associated with a smoother weaning as compared to long-term mechanical ventilation (> 3 days).
- Weaning should start soon after intubation and one should begin testing for the opportunity and should reduce the support at every opportunity. As the condition that warranted placing the patient on the ventilator stabilizes and begins to resolve, attention should be focussed on removing the ventilator as soon as possible, and patient should be assessed regularly for weaning readiness. I prefer to review my patients in the evening so that if a decision to wean is made, it can be implemented by the ICU team next morning, after the patient has had a good night's rest.
- Weaning process may be viewed as consisting of three stages. In the first, the intensivist progressively reduces, in a stepwise fashion, the level of support. In the second stage, the patient undergoes a trial of unassisted breathing. In the third stage, the patient is extubated.
- Various weaning indices have been disappointing as predictors of patient's ability to wean. In general, the indices are poor positive predictors (they do not tell us that the patient will wean), but they are strong negative predictors (they do tell us that the patient will not wean).
- Until the early 1990s, it was believed that all weaning methods were equally effective. But, results of randomized, controlled trials clearly indicate that the period of weaning is as much as three times as long with intermittent mandatory ventilation as with trials of spontaneous breathing. Performing trials of spontaneous breathing once a day is not only as effective as performing such trials several times a day, but also much simpler. Further, half-hour trials of spontaneous breathing are as effective as two-hour trials. There is currently no evidence that new modes (volume support, automatic tube compensation, and adaptive support ventilation) improve weaning outcomes over existing

modes. Two prospective, randomized, controlled trials reported that about two thirds of patients are successfully extubated after the first trial. In those who failed the first day T-piece trial, no difference in outcome (duration of ventilation) was seen between the T-piece and PSV methods.

- The spontaneous breathing trial (SBT) can be conducted either by the traditional T-piece or T-tube approach (in which the patient is removed from the ventilator, and humidified oxygen is provided to the airway), or with a low level (e.g. 5cm H_2O) of CPAP, or with a low level of PSV (e.g. 5–8 cm H_2O). For most patients, there is no evidence that a low level of CPAP is beneficial during spontaneous breathing trial, but this practice is not harmful. In patients with marginal left ventricular function, however, a low level of positive intrathoracic pressure may support the failing heart. Such patients may tolerate a CPAP trial, but may develop congestive heart failure when extubated. Those favouring low level PSV approach to the SBT argue that this overcomes resistance to breathing through the artificial airway. However, the upper airway of the intubated patient is typically swollen and inflamed because ETT has been in place for several days. The work of breathing through the swollen airways is about the same as that caused by breathing through an ETT. One study has reported a similar resistance to breathing through the upper airway after extubation as that with the ETT in place. Another study has reported similar weaning outcomes when SBT was performed with a T-piece or with 7 cm H_2O PSV.

- When patients can sustain spontaneous ventilation without undue discomfort, they are extubated. About 10–20% of such patients require reintubation. Mortality among patients who require reintubation is more than six times as high as mortality among patients who can tolerate extubation. The reason for the higher mortality is unknown. It may be that the need for reintubation itself is a marker of a more severe underlying illness.

- Studies show that steroids (dexamethasone) given 6 hours before extubation reduce the risk of post-extubation stridor in children by about 40%. However, the effect of corticosteroids in children and adults, to reduce post-extubation complications such as reintubation, is uncertain.

- Early extubation, with the back-up institution of non-invasive positive pressure ventilation as needed, may be a useful strategy in selected groups, e.g. COPD patients.

- The condition of ventilator dependent patients can vary considerably from day to day. Thus, a patient's ability to sustain spontaneous ventilation successfully, should be evaluated on a recurrent basis.

- Data available is not sufficient to support the belief that tracheostomy provides universal benefit in promoting weaning from mechanical ventilation in all ventilator-dependent patients. However, a particular group of patients may benefit from the procedure: (a) Patients, requiring sedation to assist their toleration of translaryngeal intubation, may be more comfortable and may be weaned more rapidly after tracheostomy, (b) patients with borderline levels of pulmonary mechanics may be weaned more rapidly after tracheostomy because of decreased airway resistance, especially if respiratory rates are high, and (c) tracheostomy may be helpful in weaning patients requiring long-term mechanical ventilation. It provides a psychological sense of well being because of the ability to eat orally, to communicate by artificial speech, and to provide more ambulation, which in turn contributes to enhanced recovery of muscle strength.

GUIDELINES FOR A WEANING PROCEDURE

1. Observe the patient and scan the monitoring charts.
   Look with reference to patient's drive to breathe and trigger the ventilator.

2. Explain the procedure to the patient. Allay his/her anxiety throughout the active weaning process.
   Patient's cooperation is very important. Be with the patient at the beginning of the procedure and later on, at 15-20 minute intervals, to reinforce the goals and desired outcomes.

3. Assessment for weaning readiness. Assess whether patient meets "entry level criteria".
   The "entry level criteria" include the following:
   (a) Evidence for some reversal of the underlying cause for respiratory failure.
   (b) Free from factors that increase or decrease metabolic rate.
   Factors include, temperature (>38°C), seizures, sepsis, bacteremia, hyper-/hypo-thyroid states.

   (c) Adequate haemoglobin.
   $Hb \geq 8\text{-}10$ g/dL.
   $PCV \geq 25\%$.
   (d) Adequate oxygenation.
   $PaO_2 \geq 60$ mmHg on $FiO_2 \leq 0.4$, PEEP ≤ 5 cm H_2O, and $PaO_2/FiO_2 \geq 200\text{-}300$.
   (e) Adequate mentation.
   Arousable, no continuous sedative infusions. A GCS score ≤ 8 is more likely to be associated with extubation failure and increased likelihood of complications.
   (f) Stable fluid and electrolyte status.
   pH, potassium, magnesium, phosphate, and calcium, all within normal limits.
   (g) Stable cardiovascular system.
   Heart rate ≤ 140/min, stable blood pressure, minimal (≤ 5 µg/kg/min) or no vasopressor use (such as dopamine or dobutamine). Patients with impaired left ventricular function and chronic obstructive airway disease, may suffer a combination of acute left ventricular dysfunction and acute respiratory failure, when being transferred from mechanical ventilation to spontaneous ventilation.
   (h) Stable chest wall.
   With an unstable chest wall (e.g. flail segment), weaning will only make matters worse.
   (i) Absence of massive abdominal distension, ascites.
   (j) Absence of rhonchi, wheeze, excessive secretions.
   These factors add to the resistive load.
   (k) Stable respiration.
   Absence of the use of accessory muscles of respiration, respiratory rate < 35 breaths/min.

(l)   Adequate respiratory muscle strength.

      Maximum inspiratory force greater than 20 cm H_2O.

(m) Stable breathing pattern.

      Tidal volume $\geq$ 5 mL/kg BW, respiratory rate $\leq$ 30 breaths/min.

      Minute ventilation $\leq$ 10 L/min, vital capacity $\geq$ 15 mL/kg.

4. **Evaluate the chances of success or failure of weaning.**

   A variety of physiological indices have been proposed to guide the success of the process of discontinuing ventilatory support. However, there is no evidence to suggest that one particular set of physiologic indices has a better predictability than another. The most promising weaning predictors include the following:

   - Respiratory rate < 35 breaths/min.
   - RSBI < 100-105 breaths/min/L.
   - Maximal inspiratory pressure (Pimax) < -20 cm H_2O.
   - Product of RSBI and occlusion pressure < 450 cm H_2O breaths/min/L.
   - Tracheal occlusion pressure ($P_{0.1}$).

   - A threshold value of $\leq$ 130 (RSBI) has been reported to be more appropriate in the elderly (more than 70 years of age) population.
   - RSBI must be calculated during spontaneous breathing, calculating it during pressure support markedly impairs its predictive accuracy.
   - RSBI is most helpful in patients with no underlying pulmonary disease who have been ventilated mechanically for less than 8 days.
   - In one study, measuring RSBI just before and at 30 minutes of weaning was highly predictive of weaning outcome in post-operative patients.
   - RSBI does not predict post-extubation pulmonary edema or stridor.

   Tracheal occlusion pressure is defined as the inspiratory pressure generated 0.1 seconds after airway occlusion. Values < 2 cm H_2O are good indicators of adequate central respiratory drive. (Studies show that in patients with COPD, RSBI and $P_{0.1}$ are the most accurate weaning predictors).

5. **Choose the mode of weaning.**

   One may choose between, spontaneous breathing trial, pressure support ventilation, or synchronized mandatory ventilation.

6. **Prepare the patient.**

   Explain the procedure to the patient, reassure him/her. Put the patient in a comfortable position (sitting or 45° head up position). If it is felt that the patient might splint his chest because of pain, consider administering small doses of analgesic prior to weaning.

7. **Challenge the patient for 2 hours.**

   Put the patient on the selected mode of weaning and monitor the patient at 15 minute intervals during the initial one-hour, then at 30 minute intervals in the second hour.

8. **Monitor the patient's response to challenge, in order to decide whether the trial is successful or not.**

   Criteria for successful spontaneous breathing trial include:

- Stable ventilatory pattern: respiratory rate $\leq$ 30-35 breaths/min, not varying by more than 20%.
- Haemodynamic stability: heart rate < 120-140 beats/min, not varying by more than 20%; systolic blood pressure < 180 mmHg and > 90 mmHg, blood pressure not varying by more than 20% in either direction; no vasopressor required.
- Gas exchange acceptability: $SpO_2 \geq$ 90%, $PaO_2 \geq$ 60 mmHg, pH $\geq$ 7.32, increase in $PaCO_2 \leq$ 10 mmHg.

Recognition of failed trial.

- Tachypnea (respiratory rate > 35 breaths/min for more than 5 minutes).
- Hypoxaemia (SpO_2 < 90 %).
- Tachycardia (heart rate > 140 beats/min; or sustained rate increase by more than 20%).
- Bradycardia (sustained heart rate decrease by more than 20%).
- Hypertension (systolic blood pressure more than 180 mmHg).
- Hypotension (systolic blood pressure less than 90 mmHg).
- Diaphoresis.
- Signs of increased work of breathing (e.g. use of accessory muscles of respiration, and thoracoabdominal paradox).
- Change in mental state (e.g. somnolence, coma, agitation, and anxiety).
- Onset or worsening of discomfort.

9. In case the trial is successful, consider extubation.
   See Chapter 45.

10. In case the trial fails, consider the following:
    (a) Return to prior settings. Make patient comfortable, and reassure him.
    (b) Maintain the patient in propped up position.
    (c) Document the observations.
    (d) Consider and manage remedial factors, if present (e.g. electrolyte derangement, bronchospasm, malnutrition, patient positioning, excessive secretions, and auto PEEP).
    (e) Repeat a trial of spontaneous breathing on the following day (after 24 hours). Evidence supports waiting for 24 hours because, except in cases recovering from anaesthesia, muscle relaxants and sedatives, respiratory system abnormality rarely recovers over a short period of hours. Secondly, there are data suggesting that a failed SBT (spontaneous breathing trial) may result in some degree of respiratory muscle fatigue and recovery may take any where from several hours to more than 24 hours. Thirdly, another study has provided strong evidence that SBT performed 12-hourly, offers no advantage over that performed once every 24 hours.
    - In case of repeated failures, consider performing a tracheostomy.
    - If a correctable abnormality is found, selective use of non-invasive ventilation with a ventilatory support system (BIPAP) may prevent reintubation. Pulmonary edema is the condition most approachable this way.

References

1. Brochard L, Rauss A, Benito S, et al. Comparison of three methods of gradual withdrawal from ventilatory support during weaning from mechanical ventilation. Am J Respir Crit Care Med 1994; 150:896-903.
2. Biondi JW, Schulman, DS, Wiedemann, HD and Matthay, RA. Mechanical heart lung interaction in the adult respiratory distress syndrome. Clin. Chest Med. 1990; 11:691-714.
3. Coplin WM, Pierson DJ, Cooley KD, et al. Implications of extubation delay in brain injured patients meeting standard weaning criteria. Am J Respir Crit Care Med 2000; 161:1530-1536.
4. Connors, AF, McCaffree, DR, Gray, BA. Effect of inspiratory flow rate on gas exchange during mechanical ventilation. Am. Rev. Respir. Dis. 1981; 124:537-43.
5. Dark DS, Pingleton SK, Kerby GR. Hypercapnia during weaning: a complication of nutritional support. Chest 1984; 88:141-143.
6. Dojat M, Harf A, Touchard D, et al. Evaluation of a knowledge-based system providing ventilatory management and decision for extubation. Am J Respir Crit Care Med 1996; 153:997-1004.
7. Diehl JL, El Atrous S, Touchard D, et al. Changes in the work of breathing induced by tracheotomy in ventilator-dependent patients. Am J Respir Crit Care Med 1999; 159:383-388.
8. Epstein SK, Clubotaru RL, Wong JB. Effect of failed extubation on the outcome of mechanical ventilation. Chest 1997; 112:186-192.
9. Epstein SK. Decision to Extubate. Intensive Care Med 2002; 28:535-546.
10. Esteban A, Alia I, Gordo F, et al. Extubation outcome after spontaneous breathings trials with t-tube or pressure support ventilation. Am J Respir Crit Care Med 1997; 156:459-465.
11. Esteban A, Frutos F, Tobin MJ, et al. A comparison of four methods of weaning patients from mechanical ventilation. N Engl J Med 1995; 6:345-350.
12. Girault C, Daudenthun I, Chevron V, et al. Noninvasive ventilations as a systematic extubation and weaning technique in acute-on-chronic respiratory failure: a prospective, randomized controlled study. Am J Respir Crit Care Med 1999; 160:86-92.
13. Hess DR. Liberation from mechanical ventilation: Weaning the patient or weaning old-fashioned ideas? Crit Care med 2002; 30; 2154-2155.
14. Hess D, Branson RD. Ventilators and weaning modes. Respir Care Clin N Am 2000; 6:407-435.
15. Krieger BP, Isber J, Breitenbucher A, et al. Serial measurements of the rapid-shallow-breathing index as a predictor of weaning outcome in elderly medical patients. Chest 1997; 112:1029-34.
16. Kreit, JW and Eschenbacher, WL. The physiology of spontaneous and mechanical ventilation. Clin. Chest Med 1988; 9:11-21.
17. Lemaire F, Teboul J, Cinotti L, et al. Acute left ventricular dysfunction during unsuccessful weaning from mechanical ventilation. Anesthesiology 1988; 69:171-179.
18. Lemaire F. Difficult weaning. Intensive Care Med 1993; 19:69-73.
19. MacIntyre NR, Cook DJ, Ely EW, et al. Evidence based guidelines for weaning and discontinuing ventilatory support. Chest 2001; 120:375S-395S.
20. Marik PE. The cuff-leak test as a predictor of postextubation stridor: A prospective study. Respir Care 1996; 41(6): 509-511.
21. Marini JJ, Roussos CS, Tobin MJ, et al. Weaning from mechanical ventilation. Am Rev Respir Dis 1988; 138:1043-1046.
22. Maziak DE, Meade MO, Todd TRJ. The timing of tracheotomy: a systematic review. Chest 1998; 114:605-609.
23. Namen AM, Ely EW, Tatter SB, et al. Predictors of successful extubation in neurosurgical patients. Am J Respir Crit Care Med 2001; 163:658-664.

24. Nava S, Ambrosino N, Clini E, et al. Noninvasive mechanical ventilation in the weaning of patients with respiratory failure due to chronic obstructive pulmonary disease: a randomized. Controlled trial. Ann Intern Med 1998; 128:721-728.

25. Perren A, Domenighetti G, Mauri S, et al. Protocol –driven weaning from mechanical ventilation: clinical outcome in patients randomized for a 30-min or 120-min trial with pressure support ventilation. Intensive Care Med 2002; 28:1058-1063.

26. Rivera L, Weissman C. Dynamic ventilatory characteristics during weaning in postoperative critically ill patients. Anesth Analg 1997; 84:1250-1255.

27. Saura P, Blanch L, Mestre J, et al. Clinical consequences of the implementation of a weaning protocol. Intensive Care Med 1996; 22:1052-1056.

28. Slutsky, AS. Consensus conference on mechanical ventilation (Part 2). Intensive Care Med 1994; 20:150-62.

29. Stroetz RW, Humbmayr RD. Tidal volume maintenance during weaning with pressure support. Am J Respir Crit Care Med 1995; 152:1034-1040.

30. Tobin MJ, Alex CG. Discontinuation of mechanical ventilation In: Tobin MJ (ed). Principles and Practice of Mechanical Ventilation. New York: McGrow-Hill, 1994, pp 1177-1206.

31. Tomlinson JR, Miller KS, Lorch DG, et al. A prospective comparison of IMV and T-piece weaning from mechanical ventilation. Chest 1989, 96:348-352.

32. Vallverdu I, Calaf N, Subirana M, et al. Clinical characteristics, respiratory functional parameters, and outcome of a two-hour T-piece trial in patients weaning from mechanical ventilation. Am J Respir Crit Care Med 1998; 158:1855-1862.

33. Vitacca M, Vianello A, Colombo D, et al. Comparison of two methods for weaning patients with chronic obstructive pulmonary disease requiring mechanical ventilation for more than 15 days. Am J Respir Crit Care Med 2001; 164:225-230.

34. Wood KE, Flaten AL, Reedy JS, Coursin DB. Use of a daily screen and weaning protocol for mechanically ventilated patients in a multidisciplinary tertiary critical care unit. Crit Care Med 1999; 27:A94-A94.

35. Yang KL, Tobin MJ. A prospective study of indexes predicting the outcome of trials of weaning from mechanical ventilation. N Engl J Med 1991; 324:1445-1450.

Maximal Static Respiratory Pressure Measurement in ICU

43

Introduction

- Maximal static inspiratory pressure (PImax), also known as negative inspiratory force (NIF), refers to the greatest amount of negative pressure (subatmospheric pressure) the patient can generate when inspiring against an occluded airway.
- Factors that affect the test results are, strength of the diaphragm and accessory muscles of inspiration, lung volume at which the airway is occluded, ventilatory drive, and the length of time the airway is occluded.
- PImax is used to determine (a) the weanability of a patient on ventilator and (b) to monitor the strength of patients with neuromuscular diseases.
- Normal values for spontaneously, breathing, non-intubated adult subjects, breathing from residual volume, can be predicted by the following formulae:

  Men: $143 - (0.55 \times age)$ cm H_2O. Women: $104 - (0.51 \times age)$ cmH_2O.
  The lower limit for men is -75 cm H_2O and for women is -50 cm H_2O.
- It is a strong negative predictor but a poor positive predictor.
- Maximal static expiratory pressure (PEmax) is the greatest amount of positive pressure the patient can generate when expiring from total lung capacity (TLC) against an occluded airway.
- Factors that affect the test results include, the patient's cooperation and effort, strength of the expiratory muscles, lung volumes when the airway is occluded, ventilatory drive, and the length of time for which airway is occluded.
- An effective cough is generally not possible when PEmax is less than +40 cm H_2O.
- Normal values for spontaneously breathing, non-intubated adult subjects, breathing from TLC, can be predicted by the following formulae:

  Men: $268 - (1.03 \times age)$ cm H_2O. Women: $170 - (0.53 \times age)$ cm H_2O.
  The lower limit for men is $+140$ cm H_2O and for women is $+95$ cm H_2O.
- When maximal static respiratory pressures are used for assessment of weaning potential, an inspiratory pressure less than -20 cm H_2O, and an expiratory pressure more than $+50$ cm H_2O, have been identified as predictive of the ability to wean most patients from ventilatory support. However, it should be kept in mind that the ability to breathe unassisted depends on the balance between the capacity of the respiratory muscles to perform work, and the

workload imposed on the respiratory muscles by the chest wall and lungs. Therefore, values of a single factor (i.e. maximal static respiratory pressures) should not be used in deciding about weaning potential.

GUIDELINES FOR MEASUREMENT OF MAXIMAL STATIC RESPIRATORY PRESSURES

A. Maximal Static Inspiratory Pressure

1. Explain the procedure to the patient.

    This reassures the patient and reduces anxiety. It also prepares the patient about the sensation one may experience, such as transient shortness of breath and fatigue.

2. Wash hands.

    This reduces the transmission of microorganisms.

3. Have the patient sitting upright.

    Upright posture improves efficiency. If the patient is lying down, record it in the chart.

4. Obtain the pressure gauge (Fig. 43.1) and demonstrate the procedure to the patient.

    This helps the patient in understanding the procedure and increases the chances of correct performance of the procedure. It also ensures best efforts on the part of the patient.

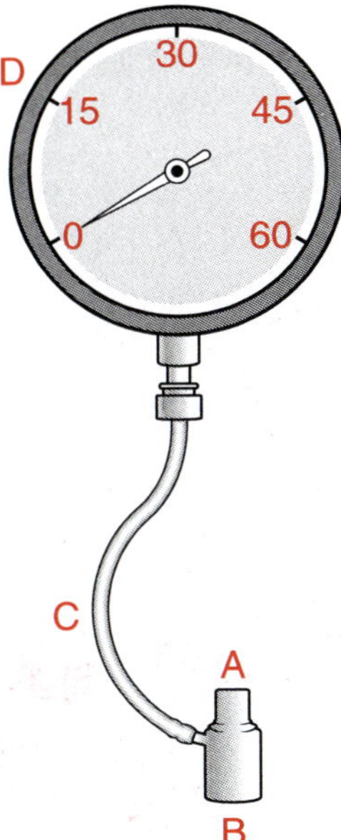

Fig. 43.1: System for measuring maximal inspiratory pressure (MIP). A: Port to be occluded during the MIP; B: Port to connect to the patient's airway; C: Connecting tubing; D: Pressure manometer.

5. Place noseclips over the patient's nose. Have the patient seal his lips and teeth around the mouthpiece and breathe through the open port.

6. Ask the patient to exhale completely. Seal the port when residual volume is reached.

    The pressure manometer is usually attached to the airway via a series of one-way valves. The valves (one for inspiration and one for expiration) are capped as necessary to ensure a closed system.

7. Ask the patient to breathe in as deeply as possible and hold the breath for 1-3 seconds.

    Observe the needle during inspiration.

8. Repeat the manoeuvre until at least three good efforts have been performed. The test can be done for 20 seconds with multiple attempts by the patients.

    The goal is to obtain the best value for a particular patient. Remember, the test can be frightening for patients because it is impossible to inhale during the manoeuvre.

9. Monitor the patient: ECG, blood pressure, SpO_2.

    Observe the patient for signs of hypoxaemia such as tachycardia, bradycardia, ventricular dysrhythmias, hypertension, hypotension, or decreasing saturation on pulse oximetry. If any of these develop, stop the procedure and record the findings.

B. Maximal Static Expiratory Pressure

1. Perform steps 1 to 5 as above.

2. Ask the patient to inhale completely. Seal the port when total lung capacity (TLC) has been reached.

3. Ask the patient to breathe out as hard as possible and hold for 1-3 seconds.

4. Perform steps 8 and 9 as above.

References

1. Black LF, Hyatt RE. Maximal respiratory pressure: normal values and relationship to age and sex. Am Rev Respir Dis 1971; 103:641.
2. Branson RD, HurstJM, Davis KJr, et al. Measurement of maximal inspiratory pressure: A comparison of three methods. Respir Care 1989; 34(9): 789
3. Clausen JL. Clinical interpretation of pulmonary function test. Respir Care 1989; 34(7): 638.
4. Hess D. Measurement of maximal inspiratory pressure: a call for standardization. Respir Care 1989; 34:857.
5. Kacmarek RM, Cycyk-Chapman MC, Young-Palazzo PJ, et al. Determination of maximal inspiratory pressure: a clinical study and literature review. Respir Care 1989; 34:868.
6. Marini JJ, Smith TC, Lamb V. Estimation of inspiratory muscle strength in mechanically ventilated patients: the measurement of maximal inspiratory pressure. J Crit Care 1986;1:32-38.
7. Multz AS, Aldrich TK, Prezant DJ, et al. Maximal inspiratory pressure is not a reliable test of inspiratory muscle strength in mechanically ventilated patients. Am Rev Respir Dis 1990;142:529-532.
8. Tobin MJ, Laghi F, Walsh JM. Monitoring of respiratory neuromuscular function. In:Tobin MJ (ed). Principles and Practice of Mechanical Ventilation, New York: McGraw-Hill, 1994, pp 945-966.

Methods of Weaning

44

Introduction

A typical weaning order could read as follows:

Method.............. FiO_2....................

Instructions: Monitor the baseline parameters. Monitor parameters every 15 minutes during the first hour, and every 30 minutes during the second hour. Obtain ABG after 30 minutes. If ABG is adequate, continue to wean. Obtain ABG after 2 hours of weaning. Assess the patient in respect of clinical picture and ABG, and decide.

GUIDELINES FOR VARIOUS METHODS OF WEANING

1. **Abrupt discontinuation.**

    Patients receiving ventilatory support for short periods, e.g. post-operative patients, can commonly be extubated without prolonged weaning trials.

2. **T-piece trial.**

    - Assemble the T-piece (Fig. 44.1). Connect a reservoir tube of about 12 inches to the expiratory port of the T-piece to prevent entrainment of room air, and to ensure that the inspired oxygen concentration is stable. Connect oxygen via venturi to the humidifier, which is connected via wide bore tubing to the patient's inspiratory end of T-piece.
    - Set the FiO_2 and adjust the flow rate between 8 and 12 L/min. Normally, the weaning FiO_2 is set 10% higher than that of the ventilator.

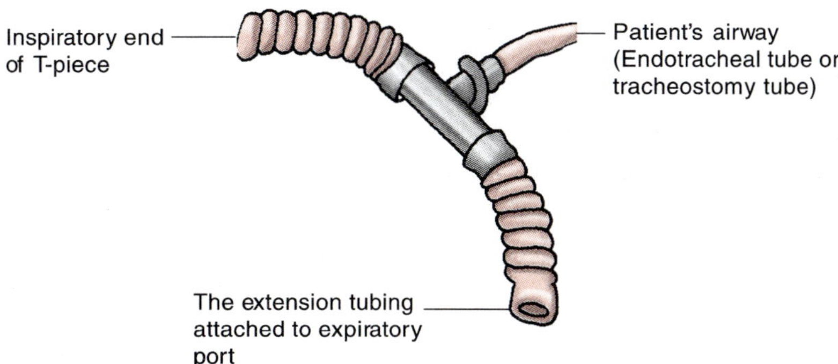

Fig. 44.1: Equipment utilized in a T-piece trial: The extension tubing is used to prevent inspiration of ambient air.

- Attach the T-piece with humidifier to the endotracheal tube or tracheostomy tube.
- Analyse the oxygen percentage. It should be within ± 2% of the ordered value.
- Maintain this for 2 hours.
- If signs of intolerance develop at any time, place the patient back on the previous ventilator settings. Give the next trial after 24 hours (since the recovery from diaphragmatic fatigue may take at least 24 hours).
- If the patient tolerates 2 hours of T-piece trial, consider extubation criteria and extubation.

3. **CPAP trial.**
- Place the patient on the desired level of CPAP (4-5 cm H_2O) while keping the FiO_2 the same as when on ventilator.
- Maintain CPAP for 2 hours, unless signs of intolerance develop.
- If signs of intolerance develop at any time, place the patient back on previous ventilator settings. Repeat the next trial after 24 hours.
- If the patient tolerates 2 hours of CPAP trial, consider extubation criteria and extubation.

4. **PSV protocol.**
- The baseline or resting PSV (and starting PSV for weaning) is set to achieve adequate tidal volume at optimal respiratory rates, with no involvement of accessory muscles of respiration.
- Decrease the pressure support by 2-5 cm H_2O/day, or more frequently, as titrated by the patient's clinical condition (Fig 44.2). Be guided by the tidal volume, respiratory rate, activity in accessory muscles of respiration, and

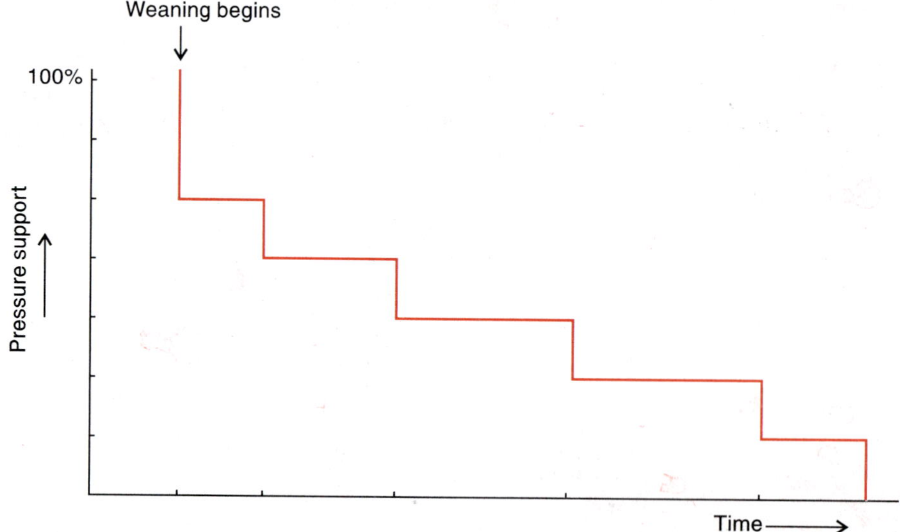

Fig. 44.2: PSV protocol for weaning involves gradual reduction of pressure support in steps of 2-5 cm H_2O depending on the patient's tolerance.

signs of intolerance. A useful predictor for stepwise reduction in mechanical support is rapid shallow breathing index (RSBI) < 65 breaths/min/L.

- Continue this process until patient reaches a PSV level of 5-6 cm H_2O.
- If at any time patient exhibits signs of fatigue or intolerance, return the pressure support level to the previous value at which patient was stable. Wait for 24 hours, assess and restart the process.
- Allow the patient's respiratory muscles to rest at night, by increasing the pressure support by 2-4 cm H_2O.
- If patient is stable at 5-6 cm H_2O pressure support for 10-12 hours, consider extubation criteria and extubation.

References

1. Brochard L, Rauss A, Benito S, et al. Comparison of three methods of gradual withdrawal from ventilatory support during weaning from mechanical ventilation. Am J Respir Crit Care Med 1994; 150:896-903.
2. Esteban A, Alia I, Gordo F, et al. Extubation outcome after spontaneous breathings trials with T-tube or pressure support ventilation. Am J Respir Crit Care Med 1997; 156:459-465.
3. Esteban A, Frutos F, Tobin MJ, et al. A comparison of four methods of weaning patients from mechanical ventilation. N Engl J Med 1995; 6:345-350.
4. Krieger BP, Isber J, Breitenbucher A, et al. Serial measurements of the rapid-shallow-breathing index as a predictor of weaning outcome in elderly medical patients. Chest 1997; 112:1029-1034.
5. MacIntyre NR, Cook DJ, Ely EW, et al. Evidence based guidelines for weaning and discontinuing ventilatory support. Chest 2001; 120:375S-395S.
6. Perren A, Domenighetti G, Mauri S, et al. Protocol –driven weaning from mechanical ventilation: clinical outcome in patients randomized for a 30-min or 120-min trial with pressure support ventilation. Intensive Care Med 2002; 28:1058-1063.
7. Saura P, Blanch L, Mestre J, et al. Clinical consequences of the implementation of a weaning protocol. Intensive Care Med 1996; 22:1052-1056.
8. Slutsky, AS. Consensus conference on mechanical ventilation (Part 2). Intensive Care Med 1994; 20:150-62.
9. Tobin MJ, Alex CG. Discontinuation of mechanical ventilation In: Tobin MJ (ed): Principles and Practice of Mechanical Ventilation. New York: McGrow-Hill, 1994, pp 1177-1206.
10. Tomlinson JR, Miller KS, Lorch DG, et al. A prospective comparison of IMV and T-piece weaning from mechanical ventilation. Chest 1989; 96:348-352.
11. Vallverdu I, Calaf N, Subirana M, et al. Clinical characteristics, respiratory functional parameters, and outcome of a two-hour T-piece trial in patients weaning from mechanical ventilation. Am J Respir Crit Care Med 1998; 158:1855-1862.
12. Vitacca M, Vianello A, Colombo D, et al. Comparison of two methods for weaning patients with chronic obstructive pulmonary disease requiring mechanical ventilation for more than 15 days. Am J Respir Crit Care Med 2001; 164:225-230.

Extubation

45

Introduction

- After the successful completion of spontaneous breathing trial, or any other mode of weaning, the patient should be assessed for a trial of endotracheal extubation. The decision to extubate is of considerable importance, as both delayed extubation and failed extubation (followed by reintubation) are associated with increased duration of mechanical ventilation and increased mortality. Moreover, the pathogenesis of extubation failure may differ significantly from that of weaning failure, and includes upper airway obstruction, inadequate cough, excessive respiratory secretions, encephalopathy, and cardiac dysfunction.
- Extubation failure is usually defined as the need for reintubation, occurring within 24 to 72 hours of planned extubation, and its incidence ranges from 2 to 25%. The risk factors include co-morbid conditions (e.g. COPD), age > 70 years, Hb< 10 g/dL, duration of ventilation prior to extubation and use of continuous intravenous sedation.
- Predictors of extubation outcome include parameters that assess airway patency and protection (in addition to the weaning parameters, as discussed in Chapter 42). These parameters are: (a) Maximal expiratory pressure, (b) peak expiratory flow rate, (c) cough strength, (d) white card test, (e) volume of secretions, (f) suctioning frequency, (g) cuff leak test, and (h) neurological function (Glasgow Coma Scale).

GUIDELINES FOR PREDICTING EXTUBATION OUTCOME

1. **Review the patient's progress charts.**

    Reviewing the progress charts helps in getting information about whether the patient has completed SBT successfully.

2. **Evaluate the chances of success or failure of extubation.**

    (a) **Assess secretion volume and suctioning frequency.**

    The amount of secretions is an independent predictor of extubation outcome. Excessive endotracheal secretions, especially in the absence of a good cough, could lead to bronchial plugging, atelectasis and/or aspiration pneumonitis, all of which in turn, can cause respiratory failure. The frequency of endotracheal suctioning gives a fair idea of the amount of secretions present. Patients requiring suction every 2 hours or less, have been reported to be 16 times as likely to have unsuccessful extubations, compared to those requiring less frequent suctioning. Similarly, patients with moderate or abundant secretions were almost nine times as likely to have unsuccessful extubation compared to those with scant or no secretions.

(b) Assess neurological function.

Brain dysfunction can contribute to extubation failure by causing hypoventilation or by decreasing the patient's capacity to protect the airway.

(c) Assess gag reflex.

Absent gag reflex could increase the chances of aspiration.

(d) Assess cough strength.
   (i)   Vital capacity.
   (ii) Maximal negative inspiratory pressure.
   (iii) Maximal expiratory pressure.
   (iv) Peak cough flow rates.

A normal cough requires a precough inspiration to about 85–90% of the total lung capacity. Glottic closure follows for about 0.2 seconds, and sufficient intrathoracic pressures are generated to obtain transient peak expiratory flows upon glottic opening that are normally 360–1000 L/min. Total expiratory volume during normal coughing is 2.3 ± 0.5 L.

The ability to take precough inspiration (deep breath) is quantified by measuring the vital capacity or the peak maximal negative inspiratory pressure (PImax.). A PI max of -20 cm H_2O usually corresponds to a vital capacity of ≥ 15 mL/kg, which is generally associated with the ability to breathe sufficiently deep to clear secretions in the presence of the other prerequisites. Glottic function can be evaluated by direct or indirect larynx examination. Expiratory muscle function (crucial for generating sufficient intrathoracic pressure or effective cough) is quantified by assessing either peak cough flow rates or maximal expiratory pressures (PEmax). According to one of the studies, successful extubation was unlikely if the peak cough flow rate (measured using peak flow meter) was less than 160 L/min. One should however, remember that bronchospasm or any condition that results in upper or lower airway obstruction also reduces peak expiratory flows. A PE max of less than +40 cmH_2O suggests severely impaired coughing ability.

(e) Perform white card test.

White card test is an objective measure of cough strength. It assesses one's ability to propel secretions onto a white index card, placed 1 to 2 cms. from the end of endotracheal tube, when asked to cough or when cough is stimulated by a catheter. Any wetness appearing on the card or secretions falling on the card is classified as WCT positive. WCT results have been reported to correlate well with cough strength. Patients with negative WCT results were three times as likely to have unsuccessful extubation as those with positive WCT results.

(f) Assess airway patency.
   (i) Qualitative cuff leak test.

      Absence of an audible air leak after deflation of the endotracheal tube balloon has been reported to be associated with an increased risk of post-extubation stridor. A leak may be defined as vocalization around the tube, or an air leak heard or felt with the patient coughing or with positive pressure inhalation.

(ii) Quantitative cuff leak test.

- Perform the test within 24 hours of planned extubation.
- Place the patient on assist-control breathing.
- Remove any endotracheal and oral secretions.
- Check whether set inspiratory tidal volume and displayed expiratory tidal volume are approximately equal.
- Deflate the balloon. Record inspiratory and expiratory tidal volumes over subsequent six to eight respiratory cycles. Take the average of the lowest three values.
- The difference between the inspiratory and expiratory tidal volumes (after deflating the balloon) is defined as the cuff leak volume.

It has been shown that a reduced cuff leak volume measured prior to extubation is associated with an increased risk of post-extubation stridor, and a volume greater than 110 mL is associated with the absence of post-extubation stridor among planned, controlled extubations. In another study, none of the 20 postoperative cardiothoracic surgery patients, with a positive cuff leak test (< 110 mL), developed stridor. These false positive test results can result from secretions adhering to the outside of the tube, or from a spuriously elevated exhaled tidal volume due to higher than expected inspiratory tidal volume (patient augmenting machine-delivered tidal volumes with spontaneous gas, inspired around the tube when the balloon is deflated).

References

1. Adderley RJ, Mullins GC. When to Extubate the croup patient: the "leak" test. Can J Anaesth 1987;34:304-306.
2. Anene O, Meert KL, Uy H, et al. Dexamethasone for the prevention of postextubation airway obstruction: A prospective, randomized, double-blind, placebo-controlled trial. Crit Care Med 1996;24:1666-1669.
3. Bach JR, Saporito LR. Criteria for extubation and tracheostomy tube removal for patients with ventilatory failure. A different approach to weaning. Chest 1996;110:1566-1571.
4. Dojat M, Harf A, Touchard D, et al. Evaluation of a knowledge-based system providing ventilatory management and decision for extubation. Am J Respir Crit Care Med 1996;153:997-1004.
5. Epstein SK, Clubotaru RL, Wong JB. Effect of failed extubation on the outcome of mechanical ventilation. Chest 1997;112:186-192.
6. Epstein SK. Decision to Extubate. Intensive Care Med 2002;28:535-546.
7. Esteban A, Alia I, Gordo F, et al. Extubation outcome after spontaneous breathings Trials with T-tube or pressure support ventilation. Am J Respir Crit Care Med 1997;156:459-465.
8. Fisher M McD, Raper RF. The 'cuff-leak' test for extubation. Anaesthesia, 1992;47:10-12.
9. Ho LI, Harn HJ, Lein TC, et al. Postextubation laryngeal edema in adults: risk factor evaluation and prevention by hydrocortisone. Intensive Care Med 1996;22:933-936.
10. Khamiees M, Raju P, Amoateng-Adjepong Y, et al. Predictors of extubation outcome in patients who have successfully completed a spontaneous breathing trial. Chest 2001;120:1262-1270.

11. Khandees M, Raja P, DeGirolamo A, et al. Predictors of extubation outcome in patients who have successfully completed a spontaneous breathing trial. Chest 2001;120;1262-1270.

12. Marik PE. The cuff-leak test as a predictor of postextubation stridor: A prospective study. Respir Care 1996;41(6):509-511.

13. Miller RL, Cole RP. Association between reduced cuff leak volume and postextubation stridor. Chest 1996;110:1035-1040.

14. Namen AM, Ely EW, Tatter SB, et al. Predictors of successful extubation in neurosurgical patients. Am J Respir Crit Care Med 2001;163:658-664.

15. Tellez DW, Galvis AG, Storgion SA, et al. Dexamethasone in the prevention of postextubation stridor in children. J Pediatr 1991;118:289-294.

16. Tobin MJ, Alex CG. Discontinuation of mechanical ventilation In: Tobin MJ (editor): Principles and Practice of Mechanical Ventilation. New York: McGrow-Hill, 1994, pp 1177-1206.

Performing Extubation and Decannulation

46

Introduction

- Extubation refers to the removal of an endotracheal tube whereas decannulation refers to the removal of a tracheostomy tube.
- Before proceeding for extubation or decannulation, ensure that the patient has been assessed for the possibility of extubation/decannulation success.
- Explain the procedure to the patient. Reassure him/her. Explain that his/her voice may be hoarse immediately following extubation or decannulation.

GUIDELINES FOR PERFORMING EXTUBATION AND DECANNULATION

1. **Wash hands, wear gloves.**
   This reduces the transmission of microorganisms.

2. **Preoxygenate, and suction the tube and pharynx.**
   See Chapter 1.

3. **Cut or remove the tape supporting the tube.**

4. **Remove the tube.**
   It can be done by one of the following methods:
   - At the peak of a deep inspiration, deflate the cuff and remove the tube in one motion,
     OR
   - Advance the suction catheter 2-4 cm beyond distal end of the tube. Release air from cuff quickly. Apply suction while withdrawing the tube,
     OR
   - Deflate the cuff. Pull the tube, asking the patient to cough while the tube is being removed.

   In a patient known to have a difficult airway, place a jet stylet (a fiberoptic bronchoscope is preferable) through the endotracheal tube, then deflate the balloon cuff, and remove the endotracheal tube over the translaryngeal jet stylet. If no difficulty with ventilation is encountered with the jet stylet still through the cords, then the jet stylet may be removed. However, if ventilation becomes laboured, reinsert the endotracheal tube into the trachea over the jet stylet. Re-assess the patient and treat the possible cause before attempting an extubation.

5. Ask the patient to take deep breaths and cough.
6. Place the patient in the semi-Fowler position.

    Respiratory muscles are more effective in this position; in addition, this position facilitates coughing.

7. Apply oxygen mask.

    Administer oxygen at a concentration higher by 10% as compared to that prior to extubation.

8. Monitor the patient and record the findings.
    - Auscultate the chest for any bronchospasm.
    - Monitor pulse, blood pressure, SpO_2, respiratory rate, sweating, chest-abdominal asynchrony and stridor, every 15 minutes for initial one hour and every 30 minutes during the second hour and then hourly till the patient is stable.

9. Measure ABG after 30-60 minutes.

10. Encourage coughing and deep breathing. Use incentive spirometer, whenever indicated. Consider steam inhalation.

    These measures prevent atelectasis and secretion accumulation. For use of incentive spirometer (see Chapter 5).

11. Extubation failure.

    Treatment of extubation failure can be divided into:
    - Specific therapy: Aimed at the approximate cause for failure, e.g. racaemic epinephrine for laryngospasm, diuretics and nitroglycerine for cardiac ischaemia and heart failure, bronchoscopy to find out any lesion in the airway.
    - Non-specific therapy: Aimed at re-establishing ventilatory support – noninvasive or invasive (following reintubation).

    As data shows higher mortality with longer time to reintubation, the intensivist should rapidly assess the response to specific therapy and not hesitate in reintubating those patients who fail to improve.

References

1. Adderley RJ, Mullins GC. When to Extubate the croup patient: the "leak" test. Can J Anaesth 1987; 34:304-306.
2. Anene O, Meert KL, Uy H, et al. Dexamethasone for the prevention of postextubation airway obstruction: A prospective, randomized, double-blind, placebo-controlled trial. Crit Care Med 1996; 24:1666-1669.
3. Bach JR, Saporito LR. Criteria for extubation and tracheostomy tube removal for patients with ventilatory failure. A different approach to weaning. Chest 1996; 110:1566-1571.
4. Dojat M, Harf A, Touchard D, et al. Evaluation of a knowledge-based system providing ventilatory management and decision for extubation. Am J Respir Crit Care Med 1996; 153:997-1004.
5. Epstein SK, Clubotaru RL, Wong JB. Effect of failed extubation on the outcome of mechanical ventilation. Chest 1997; 112:186-192.
6. Epstein SK. Decision to Extubate. Intensive Care Med 2002; 28:535-546.

7. Esteban A, Alia I, Gordo F, et al. Extubation outcome after spontaneous breathing trials with T-tube or pressure support ventilation. Am J Respir Crit Care Med 1997; 156:459-465.
8. Fisher M McD, Raper RF. The 'cuff-leak' test for extubation. Anaesthesia, 1992; 47:10-12.
9. Ho LI, Harn HJ, Lein TC, et al. Postextubation laryngeal edema in adults: risk factor evaluation and prevention by hydrocortisone. Intensive Care Med 1996; 22:933-936.
10. Khamiees M, Raju P, Amoateng-Adjepong Y, et al. Predictors of extubation outcome in patients who have successfully completed a spontaneous breathing trial. Chest 2001;120:1262-1270.
11. Khandees M, Raja P, DeGirolamo A, et al. Predictors of extubation outcome in patients who have successfully completed a spontaneous breathing trial. Chest 2001; 120; 1262-1270.
12. Marik PE. The cuff-leak test as a predictor of postextubation stridor: A prospective study. Respir Care 1996; 41(6): 509-511.
13. Miller RL, Cole RP. Association between reduced cuff leak volume and postextubation stridor. Chest 1996;110:1035-1040.
14. Namen AM, Ely EW, Tatter SB, et al. Predictors of successful extubation in neurosurgical patients. Am J Respir Crit Care Med 2001; 163:658-664.
15. Tellez DW, Galvis AG, Storgion SA, et al. Dexamethasone in the prevention of postextubation stridor in children. J Pediatr 1991; 118:289-294.
16. Tobin MJ, Alex CG. Discontinuation of mechanical ventilation In: Tobin MJ (ed). Principles and Practice of Mechanical Ventilation. New York: McGraw-Hill, 1994, pp 1177-1206.

GUIDELINES REGARDING A BASIC APPROACH FOR NUTRITIONAL SUPPORT

1. **Consider nutrition in every starving patient.**

    Like mechanical ventilation or haemodynamic support, nutritional support has progressively evolved from an adjuvant, to an essential life–saving therapy. In starving, critically ill patients, malnutrition may develop rapidly due to the presence of acute phase responses, which not only promote catabolism but also alter the response to nutritional support. Malnutrition, once established, exerts well-known deleterious effects by altering immunity, increasing susceptibility to nosocomial infection, decreasing wound healing, and by altering the function of vital organs and promoting organ failure.

2. **Decide appropriate time to start nutrition.**
    - Acknowledging that starvation is universally lethal and occurs sooner in the presence of illness without nutritional support, the timing of the latter is a crucial factor.
    - The timing of initiating nutritional support is a complex issue involving various factors which include pre-illness nutritional status, type, severity and stage of critical illness and organ failure, route of feeding and the use of special diets including immunonutrients and antioxidants. Generally speaking, the sicker the patient is, the lesser is the likelihood of his deriving benefit from nutritional support. It probably reflects the severity of the insult and the inability of the patient to effectively utilize the nutritional support.
    - It has been recommended that nutritional support should be initiated in patients with inadequate oral intake for 7-14 days, or in those patients in whom inadequate oral intake is expected over a 7-14 day period. There is no evidence that short starvation of 5-7 days is deleterious in critical care patients without pre-existing malnutrition.
    - Generally speaking, early feeding refers to beginning nutrition within 24-48 hours after an acute event, with the aim of providing at least 50% of energy requirement on day 3-4. Conventional feeding is initiating nutrition within 3-10 days, and late feeding refers to nutrition after the 10th day.
    - Early parenteral nutrition has no place in the ICU, in patients without pre-existing malnutrition. There is a reasonable evidence that early enteral nutrition is beneficial in patients with severe trauma, especially abdominal, major burns and after liver transplantation. Other indications for early

enteral feeding include acute respiratory distress syndrome, major abdominal cancer surgery and actual malnutrition. Absolute contraindications for the use of early enteral feeding are loss of bowel anatomical integrity, mechanical ileus, severe splanchnic ischaemia, shock, and generalized peritonitis. Short bowel, paralytic ileus, acute circulatory failure, and localized peritonitis could be considered as conditions where early enteral feeding is relatively contraindicated.

3. **Decide the route of providing nutritional support.**
   - Whenever possible, use enteral nutrition (EN) in preference to parenteral nutrition. Proposed advantages of EN include reduced cost, reduced infection, decreased hospital length of stay, and better maintenance of gut integrity. It is also claimed to prevent bacterial translocation and to improve patient outcome. At present, however, these assumptions are not evidence-based. Also, enteral nutrition is more time consuming.
   - Situations where enteral feeding cannot be / should not be used include patients with diffuse peritonitis, intestinal obstruction, intractable vomiting, paralytic ileus, severe diarrhoea, high-output enterocutaneous fistulas (more than 500 mL/day), severe pancreatitis, gastrointestinal ischaemia, and early stages of short bowel syndrome. These are the candidates for parenteral nutrition. Parenteral nutrition (PN) may also be of benefit in patients recovering from multiple organ failure, in whom bowel function has not yet recovered and in whom full enteral nutrition is impossible for a long period of time.

4. **Adopt a balanced, practical approach.**
   A balanced approach to the route of nutrition is appropriate. It is important to consider the nutritional support requirements of each individual patient and then to choose the most appropriate route of delivery for that patient. Guidelines for feeding critically ill patients, can be considered in the following steps:
   (a) Initiate PN and EN simultaneously.
   (b) Establish nutrient intake goals that can be achieved by combining both therapies.
   (c) Begin PN with 1.0-1.5 L of a complete formula, depending upon the volume status.
   (d) Begin EN with full strength solution at around 10-15 mL/hr.
   (e) Increase EN to goal rate as patient tolerates more.
   (f) Keeping in mind the nutrition goals, decrease PN as EN rate is increased.

References

1. Adams S, Dellinger E, Wertz M, et al. Enteral versus parenteral nutrition support following laparotomy for trauma: A randomized prospective trial. J Trauma 1986; 26:882-891.
2. Alverdy JC, Burke D. Total parenteral nutrition: iatrogenic immunosuppression. Nutrition 1992; 8:359-365.
3. Bell SJ, Borlase BC, Swails W, Dascoulias K, Ainsley B, Forse RA. Experience with enteral nutrition in a hospital population of acutely ill patients. J Am Diet Assoc 1994; 94:414-419.

4. Bozzetti F, Braga M, Gianotti L, Gavazzi C, Mariani L. Postoperative enteral versus parenteral nutrition in malnourished patients with gastrointestinal cancer: a randomized multicenter trial. Lancet 2001; 358(9292): 1487-1492.

5. Braunschweig CL, Levy P, Sheean PM, Wang X. Enteral compared with parenteral nutrition: a meta-analysis. Am J Clin Nutr 2001; 74:534-542.

6. Chiolero RL, Tappy L, Berger MM. Timming of nutritional support In: Labdarios D, Pichard C, Nestle (eds). Clinical Nutrition: Early intervention. Nutrition workshop series clinical & performance program, Kargar, 2002. Vol 7 pp 151-168.

7. GinerM, Laviano A, Meguid M, Gleason J. In 1995 correlation between malnutrition and poor outcome in critically ill patient still exists. Nutrition. 1996;12:23-29.

8. Heyland D. Nutritional support in the critically ill patient. A critical review of the evidence. Crit Care Clin 1998; 14:423-439.

9. Kehlet H. Postoperative ileus. Gut 2000;47(suppl 4) iv: 85-87.

10. Lipman TO. Grains or veins is enteral nutrition really better than parenteral nutrition? A look at the evidence. J Parenter Enteral Nutr 1998; 22:167-182.

11. Moore FA, Feliciano DV, Andrassy RJ, et al. Early enteral feeding, compared with parenteral, reduces postoperative septic complications. The results of a meta-analysis. Ann Surg 1992;216:172-183.

12. Moore FA, Moore EE, Jones TN, Mc Croskey BL, Peterson VM. TEN versus TPN following major abdominal trauma-Reduced septic morbidity. J Trauma 1989;29:916-923.

13. Marik PE, Zalogu GP. Early enteral nutrition in acutely ill patients: A systematic review. Crit Care Med 2001; 29; 2264-2270.

14. McDonald W, Sharp C, Deitch E. Immediate enteral feeding in burn patients is safe and effective. Ann Surg 1991; 213:177-183.

15. Sandstrom R, Drott C, Hyltander A, et al. The effect of postoperative intravenous feeding (TPN) on outcome following major surgery evaluated in a randomized study. Ann Surg 1993; 217:185-195.

16. Windsor AC, Kanwar S, Li AG, et al. Compared with parental feeding, enteral feeding attenuates the acute phase response and improves disease severity in acute pancreatitis. Gut. 1998;42:431-435.

Macronutrients in Parenteral Formulas

Introduction

The macronutrients in parenteral formulas include dextrose, amino acids, and lipids. The n-6 (linoleic acid) and n-3 (linolenic acid) polyunsaturated fatty acids (PUFA) are enzymatically converted into a series of oxygenated metabolites called eicosanoids. These essential fatty acids (n-6 and n-3 PUFAs) are metabolized by the same enzymes, making them competitive. While eicosanoids derived from n-6 PUFAs are generally pro-inflammatory, prothrombotic, immunosuppressive and chemoreactant, the n-3 PUFAs are able to decrease the production of pro-inflammatory cytokines and reactive oxygen species, and the reactivity of lymphocytes.

GUIDELINES FOR DECIDING MACRONUTRIENTS IN PARENTERAL FORMULAS

1. **Dextrose.**
   It is a primary source of parenteral carbohydrate. Commercial preparations are available in 2.5% to 70% concentrations. The dextrose content of parenteral formula is an important determinant of its osmolarity. Each 5% final concentration of dextrose is approximately 250 mOsm/L.

2. **Amino acids.**
   Proteins for parenteral nutrition are available as pure crystalline amino acids in a desired known composition. While choosing an amino acid product, consider the total nitrogen content of the solution, essential amino acid content, branched chain amino acid content, the aromatic amino acid content (all calculated as a percentage of the total amino acid content) and the electrolyte content of the solution. Parenteral amino acid solutions can be divided into standard solutions and modified solutions.
   (a) **Standard solutions.**
       These are used for patients with normal organ function and nutritional needs. Have a high content of essential amino acids (40-45%) and 16% to 22% branched–chain amino acids (BCAAs). Solutions are available in 3% to 15% concentrations.
   (b) **Modified solutions.**
       These products have been developed for patients with severe stress, liver and kidney failure.

- Solutions containing BCAAs in concentrations of 40% to 50% have been suggested for patients in severe stress, as BCAAs (leucine, isoleucine, and valine) are used as an energy source by muscles and are the only class of amino acids not metabolized by the liver.
- In patients with liver disease, solutions containing higher proportion of BCAAs (35%) with a concomitant decrease in the concentration of aromatic amino acids (phenylalanine, tyrosine, and tryptophan) have been suggested, with a view to normalize the abnormal serum profile, observed in most patients with severe hepatic encephalopathy.
- For patients with renal failure, products containing a higher concentration of essential amino acids or essential amino acids plus histidine, have been developed.
- For neonatal and pediatric use, standard amino acid products are modified to have a lower concentration of methionine, phenylalanine, and glycine with a higher concentration of histidine and tyrosine, which are considered essential for infants.

  Modified solutions, in general, are costly and a definite proof of their efficacy is still lacking.

3. **Lipids.**
    - Used to supply essential fatty acids and as an important source of concentrated energy.
    - Lipid emulsions, in combination with glycerol and an emulsifier (purified mixture of egg yolk phospholipids) are available in 10% and 20% concentrations. 10% emulsion provides 1.1 kcal/mL, the additional non-fat calories coming from glycerol. For all commercially available lipid emulsions of different concentrations, the phospholipid-emulsifying agent is held constant. This means, the proportion of emulsifier to triglyceride is greatest in a 10% lipid emulsion. This ratio has been suggested as the cause of hypertriglyceridemia seen with the separate administration of 10% lipid emulsions in neonates and in adults at very high rates.
    - Commercially, a number of lipids are used for lipid emulsions: polyunsaturated fatty acids as n-3 (e.g. fish oil) or n-6 (e.g. soyabean oil) long-chain triglycerides (LCTs), monounsaturated fatty acids as n-9 LCTs (e.g. olive oil), and saturated fatty acids (e.g. medium–chain triglycerides, MCTs). These oils may be used singly or in combination with others in varying proportions.
    - Intralipid is the most common lipid emulsion available and is made from soyabean oil, which has a high content of polyunsaturated fatty acids – linoleic and linolenic acids, and insufficient amounts of α-tocopherol. Its parenteral use is associated with an increased production of peroxidative catabolites and immunosuppression. A physical mixture of 50% MCTs and 50% LCTs is associated with less immunosuppression, less hepatic dysfunction, no reticuloendothelial compromise, and no interference with pulmonary haemodynamics or gas exchange. Olive oil is rich in mono-

unsaturated fatty acid, oleic acid. Lipid emulsions containing a mixture of 80% olive oil and 20% soyabean oil show benefits in terms of peroxidation, and immune function, when compared to a conventional soyabean oil emulsion. Lipid emulsions having fish oil have also shown promising results because of the immunomodulating properties of n-3 polyunsaturated fatty acids.

Forms of administration.

Several options are available for administration of the parenteral formulas:

- Separate administration of various component solutions.
- Lipid emulsion can be given separately with base solution (dextrose and amino acid combination to which electrolytes, vitamins, and minerals are added).
- Lipid emulsion, together with the base solution in a single bag (three-in-one system, total nutrient admixture).

Three-in-one system (total nutrient admixture) is associated with lesser risk of sepsis and manipulation of central line, requires lesser nursing time and equipment (bags, tubes) and is cost effective.

References

1. Alpers DH, Stenson WF, Bier DM. Manual of Nutritional Therapeutics, 4ed. Philadelphia: Lippincott, Williams & Wilkins, 2002, pp 347-393.

2. Carpentier YA, Simoens C, et al. Recent developments in lipid emulsions: Relevance to Intensive Care. Nutrition 1997;13(9) Suppl: 73S-78S.

3. Dupont I, Siderova VS, Vanweyenberg V, et al. Incorporation of alpha-tocopherol in plasma lipoproteins during and after infusion of fish oil containing emulsions. Clin Nutr 1997; 16(Suppl 2): 2.

4. Hwang TL, Huang SL, Chen MF. Effects of intravenous fat emulsion on respiratory failure. Chest 1990; 97:934-938.

5. Huang DX, Wu ZH, Wu ZG. The all-in-one nutrient solution in parenteral nutrition. Clin Nutr1992; 11:39-44.

6. Mirtallo JM. Parenteral Formulas. In: Rombeau JL, Rolandell RH (eds). Clinical Nutrition: Parenteral Nutrition, 3ed. Philadelphia: Saunders, 2001, pp 118-139.

7. Stokes MA, Hill GI. Peripheral parenteral nutrition: a preliminary report on its efficacy and safety. JPEN J Parenter Enteral Nutr 1993; 17:145.

8. Trissel LA, Gilbert DL, Martinez JF, et al. Compatibility of medications with 3-in-1 parenteral nutrition admixtures. JPEN J Parenter Enteral Nutr 1999; 23:67.

9. Warshawsky KY. Intravenous fat emulsions in clinical practice. Nutr Clin Pract 1992; 15:327.

Total Parenteral Nutrition 49

Introduction

- Total parenteral nutrition (TPN) refers to a mode of delivery of nutrients by which fluids containing nutritive elements, required to maintain proper metabolic levels within the body, are parenterally administered.
- Lipids are an important constituent of parenteral nutrition due to their high energy density and low osmolality.
- In acute illness, blood sugar levels are often increased and generally parallel the severity of stress. The management of glycaemia (usually maintained between 180 and 200 mg/dL) includes appropriate amounts of carbohydrate and insulin. A tighter control of blood sugar between 80 and 110 mg/dL by titration with intensive insulin therapy in ICU, has shown a 40% reduction in mortality rate. Although it needs confirmation, the available evidence indicates that an intensive insulin treatment aimed at maintaining level of glycaemia lower than 110 mg/dL may be an effective means to prevent infectious complications.
- At present, the preliminary evidence available supports the use of glutamine in the artificial nutrition, administered to the patients undergoing the heaviest metabolic stress i.e. trauma (including burns), sepsis and post surgical patients.
- Some amino acids, although non-essential, may become critical in diseased states, such as tyrosine for uraemic patients, glutamine and cysteine for catabolic patients, and taurine for neonates.

GUIDELINES FOR PLANNING PARENTERAL NUTRITION

1. **Define the amount of stress/trauma/catabolism and the nutritional status of the patient.**

    The nutritional status can be assessed by history and clinical examination of the patient followed by biochemical (albumin, prealbumin, transferrin, 24-hour urine and urinary urea nitrogen) and anthropometric measurements.

2. **Calculate the body weight of the patient.**

    Ideal body weight can be estimated by using the following equations:

    For Males – 106 lb for the first 60 inches of height plus 6 lb for each additional inch.

    For Females – 100 lb for the first 60 inches of height plus 5 lb for each additional inch.

For overweight persons, calculate an adjusted body weight:
Adjusted body weight = [(Actual weight – Ideal weight) × 0.24 + Ideal weight].

3. **Calculate the total energy and fluid requirement.**
    - Energy requirements can be calculated in various ways, but for all practical purposes, a calorie intake between 25 k cal/kg/24 hr (post elective surgery) and 35 kcal/kg/24hr (polytrauma, sepsis, burns), may be taken as a goal of nutritional therapy. Additional 10% calories may be added for each 1°C rise in temperature. Remember, critically ill patients should not be overfed. Baseline water requirements in adults may be taken as 30-35 mL/kg/24hr or approximately 1mL/kcal/24hr (25 ml/kg/24hr for those who are above 65 years of age). Additions must be made for fever (approximately 300-500 mL/24hr/degree centigrade above normal) and for other losses. In addition to the obvious losses with diarrhoea, vomiting, fistulae, polyuria etc, keep in mind the losses because of leakage of fluid from the vascular compartment into the interstitial space in patients with vasodilatation or low serum oncotic pressure. Fluid restriction may be indicated in certain disease states such as cardiac, liver, and renal dysfunction.
    - If a patient is getting enteral nutrition, take into account the calories and the fluid being supplied via this route.
    - During critical illness, it is better to initiate with hypocaloric nutrition, with main emphasis on supporting the metabolic response to injury rather than trying to meet the energy balance. Also, overfeeding can lead to hyperglycaemia, fluid overload, hypophosphataemia, respiratory insufficiency, hepatic steatosis, and electrolyte imbalance.

4. **Calculate the liquid necessary, as a carrier, for providing electrolytes, inotropes, heparin, sedatives, and antibiotics.**
    This volume may, at times, form a large percentage of the total volume required/ infused per day. Commonly 500-1000 mL of carrier solution is required in 24 hours.

5. **Calculate the requirement of various components of nutrient solutions: protein, fat, and carbohydrates.**
    (a) Proteins.
    While deciding amino acid requirements, the following points may be kept in mind: (i) The daily requirement for all essential amino acids should be met, (ii) a sufficient quantity of non-essential amino acids (as nitrogen donors) should be supplied so that the essential amino acids are not used as nitrogen providers, and (iii) the amino acid solution should preferably contain the non-essential amino acids arginine, histidine (semi-essential) and alanine (to improve nitrogen balance).
    The daily requirement of amino acids may vary between 0.5 to 1.6 g/kg/24hr, depending upon the amount of stress and the nutritional status of the patient, for example, 0.5 to 0.7 g/kg/24hr in patients with impaired renal or hepatic function, 0.7 to 1.0 g/kg/24hr in patients with good nutritional status and minimum stress (minor surgery), 1.0 to 1.2 g/kg/24hr in patients with poor

nutritional status and in catabolic states (major surgery, children under the age of 5 years, and patients undergoing haemofiltration), 1.2 to 1.3 g/kg/24hr in patients on haemodialysis or peritoneal dialysis, and 1.2 to 1.6 g/kg/24hr in patients with poor nutritional status and having severe catabolic stress (sepsis, burns).

The goal should not be to necessarily achieve positive nitrogen balance, but to achieve, at least, zero protein balance (amounts in and out are equal).

(b) Lipids.

Lipid emulsions should not supply more than 30% of total calories, or more than 50% of non-protein calories per day, as it does not confer any additional clinical benefits. 2% of total calories should be provided as essential fatty acids – linoleic acid (n-6) and about 0.5% of total calories from linolenic acid (n-3) to prevent essential fatty acid deficiency. In patients with renal failure, hepatic failure and in diabetic patients, maximum dose should be limited to 1g/kg/24hr with reduction in dose in case of hypertriglyceridemia.

(c) Carbohydrates.

Up to 50-60% of total calories or 70-90% of non-protein calories may be supplied as glucose, which is the most common intravenous source of carbohydrates. For ICU patients, the total glucose load may be limited to 3.5 to 5 g/kg/24hr, depending upon the severity of stress. Because the glucose in solution is hydrated, it only supplies 3.4 kcal/g of glucose.

6. Define the options available, in terms of route of infusion, for example, peripheral versus central infusion.

Peripheral parenteral nutrition (PPN) refers to nutrient supply through a peripheral vein. The maximum osmolarity that can be tolerated by a peripheral vein is 900 mOsm/L. The concentration of various solutions which can be given safely via peripheral vein /route are lipids (10% or 20% – as both concentrations are iso-osmolar), glucose (5-10%), and amino acids (2-4%). The advantages of PPN are lower cost, easier handling, fewer and less severe complications. PPN is an optimal choice for feeding patients with minimum stress, and who are not significantly malnourished e.g. in post-operative period, uncomplicated acute pancreatitis, gastric resection, etc. PPN may be used to provide nutritional support (approximately 1200-1500 kcal/24hr) for upto 2 weeks, either singly or in combination with enteral feeding. However, PPN is unsuitable for patients with poor peripheral venous access, high energy and nitrogen requirements, high fluid requirements (high output enterocutaneous fistula), and those requiring parenteral nutrition for a longer time. In these patients, central route is preferred.

7. Define the percentage of solutions required to meet the desired goals, via a particular route of infusion.

8. Determine the desired amount of sodium, potassium, chloride, calcium, phosphate, magnesium, and trace elements.

Daily requirement for electrolytes

	Enteral route	*Parenteral route*
Sodium	500 mg (22 mEq/kg)	1-2 mEq/kg
Potassium	2 g (51 mEq/kg)	1-2 mEq/kg
Chloride	750 mg (21 mEq/kg)	As needed to maintain acid-base balance
Calcium	1200 mg (30 mEq/kg)	5-7.5 mEq/kg
Magnesium	420 mg (17 mEq/kg)	4-10 mEq/kg
Phosphorus	700 mg (23 mEq/kg)	20-40 mEq/kg

Daily requirement for trace elements

	Enteral route	*Parenteral route*
Chromium	30 µg	10-15 µg
Copper	0.9 mg	0.3-0.5 mg
Fluoride	4 mg	Not well defined
Iodine	150 µg	Not well defined
Iron	18 mg	Not routinely added
Manganese	2.3 mg	60-100 µg
Molybdenum	45 µg	Not routinely added
Selenium	55 µg	20-60 µg
Zinc	11 mg	2.5 –5 mg

Because of the risk of anaphylaxis, parenteral nutrition products do not routinely contain iron. It should be supplemented separately for patients requiring long term parenteral nutrition. Further, patients with renal failure may not require some trace elements that are cleared by the kidneys (e.g. selenium and chromium).

9. **Determine the daily requirement of vitamins.**

   For most of the patients in the ICU, the requirement of the vitamins can be met by daily administration of commercially available preparations. The standard adult intravenous vitamin preparations contain all the recommended vitamins except vitamin K, which should be supplemented. The deficiency of these vitamins (if not supplemented in daily TPN) can lead to increased morbidity and mortality. The daily requirements recommended for vitamins are :

Water soluble vitamin	*Enteral route*	*Parenteral route*
Thiamine(B_1)	1.2 mg	3.0 mg
Riboflavin(B_2)	1.3 mg	3–6 mg
Pantothenic acid	5 mg	15 mg
Niacin	16 mg	40 mg
Pyridoxine(B_6)	1.7 mg	4 mg
Biotin	30 µg	60 µg
Folic Acid	400 µg	400 µg
Cyanocobalamine	2.4 µg	5 µg
Ascorbic acid (C)	90 mg	100 mg

Fat soluble vitamins

Retinoic acid (A)	900 µg	1000 µg
Ergocalciferol(D_2)	15 µg	5 µg
α-tocopherol (E)	15 mg	10 mg
Phytomenadione (K)	120 µg	1mg/24 hr (5 mg/week)

10. **Subtract the amount of electrolytes contributed by the amino acid solution from the calculated requirements.**

    Look at the amino acid product. Electrolytes are part of some amino acid products.

11. **Opt for a solution which balances the above requirements in a particular patient. Integrate nutrient supply into fluid therapy.**

12. **Add requirements of electrolytes, trace elements, and vitamins.**

    Add magnesium as magnesium sulfate, calcium as calcium gluconate, vitamins as MVI injection, and trace elements. Whenever possible, all fluid and electrolyte additions should be incorporated into the parenteral nutrition solution. This allows removal of peripheral lines and eliminates a source of sepsis. In patients with large variations in external drainage, however, it is preferable to replace these losses, as they occur with appropriate solutions infused through peripheral intravenous lines.

13. **Adopt a slowly increasing, step-by-step approach, in infusing parenteral nutrition.**

    With this approach, body metabolism gets time to adapt to the changes in energy supply, and metabolic disturbances, as described below, are less frequent.

    Glucose: Stress leads to increased levels of norepinephrine, epinephrine, cortisol and glucagon, increased insulin resistance, and elevated blood glucose levels. Moreover, since fat cannot be administered in the acute phase, glucose is the only source of energy in the early stages. Hyperglycaemia can lead to hyperosmolarity which induces intracellular dehydration, elevated lactate levels, increased risk of infection, hepatic steatosis, respiratory decompensation, and severe electrolyte disturbances. To reduce all these effects, glucose should be administered slowly and in gradually increasing amounts. Insulin may be added to drive glucose into the cells but it does not increase the rate of glucose oxidation. Further, high intracellular levels of glucose may be detrimental in areas of reduced perfusion and hypoxia.

    Amino acids: Amino acids when supplied at more than recommended dosages or at a faster rate may lead to marked increase in urea production rate (as the amino acids cannot be incorporated into the cells), increased minute ventilation, amino–aciduria, metabolic acidosis (if the amino acids in the solution are predominantly present in the form of chloride), or hyperammonemia, (when infused quickly in patients with hepatic insufficiency).

    Fat: Fat should not be administered during the acute phase of shock. In a haemodynamically stable patient, when administered at faster than recommended rate, it may lead to hypertriglyceridemia. Excessive fat administration also depresses glucose utilization resulting in elevated blood sugar levels.

14. Modify the formulation if indicated.

See Chapter 55.

15. Monitor the patient.

- Before starting TPN, obtain blood sugar, serum electrolytes (Na^+, K^+, Cl^-, HCO_3^-), blood urea, serum creatinine, albumin, magnesium, calcium, phosphorus, lipid profile, total and differential blood cell count, prothrombin time, alkaline phosphatase, aspartate aminotransferase (AST), total bilirubin, and urine analysis.
- On the first day, measure blood sugar every 6 hours for 24 hours.
- During the first week, measure serum electrolytes, blood urea, sugar, and serum triglycerides daily. Unstable patients may require blood sugar and serum electrolyte measurements as often as twice a day. Ask for serum calcium, AST, bilirubin, alkaline phosphatase, phosphorus, magnesium and blood counts, at least twice a week. Prothrombin time and albumin should be measured once a week.
- Once the desired infusion rate of TPN has been achieved, and blood chemistries are stable, monitoring may be reduced to once a week, but should never be omitted.
- Monitor the patient clinically:
  - Vital signs (temperature, blood pressure, pulse, respiratory rate).
  - Fluid balance (weight, input versus output, and edema).
  - Delivery equipment for parenteral nutrition: composition of nutrient solution, tubing, pump, filter, catheter, dressing (check skin for local infection at the time of dressing change), change of sets, hang time, accuracy of the set rate.

References

1. ASPEN Board of Directors and The Clinical Guidelines Task Force. Guidelines for the use of parenteral and enteral nutrition in adult and pediatric patients. JPEN 2002; 26(1): 22SA-24SA.
2. Beck AM, Balknas UN, Furst P, et al. Food and nutritional care in hospitals: how to prevent undernutrition-report and guidelines from the council of Europe. Clin Nutrit 2001; 20(5): 455-460.
3. Bistrian BR, Blackburn GL, Vitale J, et al. Prevalence of malnutrition in general medical patients. JAMA 1976; 235:1567-1570.
4. Bistrian BR, Blackburn GL, Hallowell E, Heddle R. Protein status of general surgical patients JAMA 1974; 230:858-860.
5. Choban PS, Burge JC, Scales D, Flancbaum L. Hypoenergetic nutrition support in hospitalized obese patients: A simplified method of clinical application. Am J Clin Nutr 1997; 66:546-550.
6. Deegan H, Dent S, Keefe L, et al. Supplemental parenteral nutrition in the critically ill patient: a retrospective study. Clinical Intensive Care 1999; 10:131-136.
7. Mirtallo JM. Parenteral formulas. In: Rombeau JL, Rolandell RH (eds). Clinical Nutrition: Parenteral Nutrition, 3ed. Philadelphia: Saunders, 2001, pp 118-130.

8. National Advisory Group on standards and practice guidelines for parenteral nutrition: safe practices for parenteral nutrition formulations. JPEN J Parenter Enteral Nutr 1998; 22:49-66.

9. Payne-James JJ, Khawaja HT. First choice for total parenteral nutrition: the peripheral route. JPEN J Parenter Enteral Nutr 1993; 17:468.

10. Shizgal HM. Parenteral and enteral nutrition. Annu Rev Med 1991; 42:549-565.

11. The Veterans Affairs Total Parenteral Nutrition Cooperative study group. Perioperative total parenteral nutrition in surgical patients. N Eng. J Med 1991; 325:525-532.

12. Van Way III CW. Nutritional support in the injured patient. Surg Clin of North Am 1991; 71(3): 537-547.

13. Wood AJJ. Nutritional support. N Engl J Med 1997; 336:41-48.

14. Worthington PH, Wagner BA. Total parenteral nutrition. Nursing Clin North Am 1989; 24(2): 355-371.

Introduction

- Adopt a step-by-step approach while initiating parenteral nutrition. Total dose and rate of infusion should be based on the patient's ability to metabolize the type and amount of energy being supplied. It is better to start at a lower dose and rate, and advance to the target rate over the next 24-72 hours.
- Parenteral nutrition solutions should be infused at a steady rate. Large changes in the infusion rate, ($\pm15\%$ or more), may lead to significant hyperglycaemia or hypoglycaemia and, if marked, to coma, convulsions, and even death.

GUIDELINES FOR INITIATION OF PARENTERAL NUTRITION

1. **Consider the indication.**
   See Chapter 47.

2. **Obtain vital information about the patient.**
   - Check vitals (temperature, blood pressure, pulse, respiratory rate).
   - Check weight, input/output balance.
   - Check baseline biochemistry.

3. **Select the route of administration.**
   See Chapter 49.

4. **Select the parenteral formula.**
   - Calculate the daily dosages of various components.
   - Decide about the form of administration – the components can be administered separately, or as premixed multi-component solutions.
   - Consider any additives to be mixed.
   - Consider any modification in the formula required, based on the patient's condition.
   - Take into account enteral nutrition, if any.

5. **Write down the instructions clearly.**
   Instructions should include: (a) Total energy, (b) substrate distribution, (c) fluid volume, (d) rate of delivery, (e) hang time, (f) any change in the rate of delivery, (g) total time frame, (h) steps to be taken, in case of accidental change in rate of delivery or in case of interruption in delivery of the solution.
   A few of these points merit further discussion:

   (i) **Rate of infusion.**
Glucose: Start slowly to a target rate of 5mg/kg/min (normal hepatic oxidation is at the rate of 5-7 mg/kg/min); check blood sugar every 6 hours; adjust the rate to keep blood sugar below 150 mg/dL, or add insulin infusion to titrate blood sugar level.
Amino acids: Start at a lower dose and rate, and increase gradually to the desired goal.
Lipids: Do not administer fat during acute phase of shock; start slowly to a target rate of 0.05 g/kg/hr. Do not exceed the maximum rate of 0.11 g/kg/hr. Remember the percentage of total calories which can be given as lipids; adjust the dose and rate by checking plasma triglyceride levels. When lipids are actually being infused, their level should neither exceed 300 mg/dL, nor show a rising trend. 12 hours after administration of the infusion, plasma triglyceride levels should not exceed 250 mg/dL (see Table 50.1).

  (ii) **Hang time.**
Lipid emulsion, when given alone, should be completely infused within 12 hours of hanging of the emulsion. Lipids when administered as total nutrient admixture and fat emulsion free TPN, are less likely to support the growth of pathogens, and may therefore be safely hung for 24 hours.

 (iii) **Accidental change in the rate of delivery.**
Simply, correct the hourly infusion rate and continue with the corrected rate. Do not try to increase or decrease the rate to meet the ordered daily volume.

 (iv) **Interruption in delivery of PN solution.**
If PN solution has to be interrupted, instructions should clearly mention the administration of 5% dextrose solution at the same rate, to prevent sudden hypoglycaemia caused by high endogenous insulin secretion that is associated with the infusion of hypertonic dextrose.

6. **Introduction and care of the catheter (central or peripheral, as applicable).**
- The catheter should be inserted under all aseptic precautions and should be used only for the purpose of parenteral nutrition. Perform it as an elective procedure.
- Always obtain a chest X-ray to confirm the position of the catheter before starting PN.
- Always use strict aseptic technique while handling the catheter-tubing connection. Clean all connections with alcohol, before any tubing changes are made.
- The catheter should be inspected daily, cleaned with an alcohol-based solution and covered with an occlusive dressing. A wet dressing, any time of the day, is an indication for an immediate change.
- Avoid drawing blood from TPN line.
- Avoid infusing medications through the TPN line.
- Prophylactic change of catheter does not reduce infection rates.

Table 50.1: The building-up of parenteral nutrition in a patient

	Day 1			Day 2			Day 3			Day 4	Day 5
Hours	1-8	8-16	16-24	1-8	8-16	16-24	1-8	8-16	16-24	1-24	1-24
Carbohydrates											
• g/kg/hr	0.05	0.10	0.12	0.16	0.16	0.20	0.20	0.20	0.20	0.20	0.20
• g/hr (assumed body weight 60 kg)	3.0	6.0	7.2	9.6	9.6	12	12	12	12	12	12
• mL/hr (% Dextrose)	30 (10%)	60 (10%)	30 (25%)	38 (25%)	38 (25%)	48 (25%)	48 (25%)	48 (25%)	48 (25%)	48 (25%)	48 (25%)
Amino acids											
• g/kg/hr	-	0.013	0.02	0.03	0.035	0.04	0.04	0.045	0.05	0.05	0.055
• g/hr (assumed body weight 60 kg)	-	0.8	1.2	1.8	2.1	2.4	2.4	2.7	3.0	3.0	3.3
• mL/hr (10% solution)	-	8	12	18	21	24	24	27	30	30	33
Fat											
• g/kg/hr	-	-	-	-	-	-	0.0125	0.0125	0.0125	0.025	0.045
• g/hr (assumed body weight 60 kg)	-	-	-	-	-	-	0.75	0.75	0.75	1.50	2.70
• mL/hr (10% emulsion)	-	-	-	-	-	-	7.5	7.5	7.5	15	27
Non-protein energy (k cal) per 60 kg/24 hr	440			850			1140			1304	1563
Total amino acids (g) per 60 kg/24 hr	18.4			50.4			65.8			72	79

Note: 1. To simplify, percentages of various component solutions have been kept constant (except a change on day 1 in case of dextrose). These need to be changed depending upon the volume and dose requirements of the patients.

2. These doses and rates may be taken as an example of how to slowly build up PN. These may be varied depending upon the patient's condition.

7. Check the pump, tubings, filters, and bag.

- Infusion sets with tubings free of plasticizer (DEHP, di-2, ethylhexylphthelate) have been recommended for use with lipid emulsions. These sets are called fat infusion sets or nitroglycerin sets.
- Administration sets should be changed every 24 hours.
- For total nutrient admixture (three-in-one system), a 1.2 µm filter, and for fat emulsion free TPN, a 0.22 µm filter has been recommended.
- Visually inspect the bag for any sign of deterioration before administration.
- Add only compatible drugs to the mixture.

8. Monitor the patient.

See Chapter 49.

References

1. ASPEN Board of Directors and The Clinical Guidelines Task Force. Guidelines for the use of parenteral and enteral nutrition in adult and pediatric patients. JPEN 2002; 26(1): 22SA-24SA.
2. Beck AM, Balknas UN, Furst P, et al. Food and nutritional care in hospitals: how to prevent undernutrition-report and guidelines from the council of Europe. Clin Nutr 2001; 20(5): 155-160.
3. Bistrian BR, Blackburn GL, Vitale J, et al. Prevalence of malnutrition in general medical patients. JAMA 1976; 235:1567-1570.
4. Bistrian BR, Blackburn GL, Hallowell E, Heddle R. Protein status of general surgical patients. JAMA 1974; 230:858-860.
5. Choban PS, Burge JC, Scales D, Flancbaum L. Hypoenergetic nutrition support in hospitalized obese patients: A simplified method of clinical application. Am J Clin Nutr 1997; 66:546-550.
6. Deegan H, Dent S, Keefe L, et al. Supplemental parenteral nutrition in the critically ill patient: A retrospective study. Clin Intensive Care 1999; 10:131-136.
7. Mirtallo JM. Parenteral formulas. In: Rombeau JL, Rolandell RH, (eds). Clinical Nutrition: Philadelphia: Saunders 2001, pp 118-130.
8. National Advisory Group on standards and practice guidelines for parenteral nutrition: safe practices for parenteral nutrition formulations. JPEN J Parenter Enteral Nutr 1998; 22:49-66.
9. Payne-James JJ, Khawaja HT. First choice for total parenteral nutrition: the peripheral route. JPEN J Parenter Enteral Nutr 1993; 17:468.
10. Shizgal HM. Parenteral and enteral nutrition. Annu Rev Med 1991; 42:549-565.
11. The Veterans Affairs Total Parenteral Nutrition Cooperative study group. Perioperative total parenteral nutrition in surgical patients. N Eng. J Med 1991; 325:525-532.
12. Van Way III CW. Nutritional support in the injured patient. Surg Clin North Am 1991; 71(3): 537-547.
13. Wood AJJ. Nutritional support. N Engl J Med 1997; 336:41-48.
14. Worthington PH, Wagner BA. Total parenteral nutrition. Nurs Clin North Am 1989; 24(2): 355-371.

Introduction

All formulas contain the macronutrients (carbohydrates, fats, proteins, and water), and the micronutrients (vitamins, minerals, trace elements and electrolytes). They differ in composition and proportion of nutrients as well as cost.

GUIDELINES FOR CLASSIFYING ENTERAL FORMULAS

1. Polymeric.
    (a) Blenderized.
    Real food; requires normal digestion and absorption, lactose/lactose-free, isotonic, nutritionally complete; time consuming; bacterial contamination more likely; do not have such excellent flow characteristics as to pass through small-caliber tubes.

    (b) Standard.
    Intact nutrients; lactose free; low residue; isotonic; nutritionally complete; requires normal digestion and absorption; most widely used; less costly; can be administered into the stomach, duodenum, or jejunum; ratio of nitrogen to non-protein calories is less than 1:130; provides approximately 1 kcal/mL; usually well tolerated.

    (c) High nitrogen.
    Intact nutrients; lactose free; isotonic; low residue; nutritionally complete; requires normal digestion and absorption; proteins more than 15% of the total calories; ratio of nitrogen to non-protein calories more than 1:130; may be enriched with branched-chain amino acids; useful in patients with high protein requirement i.e. severe trauma, healing wounds, protein losing enteropathy. Contraindicated in patients with renal failure and hepatic encephalopathy.

    (d) Fibre enriched.
    Intact nutrients; lactose free; isotonic, contains soluble and insoluble fiber; nutritionally complete; requires normal digestion and absorption; regulates bowel function and a source of short-chain fatty acids.

    (e) Calorically dense (volume-restricted).
    Intact nutrients; 1.5 to 2.0 kcal/mL; high osmolality; lactose free; nutritionally complete; requires normal digestion and absorption; useful in patients with fluid restriction i.e. renal failure, liver failure, ascites, congestive heart failure,

pulmonary edema, or the syndrome of inappropriate antidiuretic hormone (SIADH).

(f) Disease-specific.

Intact nutrients; source of fat, protein and carbohydrate varies depending on the disease state for which the formula is designed; electrolyte content and osmolality vary; requires normal digestion and absorption; expensive; efficacy controversial.

(i) Hepatic formulas.

Have low protein content, high concentration of branched chain amino acids and low concentration of aromatic amino acids to protect against hepatic encephalopathy; high osmolality (>600 mOsm/kg); high content of carbohydrate; higher cost; indicated only in those who develop hepatic encephalopathy when given standard formulations to achieve a positive nitrogen balance.

(ii) Renal formulas.

Low protein content and high percentage of essential amino acids to decrease urea production; low electrolyte content to minimize renal solute load; low or no vitamins and minerals; high osmolality (>600 mOsm/kg); high carbohydrate content; low protein content (patient's daily requirement not met), expensive; most useful for patients who have significant renal impairment but are not yet on dialysis. Those with milder renal impairment or on dialysis can be managed with standard formulas.

(iii) Diabetic formulas.

Less carbohydrate, more fat and added fibre to slow gastric emptying and delay glucose absorption in the gut (clinical effectiveness not well documented); amount of total carbohydrate provided is the most significant factor. Effectiveness of these formulas is yet to be established.

(iv) Immune-enhancing formulas.

Formulas supplemented with nucleotides, glutamine, arginine, and omega-3 fatty acids to enhance immune function. For use in critically ill septic or stressed surgical patients, have shown clinical benefits but exact role is still to be established.

2. Oligomeric (partially hydrolyzed, semi-elemental).

Hydrolyzed protein, di-, tri-peptides, free amino acids; content may vary (3-40% of total calories); lactose free; osmolality varies (250-700 mOsm/kg); nutritionally complete; digestion required; useful when capacity to digest and absorb food is diminished.

3. Monomeric (elemental/chemically defined).

Free amino acids; lactose free; variable fat (1- 15% of total calories) content; high osmolality; nutritionally complete; minimal digestion required; more expensive; has many disadvantages.

4. Modular.

Individual nutrient (carbohydrate, fat, protein) modules; used to modify pre-existing commercial formulas to increase nutrient density; requires normal digestion and absorption.

References

1. Alpers DH, Stenson WF, Bier DM. Manual of Nutritional Therapeutics, 4 ed., Philadelphia: Lippincott, Williams & Wilkins, pp 309-345.

2. Buchman AL. Glutamine: Commercially essential or conditionally essential? A Critical appraisal of the human data. Am J Clin Nutr 2001; 74:25-32.

3. Eisenberg P. Enteral nutrition: indications, formulas, and delivery techniques. Nurs Clin of North Am. 1989;24(2):315-339.

4. Gadek J, Demichele S, Karlstad M, Pacht ER, Donahoe M, Albertson TE, Van Hoozen CH. Effect of enteral feeding with eicosapentaenoic acid, Y-linolenic acid, and anti-oxidants in patients with acute respiratory distress syndrome. Crit Care Med 199; 27:1409-1420.

5. Galban C, Montejo JC, Masezo A, et al. An immune-enhancing enteral diet reduces mortality rate and episodes of bacteremia in septic intensive care unit patients. Crit Care Med 2000; 28:643-648.

6. Heyland DK, Cook DJ, Guyatt GH. Does the formulation of enteral feeding products influence infections, morbidity and mortality rates in the critically ill patient? A critical review of the evidence. Crit Care Med 1994;22:1192-1202.

7. Heyland DK, Novak F, Drover JW, Jain M, Su X, Suchner U. Should immunonutrition become routine in critically ill patients? A systemic review of the evidence. JAMA 2001; 286:944-953.

8. Heyland DK, Samis A. Does immunonutrition in patients with sepsis do more harm than good? Intensive Care Med 2003; 29:669-671.

9. Hondijk APJ, Rijnsburger ER, Jansen J, et al. Randomized trial of glutamine-enriched enteral nutrition on infections morbidity in patients with multiple trauma. Lancet 1998; 352:772-776.

10. Jones C, Palmer A, Griffiths RD. Randomized Clinical outcome study of critically ill patients given glutamine-supplemented enteral nutrition. Nutrition 1999; 15:108-115.

11. Lamache LI. Enteral nutrition in the critically ill patient. In: Ryan DW (ed) Current Practice in Critical Illness, 1996, London: Chapman & Hall, pp 1996, 89-106.

12. Matarese LE. Enteral feeding solutions. Gastrointest Endosc Clin North Am 1998;8(3): 593-609.

13. Moshe S. Enteral feeding. In: Shils ME, Olson JA, Shike M (eds). Modern Nutrition in Health and Disease, 8th ed. Philadelphia Lea and Febiger, 1994, pp 1417-1430.

14. Weinstein DS, Furman J. Enteral formulas. Nurs Clin North Am 1997; 12(4): 669-683.

Selection of Formula for Enteral Nutrition

Introduction

A number of enteral formulations with variations in specific characteristics and nutrient content are available commercially. The selection of any particular formulation should be based on the patient's digestive and absorptive capacity, organ function, specific nutrient needs, tolerance, allergies and should take into account the formula composition and total calories. Some of the nutritional considerations relating to enteral formulas are as follows:

GUIDELINES FOR SELECTING AN ENTERAL FORMULA

1. Protein source (intact protein, peptides or amino acids).
   - Formulas having intact proteins are similar to a pureed diet; they require normal levels of pancreatic enzymes to metabolize large proteins to smaller polypeptides and free amino acids. When a patient's digestion is intact, it is best to feed an intact protein diet. Formulas having partially hydrolyzed proteins have polypeptide fragments or di- and tri- peptides from protein sources and also from whey, meat, or collagen. When digestion is impaired (e.g. by pancreatic insufficiency, sepsis, multiple trauma, shock and severe malnutrition) a diet containing large amounts of smaller peptides (<10 amino acids in length) is advantageous. Peptide-based formulas are associated with numerous advantages, as compared to intact protein formulations. These include improved nitrogen absorption and protein synthesis, decreased stool output and diarrhoea, better growth and wound repair, better gut maintenance and enhanced hepatic protein synthesis.
   - Elemental formulas contain crystalline L-amino acids that do not require digestion and are readily transported across the intestinal mucosa into the bloodstream. Very few studies support the use of amino acid based diets instead of intact protein or peptide-based formulas. Reported disadvantages of amino acid-based diets include gut atrophy, bacterial translocation, decreased liver function, increased diarrhoea, decreased growth and wound healing, poor nitrogen balance and higher mortality.
   - The specific proteins used in any particular formula may also be important. In one study evaluating growth in rats, fed on diets containing different intact proteins (i.e. casein, soy, whey), growth was more in those fed on soy. Another study, evaluating growth and survival rates after methotrexate

in mice fed on diets of different protein sources (casein or soy), reported better outcome in the soy group. Lactose-free formulas are composed of soybean protein isolates, sodium, calcium or potassium caseinates, or de-lactosed or hydrolyzed lactalbumin.

2. **Carbohydrate source.**

The form and concentration of carbohydrates differ among the formulas: (a) starch (i.e. hydrolyzed cereal solids, flour, hydrolyzed corn starch); (b) glucose polymers (i.e. maltodextrins, corn syrup, glucose oligosaccharides); (c) disaccharides (i.e. sucrose, lactose, maltose); and (d) monosaccharides (i.e. glucose, fructose).

3. **Fat source.**

- Fat provides concentrated calories, essential fatty acids, enhances flavour, and serves as a carrier for fat-soluble vitamins. Digestion of fats usually requires pancreatic enzymes, bile salts, an intact intestinal wall and normal intestinal flora. However, medium-chain triglycerides (MCTs) do not require digestion by pancreatic lipase or bile salts and are transported directly to the liver for oxidation. MCTs are not carried via the lymphatic system, as long-chain fatty acids are. MCT oil containing fatty acids, primarily of 8-10 carbons in length, is useful in patients who are unable to digest or absorb fat. MCT oil does not have linoleic acid. The entry of MCTs into mitochondria is independent of carnitine, and they rapidly undergo β-oxidation. MCT oil can thus be used as a caloric supplement. However, longer-chain triglycerides should be included in the diet, as no essential fatty acids are found in MCT oil.

- Fat contained in enteral formulas is in the form of medium or long-chain fatty acids. Fat may be saturated or polyunsaturated. Examples of fats found in commercial enteral formulas include: Medium chain (usually saturated, coconut oil), Long chain (usually polyunsaturated, corn oil, safflower oil, sunflower oil, soybean oil, canola oil), Phospholipid (usually polyunsaturated, polyglycerol ester of fatty acids), and Glycerides (monoglycerides, diglycerides, triglycerides). All enteral feeds contain omega-6 and omega-3 fatty acids (linoleic and linolenic acids respectively) which must be supplied in the diet as they cannot be synthesized de novo. Unlike carbohydrates and proteins, lipids do not contribute to osmolality.

4. **Energy density (caloric density).**

Caloric density has tremendous implications in terms of patient management. Most standard formulations provide 1.0 kcal/mL. Formulas with high caloric density (1.5-2.0 kcal/mL) provide a large number of calories in a relatively small volume but such formulations tend to be hypertonic and may cause diarrhoea. Such concentrated formulas are usually given only to patients with normal renal function. Also, as the caloric density increases, gastric motility and gastric emptying decreases.

On the other hand, formulas with low caloric density (0.5 kcal/mL) provide their calories in a relatively large fluid volume; such solutions can pose problems to patients on fluid restriction.

5. **Energy distribution.**
    In most commercial formulas carbohydrates provide 50-60% of total calories. The remainder is provided by proteins (10-20%) and fats (30-40%). It is recommended that fat should make up no more than 30% of the caloric content of the diet, given as a mixture of MCTs, omega-6 and omega-3 polyunsaturated fatty acids. A balanced, fat formula could be one that contains the required amount of linoleic acid (i.e. 5% to 10% of non protein calories to prevent essential fatty acid deficiency) mixed with other lipids (i.e. MCTs, omega–3 PUFA, and saturated fats). However, the optimal ratio of each constituent is probably yet to be determined.

6. **Renal solute load.**
    Renal solute load of a formula indicates the demands placed by the nutritional product on the kidneys and should be taken into consideration while choosing a formula for patients with diminished functional capacity of the kidneys. Renal solute load is determined primarily by the protein and electrolyte content of the formula. The major contributors to the renal solute load are urea (the end-product of protein digestion) and the electrolytes (sodium, potassium, and chloride). The greater is the renal solute load, the greater would be the obligatory water loss through the kidneys. Thus, with increasing impairment of renal function and inability of the kidneys to concentrate solutes, there is increase in the obligatory water loss for a given solute load. These considerations have led to the development of renal formulas having decreased protein content (with high percentage of essential amino acids to further decrease urea production) and low electrolyte and mineral content.

7. **Fibre content and source.**
    *   Fibre is a material from plant cell walls that is resistant to digestion by enzymes of the human small intestine. Fibre is often classified according to its solubility in water. Water soluble fibres (pectin, gums, mucilages and some hemicelluloses) tend to be efficiently broken down by bacteria in the colon. Water-insoluble fibres (lignin, cellulose, and the remaining hemicelluloses) pass through the body mostly unchanged. Dietary fibre is a complex mixture of both. Insoluble fibre produces a laxative effect and increases faecal bulk. Soluble fibre ferments in the colon, producing short-chain fatty acids which are nutrients for colonic mucosal cells, have a trophic effect on mucosa, and decrease the risk of bacterial translocation. Most fibre containing commercial formulas use soy polysaccharides, which largely contain insoluble fibre and serve to increase stool bulk and regulate transit time. Some preparations contain fructo-oligosaccharides which are degraded by colonic bacteria to form short-chain fatty acids.
    *   The utility of fibre-containing enteral formulations in critically ill patients remains to be documented.
        Fibre can increase flatulence, which is sometimes distressing. Use of fibre may cause faecal impaction if adequate water is not given. Fibre also increases the potential for feeding tube obstruction, especially if small-bore tubes are used.

8. **Ratio of nitrogen to non-protein calories.**

    In a patient, consumed proteins (amino acids) are predominantly used for protein synthesis so long as enough calories are supplied for energy. Determination of the ratio of nitrogen to non-protein (fat plus carbohydrates) calories is a method of identifying calories available for energy. In normal health, this ratio approximates 1:350. During illness, trauma or stress, protein requirement increases. To allow for anabolic use of proteins, sufficient carbohydrate and fat calories must be consumed. A nitrogen to non-protein calorie ratio of 1:100 to 1:200 is believed to be adequate during illness. However, these formulations (high nitrogen formulas) may be associated with increased urea and ammonia production.

9. **Vitamin and mineral content (i.e. volume required to supply recommended dietary allowances).**

    The recommended dietary allowances (RDA) outline the levels of intake of essential nutrients judged to be adequate to meet the known nutritional needs of practically all healthy persons and therefore, do not accurately reflect potential needs of patients who are ill, injured or elderly. The RDAs should, therefore, be used only against this background. Most enteral formulas are designed to meet the RDA for vitamins in 1-3L of formula.

10. **Osmolality.**

    - Osmolality is very important in selecting appropriate enteral formula and is one of the most important piece of information regarding any formula. Isotonic formulas have approximately the same osmolality as normal plasma (i.e. 280-300 mOsm/kg). Such formulas are initially administered at full strength and the rate of administration is increased slowly, depending on the tolerance. Hypertonic formulas have osmolality in the range of 400-1100 mOsm/kg. Such formulas are initially administered either at full strength and slow rate of infusion, or at half strength and normal rate of infusion and the rate of administration is increased (as tolerated) with respect to either strength or rate. Do not increase both rate and strength at the same time.
    - Main determinants of the osmolality of a formula are carbohydrates, proteins and electrolyte content. Semi-elemental and elemental formulas have higher osmolalities. Patient receiving hypertonic formulas must be observed for delayed gastric emptying, severe diarrhoea, electrolyte depletion and severe dehydration. These problems may be further complicated by the patient's clinical condition (e.g. infection, drains, tracheostomy). In patients with jejunostomy, these formulas cause large stomal water and sodium losses.

11. **Viscosity.**

    Viscosity of an enteral formula is important in relation to the size of nasogastric tube. Most of the fine-bore tubes used in clinical practice vary from 1.4 mm (4FG) for small infants to 2.7-4.0 mm (8-12FG) for older children and adults. All commercially available feeds can be administered with good flow through an 8FG tube. However, formulas containing fibre may clog the smaller sized tubes.

12. **Palatability and patient acceptance.**

   It is more important for formulas which come as ready-to-use commercial oral (or sip) feeds.

13. **Other specific nutrients of current interest (see Chapter 55).**

References

1. Beale RJ, Bryg DJ, Bihari DJ. Immunonutrition in the critically ill: A systematic review of clinical outcome. Crit Care Med 1999; 27:2799-2805.
2. Buchman AL. Glutamine: Commercially essential or conditionally essential? A Critical appraisal of the human data. Am J Clin Nutr 2001; 74:25-32.
3. Gadek J, Demichele S, Karlstad M, Pacht ER, Donahoe M, Albertson TE, Van Hoozen CH. Effect of enteral feeding with eicosapentaenoic acid, Y-linolenic acid, and anti-oxidants in patients with acute respiratory distress syndrome. Crit Care Med 199; 27:1409-1420.
4. Galban C, Montejo JC, Masezo A, et al. An immune-enhancing enteral diet reduces mortality rate and episodes of bacteremia in septic intensive care unit patients. Crit Care Med 2000; 28:643-648.
5. Heyland DK, Novak F, Drover JW, Jain M, Su X, Suchner U. Should immunonutrition become routine in critically ill patients? A systemic review of the evidence. JAMA 2001; 286:944-953.
6. Heyland DK, Samis A. Does immunonutrition in patients with sepsis do more harm than good? Intensive Care Med 2003; 29:669-671.
7. Hondijk APJ, Rijnsburger ER, Jansen J, et al. Randomized trial of glutamine-enriched enteral nutrition on infections morbidity in patients with mulliple trauma. Lancet 1998; 352:772-776.
8. Jones C, Palmer A, Griffiths RD. Randomized Clinical outcome study of critically ill patients given glutamine-supplemented enteral nutrition. Nutrition 1999; 15:108-115.
9. Matarese LE. Enteral feeding solutions. Gastrointest Endosc Clin North Am 1998;8(3): 593-609.
10. Weinstein DS, Furman J. Enteral formulas. Nurs Clin North Am 1997; 12(4): 669-683.

Planning an Enteral Feed 53

GUIDELINES FOR PLANNING AN ENTERAL FEED

1. **Assess the patient's readiness for enteral nutrition; most patients may be ready within 24 to 48 hours of ICU admission.**
   - Patients who are on catecholamine support, heavy sedation or therapeutic neuromuscular blockade, or whose vitals are not stable and are deteriorating, are probably not ready for initiation of enteral feeding. Adequate intestinal perfusion should be restored before starting enteral nutrition, as it may induce ischaemia of the already stressed gut if mesenteric blood flow cannot be increased (a normal response to enteral nutrition is increased messenteric blood flow), either because of hypovolaemia, or catecholamine-induced vasoconstriction. There appears to be no evidence against trophic feeding (10 mL of full strength formula per hour) in a haemodynamically unstable patient.
   - Check the nasogastric aspirate in the previous 24 hours – enteral feeding may be started if the nasogastric aspirate is less than 200-300 mL/24hr. An increasing or decreasing trend may be more important than an isolated high amount of aspirate.
   - Examine the abdomen for signs of obstruction, GI tract disruption, ischaemia, abdominal distension, and tenderness.
   - Look for the presence of bowel sounds although absence of bowel sounds is not a contraindication for initiation of enteral feeding.

2. **Establish goals.**
   Feeding may be initiated at 25% of the calculated amount or even less and slowly advanced, especially in the presence of sedation or minimal vasopressor support in an adequately resuscitated patient. It is not advisable to start with 100% of the patient's caloric needs on first or second day in a critically ill patient. A feeding goal of 50 – 60% of calculated calories within the first 3-5 days is a reasonably good start, which can be slowly increased to 100% over the next 1-2 days.

3. **Choose the site for EN delivery.**
   Gastric feeding requires intact gag and cough reflexes and adequate gastric emptying. Small bowel access is indicated in clinical conditions in which tracheal aspiration, reflux oesophagitis, gastroparesis, gastric outlet obstruction, or previous gastric surgery preclude gastric feeding or when early post-operative feeding after major abdominal procedure/surgery is planned. However, studies have not consistently demonstrated the benefit of small bowel feeding over gastric feeding to prevent aspiration.

4. **Consider enteral access.**

   The nasoenteric tubes are indicated for a short-term (< 4 weeks) as they have low complication rates, are relatively inexpensive, and are easy to place. Tube enterostomies are indicated when long-term (>30 days) feeding is anticipated or when nasal obstruction makes tube placement impossible.

5. **Choose the mode of administration.**

   Bolus feeding : Refers to the administration of 200-400 mL of feed over 20-30 minutes several times a day; usually administered by gravity boluses through a syringe. It is more physiologic, requires less time for feed administration, is a preferred mode of gastric feeding and does not require a pump for administration; Bolus feeding is associated with increased incidence of diarrhoea, nausea, bloating and abdominal discomfort. It is best tolerated at a rate less than 60 mL/min and rapid administration may cause discomfort, leading to the false conclusion that patient is not tolerating the formula (instead, it may be intolerance to the method of administration).

   Intermittent feeding: Refers to administration of 200-400 mL of feed over 30-60 minutes several times a day; may be administered with an enteral pump or gravity. Intermittent feeding is associated with delayed gastric emptying when compared to continuous feeding, increased risk of aspiration, nausea, vomiting and diarrhoea.

   Continuous feeding: Refers to feed given at a continuous rate over 16-24 hours per day, is better tolerated by critically ill patients and is associated with decreased incidence of gastric distension/pooling of formula/diarrhoea and risk of aspiration. It is the preferred mode for small intestine feeding.

6. **Calculate the requirement of the patient.**
   - See Chapter 49.
   - While replacing fluids, keep the following points in mind:

   (i) Determine the amount of fluid being given orally, through tube feed, or intravenously.

   (ii) Determine the water content of the tube-feeding product being delivered. Most products contain 80–85% water (800–850 mL/L of formula); calorically dense products may contain as little as 60% water (600 mL/L of formula).

   (iii) Calculate the total amount of water being given with flushes and with medications (if they are being administered by the feeding tube).

   (iv) Subtract the patient's water intake [total of step (i) to (iii)] from the amount required (as calculated) and provide any additional fluid needed, as water flushes by the enteral tube or by intravenous route.

7. **Decide the formula.**

   On the basis of requirement, choose the formulation and the way it needs to be delivered (see Chapters 51, 52).

8. **Write the instructions/orders (the instructions should be detailed and clear):**
   (a) Name of the formula.
   (b) Mode of administartion.

(i) For bolus feeding: Begin................mL of full-strength formula every.............hours over at least...........minutes. Increase.......mL every....................hours (as tolerated). Precede and follow with 30mL flush of water. Use 50 mL syringe for feeding.

(ii) For intermittent feeding: Begin............mL of full strength formula every..............hours; infuse over 1 hour. Increase...........mL every............hours (as tolerated). Precede and follow with 30 mL flush of water.

(iii) For jejunal feeding (continuous feeding): Begin full strength formula at.............mL per hour via tube. Increase tube feeding administration rate..................mL every...hour until daily caloric requirements are met. Flush the tube every 4 hours with 30mL of water.

(c) Confirm the position of the feeding tube every time before giving feed (see Chapter 54).

(d) Elevate the head end of the bed by 30-45 degrees when feeding into stomach.

(e) Check for residual volume each time before feeding. Return residual volume to the stomach. In case of high residual volume (>200 mL), refer to Chapter 54.

(f) Take preventive measures for oral hygiene and care of the skin around gastrostomy/jejunostomy site every shift.

(g) In case of intolerance (nausea, vomiting, severe abdominal cramps), reduce the rate of infusion to 25 mL per hour (see Chapter 54). Record these, and other signs (diarrhoea, shortness of breath). Avoid airway suctioning immediately after the feed.

(h) Record number, volume, and consistency of bowel movements.

(i) Record input-output (record intake from sources other than formula, separately).

(j) Change administration tubing and feeding bag daily (wherever applicable).

9. **Monitor the patient.**

Clinical monitoring
- Vital signs (temperature, blood pressure, pulse, and respiratory rate).
- Fluid balance (input-output, weight, and edema).
- Abdominal examination for signs of intolerance.
- Delivery equipment for enteral nutrition: position of feeding tube, site around enterostomy tube, change of administration set, pump.

Laboratory monitoring
- Complete haemogram.
- Blood urea, serum creatinine, serum sodium, potassium, chloride, bicarbonate (baseline and then twice a week).
- Blood sugar, baseline, daily for 3 days – and then twice a week.
- Calcium, phophorus, magnesium, and albumin, baseline, and then once a week.
- Prothrombin time, triglycerides – as indicated.

References

1. Alpers DH, Stenson WF, Bier DM. Manual of Nutritional Therapeutics, 4 ed. Philadelphia: Lippincott, Williams & Wilkins, pp 309-346, 347-393.

2. Bell SJ, Borlase BC, Swails W. Dascoulias K, Ainsley B, Forse RA. Experience with enteral nutrition in a hospital population of acutely ill patients. J Am Diet Assoc 1994; 94:414-419.

3. Bengmark S, Andersson R, Mangiante G. Uninterrupted perioperative enteral nutrition. Clin Nutr 2001; 20(1): 11-19.

4. Booth CM, Heyland DK, Peterson WG. Gastrointestinal promotility drugs in the critical care settings: A systematic review of the evidence. Crit Care Med 2002; 30:1429-1435.

5. Buchman AL, Moukarzel AA, Bhuta S, et al. Parenteral nutrition is associated with intestinal morphologic and functional changes in humans. J Parenter Enteral Nutr 1995; 19:453-460.

6. Cerra FB, Blackburn GL, Jeejeebhoy K, et al. Applied Nutrition in ICU patients: a consensus statement of the American college of Chest Physicians. Chest 1997; 111:769-778.

7. Chpman MJ, Fraser RJ, Kluger MT. Erythromycin improves gastric emptying in critically ill patients intolerant of nasogastric feeding. Crit Care Med 2000; 28:2334-2337.

8. Cosnes J, Evard D, Beaugerie L, Gendre JP, Le Quintree Y. Improvement in protein absorption with a small-peptide-based diet in patients with high jejunostomy. Nutrition 1992; 8:406-411.

9. Eisenberg P. Enteral nutrition: Indications, formulas, and delivery techniques. Nurs Clini North Am 1989; 24(2): 315-338.

10. Frost P, Edwards N, Bihari D. Gastric Emptying in the critically ill: the way forward. Intensive Care Med 1997; 23:243-245.

11. Guenter P, Jones S, et al. Delivery systems and administration of enteral nutrition. In: Rombeau JL, Rolandelli RH (eds). Clinical Nutrition: enteral and tube feeding. Philadelphia: Saunders, 1997, pp 240-267.

12. Hadfield RJ, Sinclair DG, Houldurth PE, Evans TW. Effects of enteral and parenteral nutrition on gut permeability in the critically ill. Am J Respir Crit Care Med 1995; 152:1545-1548.

13. Hardy G and Edington J. Formulation and administration of enteral feeds. In: Nightingale JMD (ed). Intestinal Failure, pp 341-356.

14. Heitkemper M, Martin D, Hansen B, et al. Rate and volume of intermittent enteral feeding. JPEN 1981; 5:3122-316.

15. Holtz L, Milton J, Sturek JK. Compatibility of medications with enteral feedings JPEN 1987; 11:183-186.

16. Ibrahim EH, Mehunger L, et al. Early versus late enteral feeding of mechanically ventilated patients: Results of a clinical trial. JPEN 2002; 26:174-181.

17. Illig KA, Ryan CK, Hardy DJ, Rhodes J, Locke W, Sax HC. Total Parenteral nutrition induced changes in gut mucosal function: atrophy alone is not the issue. Surgery 1992; 112:631-637.

18. Klein S, Kinney J, Jeejeebhoy K, et al. Nutrition support in clinical practice: review of published data and recommendations for future research directions. JPEN J Parenter Enteral Nutr 1997; 21:133.

19. Lin HC, Van Citters GW. Stopping eneteral feeding for arbitrary gastric residual volume may not be physiologically sound: results of a computer stimulation model. JPEN 1997; 21:286-289.

20. McClave SA, Sexton LK, Spain DA, Adams JL, et al. Enteral tube feeding in the intensive care unit: Factors impeding adequate delivery. Crit Care Med 1999; 27:1252-1256.

21. McClave SA, Snider HL, Lowen CC, et al. Use of residual volume as a marker for enteral feeding intolerance: Prospective blinded comparison with physical examination and radiographic findings. JPEN J Parenter Enteral Nutr. 1992; 16:99-105.

22. Sax HC, Illag KA, Ryan CK, Hardy DJ. Low dose enteral feeding is beneficial during parenteral nutrition. Am J Surg 1996; 171:587-590.

23. Weser E, Bubbitt J, Vandeventer A. Relationship between enteral glucose load and adaptive mucosal growth in the small bowel. Dig Dis Sci 1985; 30:675-681.
24. Williams PJ. How do you keep medicines from clogging feeding tubes? Am J Nurs. 1989; 89:181-182.
25. Zaloga GP. Bedside method for placing small bowel feeding tubes in critically ill patients. Chest 1991; 100:1643-1646.

Introduction

The concept of the stomach not working is reasonable in terms of its contribution to morbidity and mortality, but gastric residual volume is probably not a good way to measure it. So far, it is not clear, what should be the "cut-off" value above which cessation of feeds should occur, whether the gastric residual volume should represent an absolute value or percent of the infusion rate, what should be the frequency of checking gastric residual volume, and whether cessation should occur after the first or second elevated gastric residual volume. At the best, certain generalizations can be made: gastric residual volume in the range of 200-300 mL should prompt careful bedside evaluation and initiation of an algorithmic approach to reduce the risk of aspiration; gastric residual volume of more than 300-400 mL or a trend of steadily increasing volumes are a cause for concern, and an abrupt cessation of feeding should occur in case of overt regurgitation or aspiration.

The fluid aspirated from the stomach contains the infused formula and digestive juices (including electrolytes) and should be reinstilled through the feeding tube (unless it is a large amount).

GUIDELINES FOR INITIATION OF ENTERAL FEEDING

1. **Wash Hands.**

    This reduces the risk of transmission of micro-organisms.

2. **Check for position of feeding tube (naso-gastric tube).**

    Check the position each time before feeding. Methods to check position include:

    (a) Aspiration of gastric juice: Use 50 mL syringe, as it exerts less negative pressure and so is less likely (than a smaller syringe) to create a vacuum and cause damage. If aspiration is negative, inject 3-5 mL of air or water into the feeding tube and re-attempt or advance the tube for a short distance (2-5 cm) and try aspirating again, or change the position of the patient (i.e. lie on one side, sit up, etc.) and attempt again.

    (b) Auscultation: Inject air into the stomach via the nasogastric tube with the help of a syringe and at the same time listen with a stethoscope over the upper abdomen – bubbling should be heard. It is not a very reliable method.

    (c) Abdominal radiography.

    (d) Laryngoscopy: Visualize the tube passing into the upper esophagus using a laryngoscope or an endoscope.

3. **Elevate the head end of patient's bed to 45 degrees from the horizontal plane.**
   See Chapter 56.

4. **Beginning with the feed.**
   - Begin with clear liquids if the patient's ability to protect airway is questionable.
   - Begin with half-strength formula if the patient is receiving hypertonic feed, is at risk for gut ischaemia, or has been NPO (nothing by mouth) for more than 2 weeks. When starting with half strength, increase to full strength formula after 24 hours.
   - Begin with full strength formula if none of the above is applicable.

5. **Calculate starting volume.**
   Bolus feeding: Calculate half the volume of full strength formula needed to meet maintenance caloric requirements, and divide it by the number of feedings per day (Usually the feeds are given every 3-4 hours).
   Continuous feeding: 5-30 mL/kg/24hr; may start at lower rates in patients at risk for gut ischaemia.

6. **Advance feeding rate.**
   Bolus feeding: Increase by 25% every 4-12 hours, as tolerated till the goal is reached.
   Continuous feeding: Increase 25-30 mL/hr every 6 hours, as tolerated.

7. **Assess tolerance.**
   Bolus feeding: Check residual volume. If more than 200 mL with a nasogastric tube located in the antrum or fundus, or more than 100 mL for surgical or endoscopic gastrostomy tubes located on the anterior wall, or more than half the previous bolus feed, look for associated symptoms and signs of intolerance:
   (a) Presence of abdominal discomfort, distension, tympany, vomiting and loss of bowel sounds – delay feeding.
   (b) Abdominal examination unremarkable:
   - Delay feeding for an hour or two and recheck the residual volume.
   - Add prokinetic agents, i.e. metoclopramide 10-20 mg, 8 hourly; domperidone 10 mg 6 hourly; cisapride 10 mg, 6 hourly; erythromycin IV, 125-250 mg 6 hourly.
   (c) Use transpyloric route for feeding with gastric decompression, as necessary in situation (a) and in situation (b) when the response to prokinetic drugs is not as expected.
   Continuous feeding: Feeding to commence at 30 mL/hr. Feed for 4 hours, rest for 1 hour, then aspirate:
   (a) Aspirated volume <200 mL – replace aspirate, increase rate by 25-30 mL/hr.
   (b) Aspirated volume >200 mL – replace 100 mL of aspirate, continue feeding at the same rate for next 4 hours and recheck aspirate.
   (c) If aspirate is still more than 200 mL – look for clinical signs of intolerance.
   - Signs of intolerance absent – return to the basic rate of infusion (i.e. 30 mL/hr), and add prokinetic agent.

- Signs of intolerance present:
  - Use transpyloric route (beyond Ligament of Treitz) for feeding with gastric decompression, if necessary.
  - If not successful, switch over to TPN (total parenteral nutrition).
  - While on TPN, make attempts to re-start enteral feeding on alternate days.
  - If successful, reduce TPN accordingly.

8. **Consider trophic feeding.**

   In a patient with non-functioning gut, with full nutritional requirements being met by parenteral nutrition, one may start with minimal enteral feeding (10 mL/hr) of full strength formula, the basis for this being that it may preserve the gut's barrier function and prevent villous atrophy; however, there is no evidence in man that it reduces bacterial translocation.

9. **While feeding through nasogastric tube, take care of certain basic points.**
   - Prefer a liquid formulation (instead of a crushed tablet), if available.
   - Do not administer thick liquids such as antacids through a tube with a diameter smaller than 10 Fr. (it may clog the tube).
   - Do not crush slow-release drugs/enteric – coated tablets, as crushing may increase the rate of absorption, expose the drug to degradation in the stomach, or may cause gastric upset.
   - Do not add medications to the feeding bag. Instead, administer these directly through the tube, then irrigate the tube.
   - Do not administer antacids beyond the pylorus.
   - Do not allow sucralfate to mix with enteral feed in the stomach or in an enteral feeding tube. It can form a solid mass.
   - Withhold tube feeding for 1 hour before and after phenytoin and ciprofloxacin administration.
   - Monitor prothrombin time in patients taking warfarin, as vitamin K in tube feeds may decrease the effect of warfarin.

References

1. Alpers DH, Stenson WF, Bier DM. Manual of Nutritional Therapeutics, 4 ed. Philadelphia: Lippincott, Williams & Wilkins, pp 309-346, 347-393.
2. Bell SJ, Borlase BC, Swails W. Dascoulias K, Ainsley B, Forse RA. Experience with enteral nutrition in a hospital population of acutely patients. J Am Diet Assoc 1994;94:414-419.
3. Bengmark S, Andersson R, Mangiante G. Uninterrupted perioperative enteral nutrition. Clin Nutr 2001;20(1): 11-19.
4. Booth CM, Heyland DK, Peterson WG. Gastrointestinal promotility drugs in the critical care settings: A systematic review of the evidence. Crit Care Med 2002;30:1429-1435.
5. Buchman AL, Moukarzel AA, Bhuta S, et al. Parenteral nutrition is associated with intestinal morphologic and functional changes in humans. J Parenter Enter Nutr 1995;19:453-460.
6. Cerra FB, Blackburn GL, Jeejeebhoy K, et al. Applied Nutrition in ICU patients: a consensus statement of the American college of Chest Physicians. Chest 1997;111:769-778.
7. Chpman MJ, Fraser RJ, Kluger MT. Erythromycin improves gastric emptying in critically ill patients intolerant of nasogastric feeding. Crit Care Med 2000;28:2334-2337.

8. Cosnes J, Evard D, Beaugerie L, Gendre JP, Le Quintree Y. Improvement in protein absorption with a small-peptide-based diet in patients with high jejunostomy. Nutrition 1992;8:406-411.

9. Eisenberg P. Enteral nutrition: Indications, formulas, and delivery techniques. Nurs Clin North Am 1989;24(2):315-338.

10. Frost P, Edwards N, Bihari D. Gastric Emptying in the critically ill: the way forward. Intensive Care Med 1997;23:243-245.

11. Guenter P, Jones S, et al. Delivery systems and administration of enteral nutrition. In: Rombeau JL, Rolandelli RH, eds, Clinical Nutrition: enteral and tube feeding. Philadelphia: Saunders, 1997, pp 240-267.

12. Hadfield RJ, Sinclair DG, Houldurth PE, Evans TW. Effects of enteral and parenteral nutrition on gut permeability in the critically ill. Am J Respir Crit Care Med 1995;152:1545-1548.

13. Hardy G, Edington J. Formulation and administration of enteral feeds. In: Nightingale JMD (ed). Intestinal Failure. pp 341-356.

14. Heitkemper M, Martin D, Hansen B, et al. Rate and volume of intermittent enteral feeding. JPEN 1981;5:3122-316.

15. Holtz L, Milton J, Sturek JK. Compatibility of medications with enteral feedings JPEN 1987;11:183-186.

16. Ibrahim EH, Mehunger L, et al. Early versus late enteral feeding of mechanically ventilated patients: Results of a clinical trial. JPEN 2002;26:174-181.

17. Illig KA, Ryan CK, Hardy DJ, Rhodes J, Locke W, Sax HC. Total Parenteral nutrition induced changes in gut mucosal function: atrophy alone is not the issue. Surgery 1992;112:631-637.

18. Klein S, Kinney J, Jeejeebhoy K, et al. Nutrition support in clinical practice: review of published data and recommendations for future research directions. JPEN J Parenter Enteral Nutr 1997;21:133.

19. Lin HC, Van Citters GW. Stopping enteral feeding for arbitrary gastric residual volume may not be physiologically sound: results of a computer stimulation model. JPEN 1997;21:286-289.

20. McClave SA, Sexton LK, Spain DA, Adams JL, et al. Enteral tube feeding in the intensive care unit: Factors impeding adequate delivery. Crit Care Med 1999;27:1252-1256.

21. McClave SA, Snider HL, Lowen CC, et al. Use of residual volume as a marker for enteral feeding intolerance: Prospective blinded comparison with physical examination and radiographic findings. JPEN J Parenter Enteral Nutr. 1992;16:99-105.

22. Sax HC, Illag KA, Ryan CK, Hardy DJ. Low dose enteral feeding is beneficial during parenteral nutrition. Am J Surg 1996;171:587-590.

23. Weser E, Bubbitt J, Vandeventer A. Relationship between enteral glucose load and adaptive mucosal growth in the small bowel. Dig Dis Sci 1985;30:675-681.

24. Williams PJ. How do you keep medicines from clogging feeding tubes? Am J Nurs 1989;89:181-182.

25. Zaloga GP. Bedside method for placing small bowel feeding tubes in critically ill patients. Chest 1991;100:1643-1646.

Modification of the Formulation in Different Clinical Situations

55

GUIDELINES FOR FINE-TUNING THE FORMULATION IN DIFFERENT CLINICAL SITUATIONS

1. Respiratory disease (e.g. COPD, ARDS).
   - (a) Avoid overfeeding.

     Increased production of excess CO_2 is the primary concern.
   - (b) Use moderate doses of each of the macronutrient. Avoid excessive glucose and lipid administration.

     When total calories are provided in moderate amounts, manipulation of the macronutrients (i.e. increasing lipid calories and decreasing carbohydrate calories, as has been suggested in the past) has little effect on CO_2 production, minute ventilation, and respiratory quotient. Rapid administration of IV lipid may cause significant increase in pulmonary vascular resistance in patients with ARDS.
   - (c) Use fluid-restricted nutrient formulation in patients whose haemodynamic status necessitates fluid restriction.

     Fluid accumulation and pulmonary edema in patients with ARDS are associated with a poor clinical outcome.
   - (d) Provide a modified (preferably enteral) formulation containing n-3 fatty acids (fish oil) in patients with early ARDS.

     Because ARDS is associated with release of inflammatory cytokines such as IL-1, IL-6, and IL-8, nutrition formulations having n-3 fatty acids and antioxidants can potentially downregulate the inflammatory response. There is evidence to suggest that patients receiving immune-modulating formula spend lesser time receiving mechanical ventilation, lesser time in the ICU, and a decreased incidence of organ failure.
   - (e) Monitor serum phosphate levels.

     Phosphate is essential for the synthesis of ATP and 2,3 DPG, and normal diaphragmatic contractility.

2. Severe metabolic stress (critical illness).
   - (a) Avoid overfeeding. Give adequate calories.

     It is still not clear if feeding at rates greater than 25 to 30 kcal/kg/24hr is of benefit to these patients. In addition, providing 1g/kg/24hr of proteins is sufficient to minimize loss of body protein during the initial 2 weeks of critical illness.

(b) **Use enteral route, whenever possible.**

Enteral nutrition is less costly and presumably safer as compared to parenteral nutrition. Parenteral nutrition should be reserved for those patients in whom enteral nutrition is not possible.

(c) **Use "immune enhancing" enteral diets containing supplemental arginine, glutamine, branched-chain amino acids, omega-3 fatty acids, RNA, and trace elements.**

Some studies have shown that use of "immune enhancing" diets reduce the risk of infection, ventilator days, and hospital length of stay without influencing mortality. Others have not confirmed these results and still others have shown increased mortality in patients receiving "immune-enhancing" diets.

3. **Congestive heart failure.**

(a) **Use enteral route, whenever possible.**

Enteral route, whenever possible, can be used safely without any adverse effect on cardiac performance. If enteral route is not possible, use parenteral route.

(b) **Energy intake.**

Adequate (25-30 kcal/kg/24hr) caloric intake is required to prevent myocardial atrophy.

(c) **Fluid and sodium intake.**

Restrict total fluid volume (i.e. 1.5 L/24hr), sodium intake (i.e. 1.5 to 2 g/24hr).

(d) **Macronutrients.**

Use concentrated solution of lipids, amino acids and glucose to decrease the fluid intake.

(e) **Take care of electrolytes.**

Loop diuretics (when used for congestive heart failure) may cause loss of sodium, potassium and magnesium. Diuretics can also cause metabolic alkalosis, which can be corrected by repletion of potassium and chloride.

4. **Acute renal failure.**

(a) **Choose route of providing nutrition.**

Whenever possible use enteral route of nutrition.

(b) **Energy**

Provide adequate calories (25-30 kcal/kg/24 hr).

(c) **Fluid and electrolytes.**

Be guided by losses. Infuse at a rate of 400 mL/24 hr plus urinary and other losses. Maintain a normal serum sodium level. There is a high possibility of developing hyperkalaemia (because of catabolism and acidosis). Decrease intake of potassium, phosphorus and magnesium, and monitor at regular intervals.

(d) **Protein.**

See Chapter 49.

High-biologic-value protein is the preferred solution. Alternatively, the amino acid solution used should have a higher proportion of essential amino acids, especially when BUN and creatinine levels are high. With dialysis (haemodialysis or peritoneal dialysis), requirement of proteins is increased.

(e) Supplement vitamins.

Water-soluble vitamins are lost during dialysis. Consider supplementation of calcium and vitamin D_3. Vitamin A status should be monitored as hypervitaminosis A is often noted in patients with end stage renal disease.

References

1. Alpers DH, Stenson WF, Bier DM, Manual of Nutritional Therapeutics. 4 ed. Philadelphia: Lippincott, Williams & Wilkins, pp 309-506.

2. ASPEN Board of Directors and The Clinical Guidelines Task Force. Guidelines for the use of parenteral and enteral nutrition in adult and pediatric patients. JPEN 2002; 26(1): 90SA-92SA.

3. Beale RJ, Bryg DJ, Bihari DJ. Immunonutrition in the critically ill: A systematic review of clinical outcome. Crit Care Med 1999; 27:2799-2805.

4. Bower RH, Cerra FB, Bershadsky B, et al. Early enteral administration of a formula (Impact ®) supplemented with arginine, nucleotides, and fish oil in intensive care unit patients: Results of a multicenter, prospective, randomized, clinical trial. Crit Care Med 1995; 23:436-439.

5. Heslin MJ Letkany L, Leung D, et al. A prospective, randomized trial of early enteral feeding arfter resection of upper gastrointestinal malignancy. Ann of Surg 1997; 226:567-580.

6. Heyland DK, MacDonald S, Keefe L, et al. Total parenteral nutrition in the critically ill patient. A meta-analysis. JAMA 1998; 280:2013-2019.

7. Heys SD, Walker LG, Snuth I, et al. Enteral nutritional supplementation with key nutrients in patients with critical illness and cancer. A meta-analysis of randomized controlled clinical trials. Ann Surg 1999; 229:467-477.

8. Horl WH, Heidland A. Enhanced proteolytic activity-Cause of protein catabolism in acute renal failure. Am J Clin Nutr 1980; 33:1423-1427.

9. Ikizler TA, Hakim RM. Renal Failure and Parenteral Nutrition. In: Rombeau JL, Rolandelli RH (eds). Clinical Nutrition: Parenteral Nutrition. Philadelphia: Saunders, 2000, pp 366-391.

10. Ishibashi N, Plank LD, Sando K, et al. Optimal protein requirements during the first 2 weeks after the onset of critical illness. Crit Care Med 1998; 26:1529-1535.

11. Lipman TO. Bacterial translocation and enteral nutrition in humans: An outsider looks in. JPEN 1995; 19:156-165.

12. Mitch WE. Dietary therapy in uremia: the impact of nutrition on progressive renal failure. Kidney Int 2000; 57(Suppl 75): S38.

13. Reynolds JV, Kanwar S, Welsh FKS, et al. Does the route of feeding modify gut barrier function and clinical outcome in patients after major upper gastrointestinal surgery? JPEN 1997; 21:196-201.

14. Sedman PC, Macfie J, Sagar P, et al. The prevalence of gut translocation in humans. Gastroenterology 1994; 107.643-649.

15. Sherman MS. Parenteral Nutrition and Cardiopulmonary Disease. In: Rombeau JL, Rolandelli RH (eds). Clinical Nutrition: Parenteral Nutrition, Philadelphia: Saunders, 2000, pp 335-352.

16. Vrees MD Albina JE: Metabolic responses to illness and its mediators. In Rombeau JL, Rolandelli RH (eds). Clinical Nutrition: Parenteral Nutrition. Philadelphia: Saunders, 2000, pp 21-34.

17. Walser M, Mitch WE, Maroini BJ, et al. Should protein intake be restricted in predialysis patients? Kidney Int 1999; 55:77.

Methods to Decrease Risk of Aspiration

56

Introduction

- Conditions predisposing patients to high risk of aspiration include depressed level of consciousness (sedation, increased intracranial pressure) (Fig. 56.1), supine position (Fig. 56.2), endotracheal intubation, vomiting, persistently high gastric residual volume, bolus or intermittent feeding, high risk disease/injury condition (neurologic disorder, major abdominal, thoracic trauma/surgery, diabetes mellitus), and advanced age. Hyperglycaemia (even in non-diabetic patients) can cause delayed gastric emptying by disrupting post-prandial antral contractions.

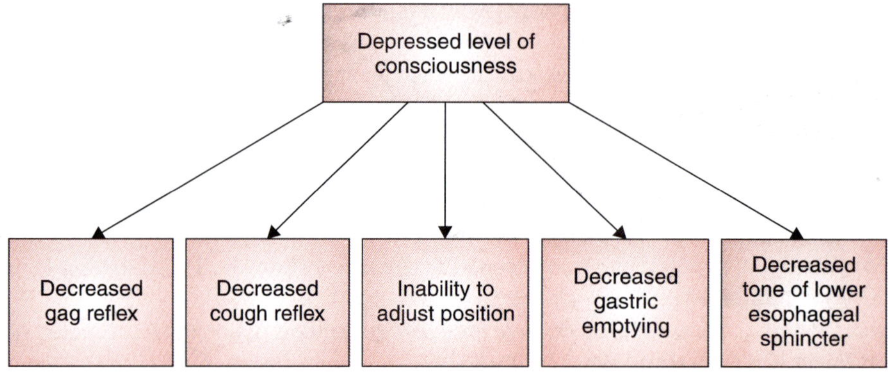

Fig. 56.1 Effects of depressed level of consciousness on predisposition for aspiration.

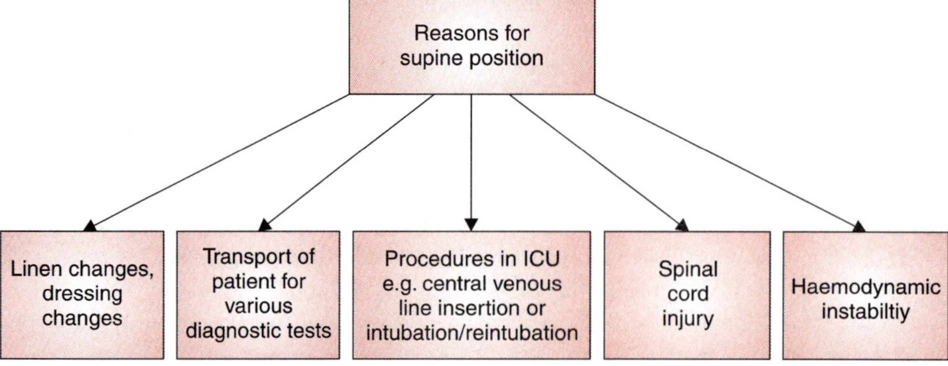

Fig. 56.2 Common reasons for maintaining supine position.

- Size of nasoenteric tube has not been shown to be an important factor for the risk of aspiration.

GUIDELINES TO DECREASE RISK OF ASPIRATION

1. **Keep the head end of the bed elevated to 30-45 degrees.**
   For ventilated patients receiving enteral feeding, the supine position has been shown to be a risk factor for gastric aspiration and pneumonia.
   The patient should be positioned in such a way that the bend of the bed is at the patient's lower back.

2. **Confirm the tip of feeding tube each time before a feed.**
   Feeding tube positioned in or near the esophagus increases the risk of aspiration.

3. **Change mode of administration.**
   Bolus feeding should preferably be limited to patients with intact cough and gag reflexes and a normal level of consciousness. Intermittent feeding is associated with a higher risk of aspiration and pneumonia when compared with continuous nasogastric tube feeding.

4. **Optimize oral health.**
   During prolonged mechanical ventilation, the oral cavity and teeth become colonized with pathogenic bacteria. Good oral care decreases the bacterial load, which gains access to the lower airway by leaking around the tracheal tube cuff.

5. **Optimize drugs.**
   Drugs such as morphine, pethidine and barbiturates predispose to aspiration by worsening the level of consciousness, lowering the lower oesophageal sphincter pressures and delaying gastric emptying. Use of paralytic agents has also been shown to be a risk for ventilator – associated pneumonia.

6. **Level of feeding.**
   Patients with high risk of aspiration or with high gastric residual volumes (> 300-400 mL) with other signs of intolerance, may preferably be fed distal to the ligament of Trietz. Simultaneous gastric decompression may be beneficial, although data confirming this are limited.

7. **Continuous suctioning of subglottic secretions.**
   Continuous aspiration of subglottic secretions has been shown to reduce the incidence of ventilator – associated pneumonias.

8. **Use of prokinetic agents: metoclopramide, erythromycin and cisapride.**
   Prokinetic agents, inspite of reducing residual gastric content, and increasing gastric emptying in mechanically ventilated patients, have not been shown to be associated with a reduced incidence of aspiration, ventilator – associated pneumonia or mortality in critically ill patients receiving enteral nutrition.

References

1. Armstrong D, Castiglione F, Emde C, et al. The effect of continuous enteral nutrition on gastric acidity in humans. Gastroenterology 1992; 102:1506-1515.
2. Atkinson S, Bihari D. The benefits of enteral feeding in critically ill patient. Curr Opinion Anesth 1994; 7:131-135.
3. Bury KD, Jambunathan G. Effects of elemental diets on gastric emptying and gastric secretion in man. Am J Surg 1974; 127:59-66.
4. Esparza J, Boivin MA, Hartshorne ME, Levy H. Equal aspiration rates in gastrically and transpylorically fed critically ill patients. Intensive Care Med 2001; 27:660-664.
5. Hopert R, Liehr RM, Riecken EO. Reduction of 24-hour gastric acidity by different dietary regimens: A randomized controlled study in healthy volunteers. J Parenter Enteral Nutr 1989; 13:292-295.
6. Jacobs S, Chang RWS, Lee B, Bartlett FW. Continuous enteral feeding: A major cause of pneumonia among ventilated intensive care unit patients. J Parenter Enteral Nutr 1990; 14:353-356.
7. Lee B, Chang RWS, Jacobs S. Intermittent nasogastric feeding: a simple and effective method to reduce pneumonia among ventilated ICU patients. Clin Intensive Care 1990; 1:100-102.
8. Payne-James JJ, Rana SK, Bray MJ, McSwiggan DA, Silk DB. Retrograde (ascending) bacterial contamination of enteral diet administration systems. J Parenter Enteral Nutr 1992; 16:369-373.
9. Rees RG, Payne-James JJ, King C, Silk DB. Spontaneous transpyloric passage and performance of 'fine bore' polyurethane feeding tubes: a controlled clinical trial. J Parenter Enteral Nutr 1988; 12(5): 469-472.
10. Winterbauer RH, Duming RB, Barron E, McFadden MC. Aspirated nasogastric feeding solution detected by glucose strips. Ann Intern Med 1981; 95:67-68.

Severe Pre-eclampsia and Eclampsia

57

Introduction

- Pre-eclampsia refers to the development of hypertension with proteinuria after the 20th week of gestation in a previously normotensive woman. Edema is not essential for the diagnosis of pre-eclampsia. Pre-eclampsia that is complicated by generalized tonic–clonic convulsions is termed eclampsia. Convulsions may occur anytime after 20 weeks of gestation and upto 10 days after delivery. 30-40% of patients with eclampsia have convulsions in the post-partum period and in this group 30% have their first convulsion 48 hours after delivery.

- Hypertension refers to a diastolic blood pressure of more than 110mmHg on one occasion, or more than 90mmHg on 2 or more occasions, recorded at an interval of at least 4 hours. The blood pressure should be measured with the patient sitting with the right arm in a roughly horizontal position at heart level, supported on a table or desk. Diastolic pressure should be defined by phase IV (muffling of sounds) Korotkoff sounds. An appropriate size cuff should be used. A regular cuff (12×23 cm) is used when the arm circumference (AC) is less than 33 cm, a larger cuff (15×33 cm) when the AC is 33-41 cm and a thigh cuff (18×36 cm) if the AC is greater than 41 cm.

- Maternal complications of severe pre-eclampsia include (i) Renal dysfunction (reduced glomerular filtration rate, elevated creatinine, acute tubular necrosis, cortical necrosis); (ii) respiratory dysfunction (ARDS, pulmonary edema); (iii) cardiac dysfunction (hypertension, cardiac failure); (iv) cerebral dysfunction (encephalopathy, ischaemia, infarction, haemorrhage, eclampsia, cortical blindness, retinal detachment); and (v) hepatic dysfunction (elevated liver enzymes, subcapsular haematoma, HELLP syndrome). Foetal complications of severe pre-eclampsia include premature delivery, abruptio placenta, and foetal distress.

- Indicators of severe pre-eclampsia/eclampsia include diastolic blood pressure of more than 100 mmHg, proteinuria 2 + or more or 5g/24hr, presence of headache, visual disturbances, upper abdominal pain, oliguria, convulsions, thrombocytopenia, hyperbilirubinemia, pulmonary edema, and elevated liver enzymes and creatinine.

- Indications of ICU admission in a patient with pre-eclampsia / eclampsia include (a) Hypertensive crisis, (b) airway protection in eclampsia, (c) aspiration pneumonia, (d) mechanical ventilation for pulmonary edema / ARDS, (e) invasive haemodynamic monitoring, (f) disseminated intravascular coagulation, (g) HELLP syndrome, and (h) persistent oliguria.

- Pulmonary edema in a pre-eclamptic patient may occur because of high pulmonary artery occlusion pressure, PAOP, (due to a very high systemic vascular resistance or secondary to left ventricular dysfunction), low oncotic pressure, leaky capillaries, and iatrogenic fluid overload. Pulmonary edema following eclamptic convulsions may be caused by aspiration pneumonitis or cardiac failure due to a combination of severe hypertension and vigorous intravenous fluid therapy.
- Convulsions are followed by an increase in the respiratory rate (due to lactic acidemia and hypoxia), cyanosis, and altered consciousness or coma. Foetal bradycardia may also follow convulsions; it usually recovers within 3-5 minutes but if it persists for longer than 10 minutes, other causes such as placental abruption or imminent delivery must be considered.
- Pulse oximetry is of great help for monitoring preeclamptic patients with oliguria who are receiving large amounts of intravenous fluids because it may detect changes in oxygen saturation before the development of overt pulmonary edema.
- Definitive treatment of pre-eclampsia/eclampsia is delivery of the body.

GUIDELINES FOR MANAGEMENT

1. **Place the patient in lateral position.**
   In the third trimester, cardiac output becomes dependent upon body position. In the supine posture, the gravid uterus can cause significant obstruction of the inferior vena cava leading to a 25% reduction in cardiac output as compared to the lateral position.

2. **Maintain the airway and oxygenation of the patient.**
   Oxygenation by facemask, intubation, and ventilation, is carried out as and when indicated.
   Maintenance of airway integrity and oxygenation is especially important during the post-ictal phase, in pulmonary edema, acute respiratory distress syndrome and pulmonary aspiration. Though upper airway obstruction due to laryngeal edema can occur at any time in pre-eclampsia, but it is most often seen after endotracheal extubation following caesarean section. These patients should be extubated only when they are fully conscious and when upper airway and facial edema has subsided sufficiently to allow the patient to breathe past the endotracheal tube with the cuff deflated.

3. **Insert an intravenous line and draw samples for baseline investigations.**
   (a) **Haemoglobin, haematocrit, total and differential blood count and peripheral smear.**
      With physiological anaemia of pregnancy, haematocrit is rarely more than 36%. Haematocrit higher than this may be due to a contracted intravascular volume. Patients with HELLP syndrome have a microangiopathic haemolytic anemia with abnormal peripheral smear.
   (b) **Platelet count.**
      Thrombocytopenia occurs in one-third of patients with pre-eclampsia. A

significant thrombocytopenia ($<100,000/mm^3$), however, occurs only in 15% of women with severe disease. This is caused by increased platelet consumption associated with low grade disseminated intravascular coagulation.

(c) **Blood urea, serum creatinine, serum electrolytes.**

Patients with pre-eclampsia have mild to moderately diminished renal perfusion and glomerular filtration with correspondingly elevated serum creatinine concentrations. Serum creatinine values more than 1.0 mg/dL, in a pregnant patient, imply significant renal dysfunction, and may be associated with delayed excretion of drugs like magnesium sulfate. In normal pregnancy, both effective renal plasma flow and glomerular filtration rate are increased by 30-50%.

(d) **Liver function tests.**

A bilirubin level greater than 1.2 mg/dL, SGOT level greater than 70 IU/L and LDH levels more than 600 IU/dL, indicate the presence of HELLP syndrome.

(e) **Coagulation profile.**

Disseminated intravascular coagulation is rare in the preeclamptic patient. It occurs most commonly in association with placental abruption or foetal death. In the absence of thrombocytopenia (less than $100,000/mm^3$), it is extremely unlikely that a woman with severe preeclampsia will have an abnormal fibrinogen or prolonged prothrombin time (PT) or partial thromboplastin time (PTT). Thus one can safely monitor only the platelet count during admission in most patients. In one study of preeclamptic patients without evidence of abruption or haemorrhage but with platelet counts less than $100,000/mm^3$, there were no abnormal PT or PTT values, and no patient had a fibrinogen concentration less than 200 mg/dL. These additional tests can probably be reserved for patients with abruption, haemorrhage, foetal death, or severe liver dysfunction.

(f) **Magnesium levels.**

Magnesium levels correlate with therapeutic response and toxicity in a patient receiving magnesium sulfate.

4. **Monitor the patient at frequent, regular intervals.**

In addition to basic clinical monitoring, fundus examination, patellar reflex, ultrasound abdomen, if indicated, strict input-output charting and monitoring of the foetus, should be done regularly.

CT scan of the head should be asked for if altered consciousness or coma is prolonged, seizures and lateralizing signs are present, or there are other concerns.

5. **Management of hypertension.**

The aim of treating hypertension is to prevent intracerebral haemorrhage and left ventricular failure without affecting the uteroplacental blood flow and maternal renal function.

(a) **General guidelines.**

- Treat diastolic pressure of more than 105 mm Hg and systolic blood pressure of more than 160 mm Hg.
- Maintain mean arterial pressure (MAP) below 125 mm Hg.

- Aim to reduce mean blood pressure to 105-110 mm Hg, but not more than 30% of baseline.
- Maintain blood pressure above 130/90 mm Hg.
- Avoid precipitous decrements in blood pressure by adequate volume expansion before the use of vasodilators (a precipitous fall can compromise placental perfusion).

(b) **Acute therapy.**

- Infuse 500 mL of colloid in 20-30 minutes, if patient has not received a colloid earlier.
- *Drugs:*
  (i) Hydralazine 5 mg IV; to be repeated at an interval of every 20 minutes till a maximum of 3 doses to bring MAP < 125 mmHg. It may cause tachycardia, flushing, headache, tremors, and nausea.
  (ii) When MAP >125 mmHg and heart rate >120 beats/min or 15 mg hydralazine has been given — use labetalol 20 mg IV followed at 15-20 minute intervals by 40, 80, 80 mg upo a total dose of 220 mg. Oral labetalol 100 mg may also be given as an initial dose. Its maximal effect is seen within 30-40 minutes. Labetalol does not have any deleterious effects on utero-placental blood flow in the above doses. It is contraindicated in asthmatic patients.
  (iii) Nifedipine 5-10 mg orally or sublingually. Oral nifedipine can be repeated after 30 minutes, if required. If no side effects occur, it may be given in a 10 or 20 mg dose every 4 to 6 hours, according to the blood pressure response. Nifedipine when used sublingually may lead to a precipitous fall in blood pressure with consequent foetal distress. When it is given to a patient receiving magnesium sulfate, it may lead to a profound hypotension.
  (iv) Sodium nitroprusside or nitroglycerin may be started as a continuous infusion at an initial rate of 5 µg/kg/min and titrated with the response. It should be used only if there is no response to nifedipine.

(c) **Maintenance therapy.**

- Heart rate < 120/min, no side effects with bolus hydralazine—start an infusion. Dilute 40 mg in 40 ml N-saline. Start at 10 mg/hr and double every 30 minutes until satisfactory response or dosage of 40 mg/hr is reached.
- Heart rate > 120/min or side effects with hydralazine — start labetalol infusion. Dilute 200 mg in 50mL N-saline. Start at 40 mg/hr and double every 30 minutes until satisfactory response or dosage of 160 mg/hr is reached.
- Oral methyldopa, given initially at 1g/24 hr in three to four divided doses, may be increased to 3 to 4 g/24 hr.
- Oral nifedipine.
- ACE inhibitors are associated with toxic effects in the foetus and are therefore contraindicated.

(d) Persistent severe hypertension in immediate postpartum period.
   - Add thiazide diuretic or oral labetalol.
   - The persistence of hypertension is because of at least two mechanisms:
     (i) Mobilization of edema fluid with redistribution into intravenous compartment, and
     (ii) Underlying chronic hypertension.

(e) Role of furosemide and mannitol.

   Furosemide is recommended only in cases of pulmonary edema. Routine use simply adds on to the already depleted intravascular volume and compromises the placental perfusion.

   Hyperosmolar agents like mannitol, can leak through leaky capillaries into the lungs and brain and promote accumulation of edema at these sites.

6. **Fluid management and management of oliguria.**

   Pre-eclampsia is associated with a reduction in intravascular volume, haemoconcentration and hypoproteinemia. Hypoproteinemia causes a decrease in the colloid osmotic pressure (COP) which may become as low as 15 mmHg in severe pre-eclampsia, compared to a value of 22 mmHg in a normotensive patient at term. After delivery, COP further decreases as a result of fluid shifts and may reach as low as 13.8 mmHg in pre-eclamptic patients. Simultaneously, the hydrostatic pressure in the capillaries (PAOP) increases significantly, owing to mobilization of the extravascular edema fluid, iatrogenic fluid overload, and diminished renal output. The lowering of COP with the simultaneous elevation of PAOP narrows the COP-PAOP gradient. The decrease in this gradient, along with the increased capillary permeability associated with pre-eclampsia, may increase the risk of development of pulmonary edema. Fluid administration should be based on this background along with strict fluid balance (input/output), selective haemodynamic monitoring, and selective plasma colloid expansion.

7. **Guidelines for fluid administration.**

   (a) Check urine output.
     (i) If >0.5 mL/kg/hr
         Administer Ringer lactate at the rate of 80-90 mL/hr. Continue monitoring of urine output.
     (ii) If < 0.5 mL/kg/hr
         Administer 1000 mL of Ringer lactate at the rate of 80-120 mL/hr. If urine output does not improve, insert CVP catheter.

   (b) Check CVP (central venous pressure).
     (i) Initial CVP ≤ 4 mm Hg.
       - Give 500 ml of colloid over 5-10 minutes.
       - If urine output improves to more than 0.5 mL/kg/hr; switch over to Ringer lactate at a rate of 80-90 mL/hr.
       - If urine output remains less than 0.5 mL/kg/hr, check CVP again.
       - If CVP ≤ 4 mm Hg, give 500 mL of colloid over 10-30 minutes. Do not give more than 1000 mL of colloid without monitoring PA pressure.
       - If CVP becomes = 5 to 10 mmHg, start Ringer lactate, monitor.

(ii) Initial CVP = 5-10 mm Hg.

Continue with Ringer lactate at the rate of 80-90 mL/hr.

- If urine output improves, continue with Ringer lactate.
- If urine output remains < 0.5 mL/kg/hr, administer 200 mL of colloid over 5-10 minutes. Recheck CVP. If CVP increases to more than 10 mm Hg or increases by more than 2 mm Hg, and oliguria persists, then start dopamine at the rate of 1-5 µg/kg/min, and send samples for urea/creatinine/electrolytes.
- If urine output improves, continue dopamine and Ringer lactate.
- If oliguria persists and creatinine and potassium levels increase, then
  - Add nifedipine, 10 mg orally, every 4 hours, check blood pressure.
  - Consider fluid and potassium restriction.
  - Add furosemide in a single dose of 80-100 mg.
  - Perform pulmonary artery catheterization and optimize PAOP (preload) to 12-14 mm Hg and systemic vascular resistance to 1000-1200 dynes.sec cm^{-5}.
  - Screen for hepatitis, HIV prior to dialysis.
  - Send a referral to the nephrologist.

(iii) Initial CVP > 10 mmHg.

- Look for signs of pulmonary edema—presence of basal crepitations, SpO_2 < 92%. If signs of pulmonary edema are absent and oliguria persists, add dopamine and follow the guidelines as mentioned above (from addition of dopamine onwards).
- If signs of pulmonary edema are present, then
  - Add furosemide 20 mg, followed by 40 mg (if no diuresis).
  - Ask for x-ray chest.
- If oliguria and hypoxaemia persist, then
  - Continue dopamine.
  - Consider fluid and potassium restriction.
  - Consider pulmonary artery catheterization.
  - Add ventilatory support, (non invasive/invasive) as indicated.
  - Proceed to next step.

8. Pulmonary edema.

(a) PCWP > 20 mm Hg.

Probable causes of pulmonary edema are pump failure and fluid overload.

- Continue with furosemide.
- Maintain strict fluid balance and monitor potassium levels.
- Consider rapid digitalization.
- Provide adequate respiratory support.

(b) PCWP normal or below normal.

Probable cause is capillary leakage of high-protein fluid into the alveoli.

- Provide adequate respiratory support. Antepartum pulmonary edema may be an indication (in consultation with the obstetrician) to initiate the process of delivery, after haemodynamic stabilization of the patient.

9. Guidelines for seizure prophylaxis.
    (a) Dose schedule.
         (i)   Magnesium sulfate 4 g (20 mL of 20% solution or 8 mL of 50% solution) IV over 5 minutes.
               PLUS
         (ii) 10 g of 50% magnesium sulfate, one-half (5 g) injected deep in the upper outer quadrant of each buttock with a 3-inch-long, 20-gauge needle (add 1.0 mL of 2% xylocaine to minimize discomfort).
         (iii) Give additional $MgSO_4$ 2g IV (20% solution) if seizures persist longer than 15 minutes.
         (iv) Give $MgSO_4$, 5g deep IM every 4 hours, starting 4 hours later.
         (v)   If convulsions still persist, add thiopentone infusion (see Chapter 66).
               - Magnesium acts primarily by relieving vasospasm. Maintenance magnesium sulfate therapy is continued for 24 hours after delivery. In casc cclampsia develops post-partum, administer magnesium sulfate for 24 hours after the onset of convulsions.
               - Pre-treatment plasma levels of magnesium are less than 2.0 mEq/L (1mEq/L = 1.2 mg/dL). With the above mentioned dosage schedule, therapeutic levels sufficient enough to prevent convulsions are maintained between 4 to 7mEq/L (4.8 to 8.4 mg/dL or 2.0 to 3.5 mmol/L). Pateller reflexes disappear (first sign of magnesium toxicity) when the plasma levels reach 10 mEq/L (10-12 mg/dL).
               - Do not use magnesium sulfate to treat hypertension.
               - Reduce the intramuscular dose to half, if serum creatinine is more than 1.3 mg/dL (upper limit of serum creatinine and BUN, in normal pregnancy, is 0.8 mg/dL and 15 mg/dL, respectively.)
    (b) Monitor vital signs, patellar reflexes, fluid intake, urine output, foetal heart rate, and magnesium levels.
         - Decrease in or absence of foetal heart rate variability is a sign of potential fetal compromise.
         - Respiratory rate of less than 13-14 per minute in the patient may be associated with magnesium toxicity.
         - Urine output should be at least 0.5 mL/kg/hr. (Magnesium is excreted by the kidneys).
    (c) Treat magnesium toxicity (or hypermagnesemia $\geq$15mg/dL).
         - Withhold magnesium sulfate therapy.
         - Infuse calcium gluconate, 1gm IV slowly.
         - Consider intubation and assisted ventilation, if indicated.
    (d) Management of a convulsive episode (also see Chapter 66).
         - Maintain patent airway. If seizures are repetitive, consider intubation.
         - Maintain oxygenation.
         - Avoid maternal injury, e.g. by inserting a padded tongue blade between teeth.
         - Minimize risk of aspiration.

- Start magnesium sulfate.
- Think before giving diazepam as most eclamptic convulsions resolve within 60-90 seconds. Rapid administration of diazepam may not only produce apnea and lead to aspiration, but may also accumulate in the foetus causing respiratory depression at birth.
- Immediately after convulsions,
  - (i) Maintain the patient in lateral position.
  - (ii) Monitor vitals and foetal condition.
  - (iii) Obtain ABG.
  - (iv) Consider X-ray chest at an appropriate time to rule out aspiration.

10. Consider inserting CVP catheter.

- The common indications for CVP catheter insertion include: (i) Oliguria, (ii) impending or established pulmonary edema, (iii) signs of severe pre-eclampsia, or (iv) blood loss of more than 500 mL.
- Since these patients may have coagulation abnormalities, it may be preferable to insert the central venous catheter via a peripheral site such as the antecubital fossa.
- It has been shown that there is no correlation between CVP and PCWP when the CVP exceeds 6mm Hg, thus justifying the use of pulmonary artery catheterization whenever indicated.

11. Consider inserting pulmonary artery catheter.

Pulmonary artery catheterization is indicated in cases of pre-eclampsia associated with persistent oliguria and pulmonary edema.

References

1. Barton JR, Hiett AK, Conover WB. The use of nifedipine during the postpartum period in patients with severe preeclampsia. Am J Obstet Gynecol. 1990;162:788-792.
2. Belfort MA, Anthony J, Kirshon B. Respiratory function in severe gestational proteinuric hypertension: the effects of rapid volume expansion and subsequent vasodilation with verapamil. Br J Obstet Gynaecol 1991; 98:964-972.
3. Benedetti TJ, Kates R, Williams V. Hemodynamic observations in severe pre-eclampsia complicated by pulmonary oedema. Am J Obstet Gynecol 1985; 152:330-334.
4. Clark SL, Cotton DB. Clinical indications for pulmonary artery catheterization in the patient with severe pre-eclampsia. Am J Obstet Gynecol 1988;158:453-458.
5. Clark SL, Greenspoon JS, Aldahl D, et al. Severe pre-eclampsia with persistant oliguria: Management of hemodynamic subsets. Am J Obstet Gynecol 1986; 154:490-494.
6. Fenakel K, Fenakel G, Appelman Z, Lurie S, Katz Z, Shoham Z. Nifedipine in the treatment of severe pre eclampsia. Obstet Gynecol 1991;77:331-337.
7. Fox DB, Troiano NH, Graves CR. Use of the pulmonary artery catheter in severe pre eclampsia: a review. Obstet Gynecol Surv 1996; 51:684.
8. Hawkins J. Anesthesia and preeclampsia/eclampsia. In: Norris MC (ed).Obsteric Anesthesia 2edn, Philadelphia: Lippincott, Williams & Wilkins., 1999, pp 501-523.

9.   Kirshon B, Lee W, Maner MB, Cotton DB. Effects of low dose dopamine therapy in the oliguric patient with preeclampsia. Am J Obstet Gynecol 1988; 159:604-607.

10. Leduc L, Wheeler JM, Kirshon B, et al. Coagulation profile in reverse preeclampsia. Obstet Gynecol 1992; 79:14.

11. Lindheimer MD, Katz AL. Preeclampsia: Pathophysiology, diagnosis, and management. Ann Rev Med 1989;40:233.

12. Linton DM, Anthony J. Critical Care management of severe pre-eclampsia. Intensive Care Med 1997;23:248-255.

13. Mushambi MC, Hallingan AW, Williamson K. Recent developments in the pathophysiology and management of pre-eclampsia. Br J Anesth 1996; 76:133-148.

14. Potgieter PH, Hammond JMJ. Cuff test for safe extubation following laryngeal oedema. Critical Care Medicine 1988; 16:818.

15. Prieto JA, Mastrobattista JM, Blanco JD. Coagulation studies in patients with marked thrombocytopenia due to severe preeclampsia. Am J Perinatol 1995; 12:220.

16. Redman CWG, Reberts JM. Management of pre-eclampsia. Lancet 1993; 341:1451-1454.

17. Richards AM, Moodley J, Graham DI, Bullock MRR. Active management of the unconscious eclamptic patient. Br J obstet Gynaecol 1986;93:554-562.

18. Sibai BM, Villar MA, Mabie BC. Acute renal failure in hypertensive disorders of pregnancy. Am J Obstet Gynecol 1990; 162:772-783.

19. Zinaman M, Rubin J, Lindheimer MD. Serial plasma oncotic pressure levels and echoencephalography during and after delivery in severe pre-eclampsia. Lancet 1985;1:1245-1247.

Sepsis, Severe Sepsis, and Septic Shock

58

Introduction

- *Sepsis* is defined as the host response to infection, occurring as a result of the release of cytokines and other mediators.
- Possible signs of sepsis include:
  General parameters: Hyperthermia (core temperature > 38.3°C), hypothermia (core temperature < 36°C), chills, tachypnea > 30 breaths/min, altered mental status, significant edema or positive fluid balance (>20 mL/kg over 24 hours), hyperglycaemia (plasma glucose > 110 mg/dL).
  Inflammatory parameters: Leucocytosis (white blood cell count > 12,000/µL), Leucopenia (white blood cell count < 4000/µL), normal white blood cell count with > 10% immature forms, increased plasma C reactive protein and procalcitonin levels.
  Haemodynamic parameters: Tachycardia (heart rate>90/minute), arterial hypotension (systolic blood pressure < 90mmHg, mean arterial pressure < 70 mmHg, or a decrease in systolic blood pressure by > 40 mmHg in adults), cardiac index > 3.5L/min/m^2.
  Organ dysfunction parameters: Arterial hypoxaemia (PaO_2/F_iO_2 < 300), acute oliguria (urine output < 0.5 mL/kg/hr for at least 2 hours), creatinine increase $\geq$ 0.5 mg/dL, ileus (absent bowel sounds), thrombocytopenia (platelet count < 100,000/µL), coagulation abnormalities (international normalized ratio > 1.5 or activated partial thromboplastin time > 60 sec), hyperbilirubinemia (plasma total bilirubin > 4 mg/dL).
  Tissue perfusion parameters: Hyperlactatemia (>3 mmol/L), decreased capillary refill or mottling.
- *Severe sepsis* is defined as sepsis complicated by organ dysfunction.
- *Septic shock* in adults refers to a state of acute circulatory failure characterized by persistent arterial hypotension, despite adequate volume resuscitation and unexplained by other causes.
- Approximately 60% of patients with sepsis have a microbiologically confirmed infection. Most likely sites of infection (when they can be identified) are the lung (46%) followed by abdominopelvic region (15%) and urinary tract (10%). An infection from any type of microorganism can result in sepsis with the clinical progression of the sepsis syndrome being similar regardless of the cause.
- In gram-negative infections, endotoxin, a lipopolysaccharide (LPS) that is a major part of the cell wall of gram-negative bacteria is associated with the

development of sepsis. Following infection, LPS interacts with CD14 (a cell surface receptor) that is expressed by white blood cells. The LPS then activates both the classical and alternative complement pathways. On the other hand, in gram-positive infections it is lipoteichoic acid that activates the CD14 receptor on the white blood cells. Amongst fungal infections, candida, which is most commonly implicated in the development of sepsis, is associated wtih a high mortality rate.

- Inflammation is an essential part of the body's response to infection with the host mounting and then downregulating the inflammatory response. A healthy endothelium is essential for the maintenance of equilibrium between coagulation and fibrinolysis. In sepsis, the regulatory function of the endothelium fails, thus leading to an imbalance between activation and downregulation. An excessive amount of pro-inflammatory cytokines are released, which lead to systemic endothelial damage. In response to the pro-inflammatory mediators, anti-inflammatory mediators are also released, which cause immune suppression, followed by secondary infection. Hence the sequelae of sepsis are: endothelial damage, inflammatory changes, alteration of coagulation and immune suppression.

- Patients with severe sepsis are prone to develop thromboses in the microvasculature which can lead to organ failure. As the sepsis syndrome progresses, the following clinical picture develops: excessive vasodilatation, hypoperfusion, generalized tissue damage, inappropriate cytokine response, coagulopathy, and microthrombi formation.

- In hypovolaemic, cardiogenic, and obstructive shock, hypotension occurs as a result of decreased cardiac output, with consequent anaerobic metabolism. Septic shock, however, typically results from distributive alterations, so that alterations in tissue perfusion result from abnormal control of the microvasculature with abnormal distribution of a normal or increased cardiac output. Cellular alterations in sepsis also result from the important inflammatory response, with the involvement of many mediators. Hence, the endpoints of therapy are much more difficult to define with certainity in septic shock than in other forms of shock, in which a reduction in blood flow is the dominant problem.

- Septic shock is characterized by hypotension, which in adults generally refers to a mean arterial pressure (MAP) below 65-70 mmHg. The adequacy of regional perfusion is usually assessed clinically by evaluating indices of organ function, although none of these parameters has been validated as a reliable indicator of adequate resuscitation. These parameters include: CNS dysfunction indicated by a clouded sensorium, altered renal function with increased blood urea nitrogen and creatinine, coagulation abnormalities (DIC), altered liver parenchymal function with increased serum levels of transaminases, lactic dehydrogenase, and bilirubin, and altered gut perfusion, manifested by ileus and malabsorption.

- Clinical management of sepsis syndrome includes: oxygen support, cardiovascular support, treatment of infection (including surgical debridement or other interventions, wherever required), monitoring and supportive care of all organs, and anti-microbial therapy. A small percentage of patients might require dialysis for acute renal failure.

- Norepinephrine (NE) increases glomerular filtration rate and urine output as well as, dopamine and probably is more effective than dopamine at reversing hypotension in septic shock patients. There is no difference in adverse effects between dopamine and norepinephrine. Norepinephrine can be used (in the therapy of septic shock) either as a sole vasopressor or in conjunction with dopamine. The well-documented negative effects of NE on kidney function in non-septic patients do not seem to be present in septic patients with adequate volume resuscitation. NE (0.01-$3\,\mu g/kg/min$) should be used to restore normal values (lower values of the normal range) of mean arterial blood pressure and systemic vascular resistance. There is strong evidence suggesting that as long as cardiac output is maintained, treatment with NE alone has no negative effects on splanchnic tissue oxygenation and that when contemplated in the treatment of patients with septic shock, NE should be used early and not merely as a last resort.

- Dobutamine is the agent of choice for increasing the cardiac output in patients with septic shock. Though direct measurement of cardiac output by invasive haemodynamic monitoring is preferable, other end-points of global perfusion including mixed venous oxygen saturation (SvO_2) and serial blood lactate levels may also be monitored.

- Epinephrine may achieve haemodynamic stability in patients unresponsive to other inotropic agents, but it compromises regional hepatosplanchnic perfusion and causes profound metabolic alterations as shown by lactic acidosis. Therefore, its use should be limited.

- Early aggressive therapy (during the first six hours) to optimize cardiac output, afterload, and contractility improves the likelihood of survival of ptients with severe sepsis and septic shok. In one study, mortality was 30.5% in the group receiving early goal directed therapy as compared to 46.5% in the control group. Thus, early therapeutic intervention to restore the balance between oxygen delivery and oxygen demand improves survival among patients with severe sepsis. Monitoring of objective parameters including serum lactate concentration, base deficit, pH, and possibly central venous oxygen saturation, is advisable in patients receiving resuscitation therapy.

- Early and effective antimicrobial therapy is of crucial importance in managing septic shock and its complications. Since the prognosis of these patients depends mainly on the success of the initial antimicrobials used, a "hit hard" strategy employing two or three appropriate antimicrobials is preferred to using one antimicrobial.

- The initial empirical antimicrobial therapy (when a possible source is not found) should provide broad-spectrum coverage against Staph. aureus, commoner gram-negative bacilli such as Escherichia coli and Klebsiella spp, group A β-hemolytic streptococci, Strept. pneumoniae, and Neisseria meningitides. A third-generation cephalosporin may be advised for this purpose. But before a final prescription, a few other consideration should also be kept in mind:

(i) If CNS infection is suspected, a drug with good CNS penetration and covering a somewhat different range of organisms (e.g. Strept. pneumoniae, Meningococcus, Listeria monocytogenes, H. influenzae, Enterobacteriacae, Bacterioides spp. and other anaerobes, and Staph. aureus) should be selected. Options may include a suitable combination of ceftriaxone, cefotaxime, ampicillin, chloramphenicol, and metronidazole.

(ii) If involvement of B.fragilis and other anaerobic bacteria in the infectious process is a possibility (e.g. intra-abdominal infection, female genital tract infection, necrotizing cellulitis, infected decubitus ulcers), antimicrobials such as metronidazole, clindamycin, piperacillin/tazobactum, or imipenum/cilastatin may be considered.

(iii) If a patient is at a risk of being infected with Pseudomonas spp. (e.g. prolonged hospitalization, chronic complicated urosepsis, severe immuno-suppression, recent broad-spectrum antimicrobial treatment, history of intravenous drug abuse), antibiotic coverage should include antimicrobial agents against Pseudomonas e.g. ceftazidime, ciprofloxacin, piperacillin/tazobactum, imipenum/cilastatin, cefoperazone/sulbactum.

(iv) If the patient needs to be covered against Legionella spp. and Mycoplasma, addition of a macrolide or a fluroquinolone drug needs to be considered.

(v) In case of ventilator associated pneumonia (VAP), the time of onset of the pneumonia is a major determinant of its etiology. In early onset cases, usually "normal flora" (i.e. Streptococcus pneumoniae and other Streptococci, H. influenzae, Staph. aureus and possibly anaerobes in selected circumstances) are involved and there is no need for administration of an antipseudomonal, broad-spectrum penicillin combined with a β-lactamase inhibitor or of ciprofloxacin. Late onset VAP is frequently caused by antibiotic-resistant pathogens (i.e. methicillin-resistant Staph aureus, Pseudomonas aeruginosa, Acinetobacter spp. and Enterobacter species). It is very difficult to pinpoint the microorganism and the empirical antimicrobial therapy should include a combination of a β-lactam, an aminoglycoside and a glycopeptide.

(vi) Consider the presence of liver and renal impairement, if any.

(vii) Before deciding the final strategy, local differences in antimicrobial susceptibility of organisms should be taken into account. Prevalence and resistance pattern of relevant pathogens (e.g. macrolide-resistant Pneumococci, MRSA, VRE, ESBL-producing Klebsiella) differ not only between countries and hospitals but even between different intensive care units within the same hospital.

(viii) In case of a high local prevalence of MRSA or VRE (>20% of staph. aureus), the initial therapy should include a glycopeptide.

(ix) Crop rotation/antibiotic cycling has been shown to reduce the emergence of resistance among microorganisms.

(x) The inflammatory response associated with sepsis results in a rapid decrease in serum albumin levels, large fluid shifts and third space losses initially with a high cardiac output. These changes result in increased creatinine clearance and increased renal drug clearance and therefore, higher antibiotic dosages are required. Later in the disease process, organ dysfunction may necessitate re-evaluation and reduction of dosing requirements.

- Once microbiological results become available, the initial broad-spectrum therapy may be adjusted to a more specific antibiotic with a narrower spectrum (and usually a cheaper one).

- Fever may take 4-6 days to respond to anti-microbial therapy. However, before concluding that the initial antimicrobial therapy is ineffective, the clinician should re-evaluate all the manifestations of sepsis, including, directional trends in white blood cell count, platelet count, temperature, level of consciousness, haemodynamic stability, and clinical findings at the site of infection.

- The important causes of antimicrobial treatment failure include incorrect initial choice of drugs, lack of penetration of the antimicrobial to the site of infection (e.g. poor penetration of aminoglycosides into lung tissue), absence of blood supply to the site of infection (abscess, necrotic tissue, bony sequestra), and development of secondary antimicrobial resistance (quite common in complicated intrabdominal sepsis). Modification of antimicrobial therapy is considered based on cultures from the site of wound or from surgical drain, if the patient continues to have signs of infection.

- Examine the patient at frequent intervals. Check all drains and tubes to make sure that they are functioning and have not been dislodged. The surgical wound (e.g. abdominal sepsis) should be examined daily. Drainage of fresh serosanguinous fluid or wound dehiscence (most common on post-operative day 4 to 5 but may occur any time) should be noted and the fluid sent for microbiological examination.

- Look for adequate functioning of the gastrointestinal tract. It is no longer recommended to wait for appearance of bowel sounds before starting feeds in a sedated and ventilated patient. It is frequently necessary to challenge the patient by starting tube feeding and simply checking the gastric residual volume every 4 hours.

- If the patient is not improving following laparotomy for intra-abdominal sepsis, or if the patient begins to deteriorate after initial improvement, an ultrasound or CT scan of the abdomen is indicated to exclude possible fluid collection. However, a scan is not helpful until 5 days after the laparotomy. Any evidence of persistent or recurrent infection (as evidenced by fluid collection) usually requires a repeat laparotomy and sending the fluid/sample for microbiological examination.

- Some patients do not become febrile when sepsis develops, for example, elderly patients or patients with uraemia, etc. The lack of an appropriate acute-phase response is associated with high mortality and may reflect the immunosuppressive phase of sepsis. Early manifestations of sepsis include subtle changes in mental status, minor increase or decrease in white-cell count or neutrophil percentage, and elevated blood glucose levels. Early recognition of sepsis is the key to a successful outcome.

- For blood culture, blood should be obtained by fresh venipuncture, after swabbing the skin twice, either with 70% isopropyl alcohol or with an iodine containing solution. The needle used for venipuncture should be changed prior to inoculation of blood into culture bottles.

GUIDELINES FOR THE MANAGEMENT OF A PATIENT WITH SEVERE SEPSIS AND SEPTIC SHOCK

1. **Confirm the presence of shock.**

   Empiric criteria for diagnosis of shock are: patient appears ill or has altered mental status, heart rate > 100 beats/min, respiratory rate > 25 breaths/min, $PaCO_2$ < 32 mmHg, arterial base deficit < -5 mEq/L or lactate > 4 mmol/L, urine output < 0.5 mL/kg/hr, arterial hypotension > 20 minutes duration. Of these, regardless of the cause, at least four criteria should be met.

2. **Confirm whether it is a low cardiac output shock or a high cardiac output shock. Take a history and perform clinical examination.**

   Low cardiac output shock is commonly due to cardiogenic or hypovolaemic shock and is signalled by cool extremities, poor nailbed return, small pulse pressure and muffled heart sounds. A high cardiac output hypotension is signalled by warm extremities, good nailbed return, fever/ hypothermia, large pulse pressure, low diastolic blood pressure, leucocytosis/leucopenia. In septic shock, a low blood pressure is accompanied by a large pulse pressure because the stroke volume is large and diastolic pressure very low because stroke volume has a rapid peripheral runoff through dilated peripheral arterioles.

3. **Establish an IV access, take blood samples for investigations. Monitor ECG, blood pressure, SpO_2, CVP, respiratory rate, urine output, every hourly.**

   Establish an IV access with a large bore cannula (two 18 gauge or one 16 gauge). Send samples for complete blood count, including platelet count, electrolytes, urea, creatinine, sugar, coagulation study, serum lactate, calcium, magnesium, phosphorus, and arterial blood gas for analysis. Get a chest radiograph, ECG and urine analysis done.

   Before starting antibiotic therapy, send appropriate cultures, including blood culture for microbiological examination.

4. **Maintenance of airway and breathing.**
   Consider early intubation and ventilation.
   Indications for intubation in patients with shock include hypoxaemia, ventilatory failure (high $PaCO_2$, laboured breathing, tachypnea, use of accessory muscles, abdominal paradoxical respiratory motion), vital organ hypoperfusion, airway compromise, profound acidosis, and obtundation.

   Transport of a shocked patient should be preceded by intubation.

   Altered mental status is common in septic shock and patients may require rapid airway protection. Patients with a respiratory rate greater than 30 breaths per minute are likely to develop respiratory collapse, irrespective of arterial oxygenation. It has been reported that 85% of patients with "severe sepsis" will require mechanical ventilation during the course of their hospital stay. Intubation and mechanical ventilation prevents aspiration, reduces the work of breathing, increases oxygenation and helps in management of acute respiratory and metabolic failure. Strenuous use of accessory respiratory muscles can increase oxygen consumption by 50% to 100% and decrease cerebral blood flow by 50%. Moreover, with a decrease in lung compliance, a more negative intrathoracic pressure must be generated to fill the lungs with each inspiration during spontaneous breathing. The greater suction effect exerted on the left ventricle, thus impedes its ability to eject and increases functional afterload. Positive pressure ventilation by removing this impedence can improve ventricular function and cardiac output by 30%. Intubation and positive pressure ventilation frequently reduces venous return in patients with hypovolaemic shock. A greater volume resuscitation and selection of an adequate but small tidal volume (8 mL/kg) minimizes this problem. 3-5 cmH$_2$O PEEP is required to prevent alveolar collapse, thereby preventing severe ventilation/perfusion mismatch and hypoxaemia.

For further ventilatory management, see Chapter 59.

5. **Monitor the patient at frequent intervals.**

    Monitoring includes continuous ECG, pulse oximetry, central venous pressure, arterial blood pressure, urine output, pulmonary artery pressure, and central venous oxygen saturation (ScvO$_2$), if available.

    In shock states, the measurement of blood pressure using a cuff is often unreliable and inaccurate. Therefore, an invasive arterial catheter for continuous blood pressure monitoring is preferable.

6. **Haemodynamic support.**

    Resuscitate to target values:
    -MAP $\geq$ 65 mmHg.
    -CVP 8-12 mmHg.
    -SpO$_2$ $\geq$ 95%.
    -Mixed venous PO$_2$ > 30 mmHg.
    -ScvO$_2$ $\geq$ 70%.
    -PCWP > 10 but < 20 mmHg.
    -Cardiac index > 3L/m^2/min
    -Blood lactate conc < 2 mmol/L.
    -Urine output > 1 mL/kg/hr.

    Crystalloids and colloids are equally effective when titrated to the same haemodynamic end points. There is no evidence-based support for one type of fluid over another.

    When CVP increases, a pulmonary artery catheter is probably required, although its role has recently been questioned.

    - The first step for providing haemodynamic support in patients with septic shock, is fluid resuscitation with a goal to restore tissue perfusion and normalize cellular metabolism. Requirements of fluid infusion cannot be easily determined and therefore, a fluid challenge technique titrated to the clinical end points of mental status, blood pressure, heart rate, and urine output has been recommended. CVP should be monitored. Initial fluid: 20-30 mL/kg crystalloid (N-saline or Ringer lactate) over 30 minutes followed by 500 mL bolus of crystalloid every 30 min. Use blood or red cells to restore haematocrit to at least 30% to 35%. Therapy with crystalloids may decrease haemoglobin concentration by 1-3 g/dL. Flow rigidity of red blood cells is known to increase with increased duration of storage. Based on pathophysiological changes in sepsis at the microcirculatory level, it must be assumed that transfusion of old red blood cells (stored for more than 15 days) may lead to further impairment of the microvasculature and a decrease in gastric pH.

- Fluid administration alone may restore haemodynamic stability in 30-40% of septic patients who develop arterial hypotension. When fluid challenge fails to restore an adequate arterial pressure and organ perfusion, therapy with vasoactive agents should be started.

  (a) MAP<70, cardiac index (CI) >5 L/min/m^2 (associated with SVR < 400 dynes/sec/cm^5), start vasopressor (e.g. dopamine, noradrenaline)

  (b) CI < 3.5 L/min/m^2 (associated with SVR > 800 dynes/sec/cm^5) and evidence of hypoperfusion, start dobutamine.

  (d) If the haemodynamics is mixed (as is common), dopamine or noradrenaline are suitable first line drugs. When pulmonary artery cathcterization facilities are not available, dopamine is the standard first line drug. If there is no response to a dose of about 20 µg/kg/min, noradrenaline may be added or therapy may be started with noradrenaline as the drug of first choice. Dobutamine should be added to either of the above regimens, whenever there is evidence of reduced perfusion inspite of adequate volume expansion and vasopressor therapy. Dobutamine is the drug of choice when oxygenation to the tissues is limited due to myocardial depression despite a normal or high cardiac output. It increases the myocardial contractility without increasing mean arterial pressure or heart rate.

  (d) If ScvO$_2$ < 70%, transfuse red cells to reach a haematocrit of > 30%.

7. Monitor blood sugar every 1 to 2 hours and maintain normoglycaemia (80-110 mg/dL).

   - Initial blood sugar 110-220; start insulin at 1-2 IU/hr; if > 220, start at 2-4 IU/hr.
   - Measure blood sugar every 1-2 hours till it is within normal range; if > 140, increase insulin dose by 1-2 IU/hr; if 110-140, increase insulin dose by 0.5-1 IU/hr; if approaching normal range, adjust insulin dose by 0.1-0.5 IU/hr.
   - Once it is within normal range, measure blood sugar every 4 hours.
   - If blood sugar falls steeply, reduce insulin dose by half and check every 1-2 hours. Avoid hypoglycaemia.
   - Maintain continous supply of intravenous glucose 8-10 g/hr till feeding (parenteral or enteral) is started.
   - If corticosteroids need to be added, increase the dose of insulin. Steroids are preferably given as a continuous infusion to avoid fluctuations in insulin requirements ocurring with intermittent bolus injections.

- Hyperglycaemia, caused by insulin resistance in the liver and muscle, is a common finding in ICU patients and is thought to be an adaptive response, for providing glucose to the brain and red cells, and for wound healing. It is generally treated only when blood sugar increases more than 215-220 mg/dL. However, recent studies have shown that maintaining blood glucose levels between 80-110 mg/dL in critically ill patients reduces the frequency of episodes of sepsis by 46% and reduces the mortality to 12.5% (vs 29.5 % in the conventional therapy group). Insulin therapy reduces the rate of death from multiple organ failure among patients with sepsis, regardless of whether the patient had a prior history of diabetes mellitus or not. The exact protective mechanism by which insulin acts in sepsis is unknown, but it seems reasonable to control blood sugar more tightly in critically ill patients.

8. **Role of corticosteroids.**
   Add 50-100 mg hydrocortisone IV bolus every 8 hours.

   There is now preliminary evidence to support the use of supplemental corticosteroids in patients with established septic shock, especially in those with biochemical evidence of functional hypoadrenalism. Patients receiving mechanical ventilation and having hypotension not responding to fluids and 6-8 hours of vasopressor therapy, should be started with 50-100 mg hydrocortisone IV bolus every 8 hours with or without 50 mg of fludricortisone daily for 7 days.

9. **Stress ulcer prophylaxis.**

   See Chapter 22.

   There is abundant data recommending stress ulcer prophylaxis (SUP) in patients with prolonged mechanical ventilation, hypotension, and coagulopathy. For other septic patients in whom these factors are not present, SUP is recommended on the basis of small randomized trials in which SUP has proven efficacious in preventing bleeding and therefore, in reducing morbidity in critically ill patients.

10. **Take care of the nutrition.**

11. **Consider bicarbonate therapy.**

    Bicarbonate supplementation was previously the standard therapy for those with presumed lactic acidosis. Current consensus is to delay therapy till there is severe acidaemia (pH < 7.15), as there may be a paradoxical decrease in intracellular pH as a result of diffusion of soluble CO_2 across the cell membrane after bicarbonate administration. Alternatively, hyperventilation has been suggested to help increase systemic pH.

12. **Deep vein thrombosis prophylaxis.**
    Use either low dose unfractionated heparin (5000 U bd or tds) or low molecular weight heparin (in recommended dosages). When heparin is absolutely contraindicated (i.e. thrombocytopenia, severe coagulopathy, active bleeding, recent intracerebral hemorrhage), use a mechanical prophylactic device.

    Septic patients, especially those with multiple organ failure have less cardiopulmonary reserve, and the impact of a minor thromboembolic event could further compromise them. These patients have several risk factors for thromboembolic phenomena, which include bed rest (> 5 days), major surgery, use of central venous catheter, neuromuscular blockade, deep sedation, presence of coagulopathy, age (> 40 years) and a history of venous thromboembolism.

13. Activated protein C.

Recombinant Human Activated Protein C (rhAPC) is recommended in patients at high risk of death (Acute Physiology and Chronic Health Evaluation II > 25, sepsis-induced multiple organ failure, septic shock or sepsis-induced acute respiratory distress syndrome), and with no absolute contraindication related to bleeding risk.

Recombinant human activated protein C inactivates factor Va and VIIIa, thereby preventing the generation of thrombin. Inhibition of thrombin generation by activated protein C decreases inflammation by inhibiting platelet activation, neutrophil recruitment and mast-cell degranulation. Activated protein C has direct anti-inflammatory properties which include blocking of the production of cytokines by monocytes and blocking of cell adhesion. Currently, activated protein C is approved for use in patients of sepsis with severe organ compromise and a high likelihood of death. Risk assessment is best determined by bedside clinical evaluation and Judgement. Once a patient has been identified at a high risk of death, treatment should begin as soon as possible.

References

1. Bodi M, Ardanuy C, Olona M, Castander D, Diaz E, Rello J. Therapy of ventilator-associated pneumonia: the Tarragona strategy. Clin Microbiol Infect 2001; 7:32-3.
2. Bodi M, Ardanuy C, Rello J. Impact of Gram-positive resistance on outcome of nosocomial pneumonia. Crit Care Med 2001; 29:N82-N86.
3. Brun-Buisson C. Antibiotic therapy of ventilator-associated pneumonia: in search of the magic bullet. Chest 2003; 123:670-3.
4. Burke JP. Patient safety: infection control-a problem for patient safety. N Engl J Med 2003; 348:651-6.
5. Dellinger RP, Carlet JM, Masur H, et al. Surviving Sepsis Campaign guidelines for management of severe sepsis and septic shock. Crit Care Med 2004;32(3):858-870.
6. Gunnar R et al: Hemodynamic measurements in bacteremia and septic shock in man. J Infect Dis 128:295-298, 1973.
7. Herbrecht R, Denning DW, Patterson TF, et al. Voriconazole Versus amphotericin B for primary therapy of invasive aspergillosis. N Engl J Med 2002; 347:408-15.
8. Hoffken G, Niederman MS. Nosocomial pneumonia: the importance of a de-escalating strategy for antibiotic treatment of pneumnia in the ICU. Chest 2002; 122:2183-96.
9. Ibrahim EH, Scherman G, Ward S, Fraser VJ, Kollef MH. The influence of inadequate antimicrobial treatment of bloodstream infections on patient outcomes in the ICU setting. Chest 2000; 118:146-55.
10. Karam GH, Niederman MS. How do we achieve adequate therapy for severe infection? Crit Care Med 2003; 31:648-50.
11. Kollef M Niederman M. Antimicrobial resistance in the ICU: the time for action is now. Crit Care Med 2001; 29:N63.

12. Kollef MH, Sherman G, Ward S, Fraser VJ. Inadequate antimicrobial treatment of infections: a risk factor for hospital mortality among critically ill patients. Chest 1999; 115:462-74.

13. Kollef MH. Antimicrobial therapy of ventilator-associated pneumonia: how to select an appropriate drug regimen. Chest 1999; 115:8-11.

14. Kollef MH. Inadequate antimicrobial treatment: an important determinant of outcome for hospitalized patients. Clin Infect Dis 2000; 31(Suppl 4): S131-8.

15. Kollef MH. Is there a role for antibiotic cycling in the Intensive Care Unit? Crit Care Med 2001; 29:N135-42.

16. Kollef MH. The prevention of ventilator-associated pneumonia. N Engl J Med 1999; 340:627-34.

17. Luna CM, Blanzaco D, Niederman MS, et al. Resolution of ventilator-associated pneumonia: prospective evaluation of the clinical pulmonary infection score as an early clinical predictor of outcome. Crit Care Med 2003; 31:676-81.

18. Martinez JA, Horcajada JP, Almela M, et al. Addition of a macrolide to a beta-lactam-based empirical antibiotic regimen is associated with lower in-hospital mortality for patients with bacteremic pneumococcal pneumonia. Clin Infect Dis 2003; 36:389-95.

19. Mora-Duarte J, Betts R, Rotstein C, et al. Comparison of Caspofungin and Amphotericin B for invasive candidiasis. N Engl J Med 2002; 347:2020-29.

20. Murray BE. Vancomycin-resistant enterococcal infections. N Engl J Med 2000; 342:710-21.

21. Perez J, Dellinger RP. Other supportive therapies in sepsis. Intensive Care Med 2001; 27:S116-S126.

22. Reinhart K, Sakka SG, Meier-Hellmann A. Haemodynamic management of a patient with septic shock. Eur J Anaesth 2000; 17:6-17.

23. Rello J, Ollendrof DA, Oster G, et al. Epidemiology and outcomes of ventilator-associated pneumonia in a large US database. Chest 2002; 122:2115-21.

24. Rello J, Paiva JA, Baraibar J, et al. International conference for the development of consensus on the diagnosis and treatment of ventilator-associated pneumonia. Chest 2001; 120:955-70.

25. Russell JA, Singer J, Bernard GR, et al. Changing pattern of organ dysfunction in early human sepsis is related to mortality. Crit Care Med 2002; 28:3405-11.

26. Sandiumenge A, Diaz E, Bodi M, Rello J. Therapy of ventilator-associated pneumonia. A patient-based approach based on the ten rules of 'The Tarragona Strategy'. Intensive Care Med 2003; 29:876-83.

27. Singh N, Rogers P, Atwood CW, Wagener MM, Yu VL. Short-course empiric antibiotic therapy for patients with pulmonary infiltrates in the intensive care unit. A proposed solution for indiscriminate antibiotic prescription. Am J Respir Crit Care Med 2000; 162:505-11.

28. Trouillet JL, Chastre J, Vuagnat A, et al. Ventilator-associated pneumonia caused by potentially drug-resistant bacteria. Am J Respir Crit Care Med 1998; 157:531-9.

29. Valles J, Rello J, Ochagavia A, Garnacho J, Alcala MA. Community-acquired bloodstream infection in critically ill adult patients: impact of shock and inappropriate antibiotic therapy on survival. Chest 2002; 28:1030-5.

30. Vincent JL. Hemodynamic support in septic shock. Intensive Care Med 2001; 27:S80-S92.

31. Weber DJ, Raasch R, Rutala WA. Nosocomial infections in the ICU: the growing importance of antibiotic-resistant pathogens. Chest 1999; 115:34S-41S.

32. Wood MJ. Comparative safety of teicoplanin and vancomycin. J Chemother 2000; 12(Supp) 51:21-5.

33. Martin C et al. Norepinepherine or dopamine for the treatment of hyperdynamic septic shock. Chest 1993; 103:1826-1831.

Acute Respiratory Distress Syndrome

59

Introduction

- The term acute respiratory distress syndrome (ARDS) is applied to acute, diffuse infiltrative lung lesions of diverse etiologies associated with severe arterial hypoxaemia. A variety of cytokines and other molecular mediators are involved in the pathogenesis of ARDS.
- ARDS occurs due to a wide variety of insults but is considered to have two main causes. Direct or pulmonary ARDS is secondary to a primary pulmonary insult and is manifested by pulmonary consolidation, reduced pulmonary compliance, and normal chest wall compliance. Indirect or extrapulmonary ARDS is secondary to trauma or sepsis and is manifested by diffuse interstitial edema, alveolar collapse, reduced pulmonary compliance, and reduced chest wall compliance.
- Regardless of the initiating process, there is a systemic inflammatory response, leading to injured pulmonary capillaries and release of immunologic mediators. Alveolar flooding leads to atelectasis and consolidation, which manifests clinically as low functional residual capacity (FRC), refractory hypoxaemia, and low lung compliance.
- Surfactant production is usually impaired in ARDS, and this also contributes to atelectasis, compromised gas exchange and a further decrease in compliance. There is increased ventilation/perfusion mismatch (because of excessive blood flow to alveoli with atelectasis or consolidation), increased right-to-left shunting (perfusion through areas of alveolar edema and atelectasis), and increased dead space (because of microvascular obstruction by fibrotic thrombi, aggregation of platelets or polymorphonuclear leucocytes). Dead space may increase to over twice the normal levels in ARDS, and interfere with efficiency of CO_2 elimination.
- The disease process is patchy and uneven, and the affected lung may be divided into three zones: an upper, non- dependent zone that remains normal, a middle zone with low compliance that is diseased but recruitable, and a lower dependent zone that is consolidated and not recruitable. This, in effect, means that only a small portion of the lung is recruitable and involved in gas exchange. Therefore, in early ARDS, the lung is 'small' rather than 'stiff'. Use of traditional tidal volumes (10-12 mL/kg) in these patients will, therefore, result in high inspiratory pressures with overdistention of the normally aerated lung units. Therefore, at this stage, a 'lung-protective strategy' for respiratory support is appropriate (Fig. 59.1). In the later states of ARDS, the lung is 'stiff' rather

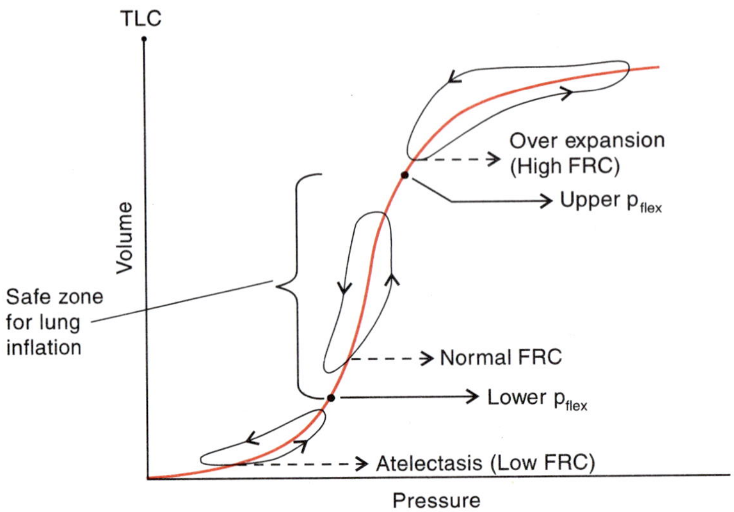

Fig. 59.1: Pressure-volume relationship in ARDS. Upper p_{flex}– Upper inflection point; Lower p_{flex}– Lower inflection point. Patients with ARDS demonstrate areas of overinflated, anteriorly placed areas, diseased but recruitable areas, and the areas of consolidated and collapsed lung predominantly distributed in the dependent areas, participating minimally in gas exchange. The compliance of each region varies as reflected by its location on the pressure-volume curve. Tidal volume should be limited so that it lies on the straight part of the pressure-volume curve between the lower and upper inflection points.

than 'small', and a traditional approach for respiratory support may be appropriate.

- ARDS differs from classical causes of acute respiratory failure (i.e. atelectasis, pneumonia, and bronchospasm) in many respects. In classical acute respiratory failure (ARF), problems related to gas exchange are less severe, pulmonary architecture is intact, pulmonary vascular resistance (PVR) is normal and prognosis is more favourable. On the other hand, in ARDS, gas exchange problems are more severe, basal pulmonary architecture is destroyed, PVR is increased, and prognosis is less favourable. However, in both (ARDS and classical ARF), hypoxaemia and reduced FRC are common features.

- Common features of ARDS and cardiogenic pulmonary edema include dyspnea, tachypnea, refractory hypoxaemia and diffuse bilateral infiltrates. However, in ARDS, pulmonary artery wedge pressure is usually normal, pulmonary vascular resistance is increased, and cardiac output is either normal or increased. In cardiogenic pulmonary edema, on the other hand, pulmonary artery wedge pressure is increased, pulmonary vascular resistance is normal, and cardiac output is decreased.

- Most patients with ARDS do not die of hypoxaemia during the early phase of disease but mortality increases over days to weeks, frequently with evidence of hypermetabolism, nosocomial infection, and multiple organ dysfunction.

- Circulatory management of these patients has been described as a therapeutic dilemma. On the one hand, judicious volume reduction may improve lung function, while on the other, hypoperfusion and multiple organ failure may occur. A balanced approach is thus indicated, which seeks to attain lowest pulmonary vascular pressure compatible with an adequate cardiac output and oxygen delivery. There is some evidence to presume that if edemagenesis could be diminished early after lung injury, the duration of potentially dangerous ventilation, PEEP, and oxygen therapy could be reduced and the outcome improved.

- Ventilator-induced lung injury (VILI) results from regional hyperinflation, excessive airway pressures, high tidal volumes, and repeated opening and closing of alveoli. Limiting plateau pressure (<30 cm H_2O) and adjusting PEEP appropriately are important factors to prevent VILI. Regional hyperinflation also reduces capillary perfusion, increases dead space, and further exacerbates ventilation/perfusion mismatch.

- In the setting of extrapulmonary ARDS, such as a patient with multiple injuries who has undergone massive blood and fluid resuscitation, transpulmonary pressures are reduced due to a decrease in chest wall compliance. In these patients, higher plateau pressures (>30cm H_2O) and PEEP will be required to recruit collapsed alveoli.

- Pulmonary ARDS, i.e. secondary to consolidation, is not particularly responsive to lung recruitment manoeuvres such as PEEP or prone positioning, predisposing the patient to barotrauma due to regional hyperinflation, and requiring careful manipulation of plateau pressure. On the other hand, edema and alveolar collapse in extrapulmonary ARDS are more responsive to recruitment manoeuvres and the non-compliant chest wall may reduce the risk of barotrauma. However, the stiff chest wall increases the risk of haemodynamic compromise. Extrapulmonary ARDS requires early application of recruitment manoeuvres including PEEP of 10-15 cm H_2O and allows for a higher safe limit of inspiratory plateau pressure.

- In early ARDS, edema, alveolar collapse, and hypoxaemia predominate. In late ARDS (10-14 days), fibrosis, cyst formation, and hypercarbia are prevalent. In early ARDS, alveolar recruitment is the mainstay of treatment. In late ARDS, attempts at alveolar recruitment may worsen ventilation/perfusion mismatch and hypercarbia.

- No particular mode of ventilation has been proven to be superior to others in terms of outcome, although complete ventilatory support is appropriate immediately after institution of mechanical ventilation. Volume-cycled ventilation using the "assist-control" mode is an appropriate mode to choose at the outset. Similar degree of respiratory support can probably be achieved with synchronized intermittent mandatory ventilation or pressure-regulated volume-controlled ventilation.

- Pressure-regulated volume-controlled (PRVC) ventilation incorporates the positive attributes of both pressure controlled and volume-controlled ventilation. With this mode, the clinician sets a target TV and inspiratory time, and the ventilator automatically determines the initial flow rate, flow waveform (angle of deceleration), and peak inspiratory pressure. The inspiratory pressure varies in each breath due to changes in compliance, resistance and/or patient effort to keep the tidal volume constant. This mode is analogous to having a clinician at the bedside watching the delivered TV and increasing or decreasing the pressure to maintain a constant tidal volume.

- Whether PEEP is best adjusted using PaO_2/FiO_2 values or the lower inflection point remains uncertain.
- Permissive hypercapnia is a clinical strategy that allows the $PaCO_2$ to increase above normal values, provided the pH is within a specified range. The aim is to provide adequate oxygenation and minimize the risk of volutrauma by accepting a level of hypoventilation that is felt to be safely tolerated by the human body.
- Various, comparatively new, approaches ($ECMO/ECCO_2R$, high frequency ventilation, surfactant, partial liquid ventilation, aerosolized prostacyclin, corticosteroids for early phase of ARDS, non-steroidal anti-inflammatory drugs, ketoconazole, and antioxidants) have been used in the management of ARDS, but their role is still not well defined. Nitric oxide has been used for two reasons: i) as a selective pulmonary vasodilator, and ii) as a selective dilator of only those pulmonary vessels, which are in contact with ventilated alveoli. This leads to reduction in pulmonary artery pressure and an increase in arterial oxygenation. Use of nitric oxide remains experimental and clear benefits are unproven.

GUIDELINES FOR THE MANAGEMENT OF A PATIENT WITH ARDS

1. **Suspect ARDS.**

    Have a high index of suspicion for any patient with direct or indirect pulmonary insult, presenting with dyspnea, tachypnea, anxiety, cyanosis, and refractory hypoxaemia (i.e. $PaO_2 < 60$ mmHg on $FiO_2 > 0.35$). Bilateral rales, worsening hypoxaemia, as indicated by low oxygen saturation and $PaO_2/FiO_2 \leq 200$, or $PaO_2/PAO_2 < 0.2$ (or $PaO_2 < 50$ mmHg on $FiO_2 > 0.6$), no clinical evidence of elevated left atrial pressure (i.e. CHF), PCWP ≤ 18 mmHg, and bilateral pulmonary infiltrates on x-ray chest are other indicators of possible ARDS. A hypoxic patient will also have increased serum lactate levels (indicator of the imbalance between tissue oxygen demand and supply).

2. **Diagnose and treat the primary insult initiating ARDS; control any source of infection.**

    Common causes of ARDS are

    (a) *Direct lung injury:* Pneumonia, aspiration pneumonitis, trauma (lung contusion), near-drowning, fat embolism. ARDS may also occur after lung re-expansion, after relief of upper airway obstrucion, and after bone marrow and lung transplantation.

    (b) *Indirect lung injury:* Sepsis, severe trauma with shock and multiple transfusions, acute pancreatitis, after cardio-pulmonary bypass, neurogenic (intracerebral bleed, seizures), and drug overdose (tricyclic antidepressants, cocaine). Initial antibiotic therapy should have broad-spectrum coverage for both Gram-negative (including Pseudomonas spp.) and Gram-positive (including Staphylococcus aureus) organisms. Antibiotic coverage can be changed when microbiological results are available.

3. Supportive care.
    (a) Minimize edema formation.
    - Loss of alveolar-capillary membrane integrity allows the formation of pulmonary edema in large quantities, even at low hydrostatic pressures. The goal is to maintain intravascular volume at the lowest level that is consistent with adequate systemic perfusion, as assessed by the metabolic status, acid-base balance, and renal function. Fluid intake is kept at approximately 70% of daily requirement and increased as required for optimal cardiac, renal, and nutritional support. Haemodynamic monitoring is essential. Nutritional support should usually not be reduced in a bid to restrict fluids. If needed, intravascular volume status may be adjusted with diuretics. However, diuretics are not strongly indicated, as these drugs do not necessarily decrease lung water significantly since lung infiltration in ARDS is an inflammatory process, and diuretics do not reduce inflammation. Rather, diuretics can result in inadequate systemic circulation to the tissues. Use of furosemide may also confound interpretation of renal function as an indicator of the adequacy of perfusion. Debate regarding crystalloids vs colloids is ongoing. Judicious use of crystalloids has been recommended with colloid solutions which are considered in hypo-oncotic patients. Packed red blood cells may be used in patients with low hematocrit or a low PCWP. Packed RBCs not only increase the oxygen carrying capacity, they also expand the intravascular volume by being retained in the vascular space.
    - If pulmonary artery catheter is not available, optimization of oxygenation may be done by ensuring that blood pressure is adequate (i.e. systolic blood pressure >90mmHg and mean blood pressure >60mmHg), urine output is adequate, mental status is normal, and lactic acidosis does not develop. However, these non-invasive measures are not always reliable indicators of the adequacy of cardiac output.
    - In selected patients, particularly those with manifest systolic dysfunction, dobutamine may be used to maintain perfusion at a reduced pulmonary capillary wedge pressure.
    (b) Ensure adequate tissue oxygenation.
    (i) Minimize demand.
    (ii) Optimize supply.
    Control pain, anxiety, fever.
    - Maintain haemoglobin $\geq$10 g%, PCV $\geq$30%. If haemoglobin is low, transfuse packed red cells.
    - Support cardiovascular system-maintain systolic blood pressure >90 mmHg and mean blood pressure > 60 mmHg, maintain urine output.
    - Use inotropes/vasopressors to maintain blood pressure.
    - Use vasodilators to lower systemic afterload and thereby improve cardiac output while maintaining low pulmonary vascular pressures. If blood pressure falls, add inotropes to maintain blood pressure.

(c) Maintain oxygen saturation $\geq$90% and $PaO_2 \geq 60$ mmHg.

- In the early stages of ARDS, supplemental oxygen by mask at varying and increasing FiO_2 may be the only form of therapy required to maintain PaO_2 or SpO_2. The goal should be to attain adequate oxygenation with the lowest possible FiO_2 so as to avoid the toxic effects of high concentrations of oxygen. Oxygen toxicity can lead to injury if more than 60% oxygen is administered for more than 24 hours. However, maintaining oxygen delivery or tissue oxygenation at any FiO_2 is the primary objective.
- When ARDS is fully developed, with stiff, non-compliant lungs, patient may have increased work of breathing, progressive refractory hypoxemia, increasing respiratory failure (respiratory rate >35 breaths/min, use of accessory muscles, altered mental status, and/or severe refractory hypoxaemia despite supplemental oxygen) and may require ventilatory support.

4. Consider initiating mechanical ventilation.

In ARDS, the work of breathing may consume 25-50% of the body's total oxygen consumption (normal 3-5%). Mechanical ventilation can reduce the work of breathing, thereby allowing redirection of oxygenated blood from the respiratory muscles to vital organs.

(a) Non-invasive positive pressure ventilation (NIPPV).

From the available literature, it appears that patients with ARDS are more likely to fail this therapy. NIPPV is most effective in selected patients (with normal or near normal mental status and without significant respiratory secretions) with expected resolution of respiratory failure within 72 hours - a rare situation in ARDS. Although use of NIPPV may avoid mechanical ventilation (and its attendent risks) in a small population of ARDS patients, the delay in institution of mechanical ventilation may result in untoward complications in the majority of patients.

(b) Initiation of invasive mechanical ventilation.

(c) Use judicious sedation and paralysis (see Chapters 7 and 8)

(i)   Calculate predicted body weight.

(ii) Set goals of ventilation.

FiO_2 goal: The lowest that maintains PaO_2 60-80 mmHg and SpO_2 90-95%.

Pplat goal: $\leq$ 30 cm H_2O

pH goal: 7.30-7.45.

(iii) Initial ventilator settings.

Volume ventilation in assist-control mode, TV 8mL/kg, decelerating flow pattern, PEEP 10±2 cmH_2O, PIFR $\geq$80L/min. FiO_2 to maintain $SpO_2 \geq$ 90%, and $PaO_2 \geq$ 60mmHg. PIFR should be set above the patient demand. Adjust flow rate to achieve goal of 1:E ratio of 1:1.0-1.3. Slowly reduce TV by 1 mL/kg at intervals of $\leq$2 hours until TV= 6mL/kg.

(iv) Monitor the patient at regular intervals.

Check Pplat (use 0.5 sec inspiratory pause], SpO_2, total respiratory rate, TV, and ABG at least every 6 hours and after each change in PEEP or TV.

(v) Plateau pressure goal.
- If Pplat > 30cmH2O: decrease TV by 1 mL/kg steps to a minimum of 4 mL/kg, accept rise in $PaCO_2$ (permissive hypercapnia) if any.
- If Pplat < 25 cmH$_2$O and TV< 6mL/kg: increase TV by 1mL/kg until Pplat >25 CmH$_2$O and TV=6 mL/kg.
  If Pplat < 30cmH$_2$O and breath stacking present: may increase TV in 1mL/kg increments, to a maximum of 8 mL/kg.

(vi) pH goal.
- pH 7.15-7.30: increase respiratory rate until pH>7.30 or $PaCO_2$ <25 mmHg (maximum respiratory rate 35/min). If respiratory rate is 35/min and $PaCO_2$ < 25mmHg, may give $NaHCO_3$.
- pH < 7.15 and $NaHCO_3$ already infused: TV may be increased in 1mL/kg steps until pH > 7.15 (Pplat goal may be exceeded)
- pH >7.45: decrease respiratory rate.

(vii) Oxygenation goal.
See Chapter 39.
Use the following incremental FiO_2-PEEP combinations to achieve oxygenation goal: FiO_2 (PEEP in cm) – 0.3 (5), 0.4(5), 0.4(8), 0.5(8), 0.5(10), 0.6(10), 0.7(10), 0.7(12), 0.7(14), 0.8(14), 0.9(14), 0.9(16), 0.9(18), 1.0(20), 1.0(22), 1.0(24).

5. With the strategy as mentioned, goals are being met, and condition of the patient improving.
    Slowly decrease the support and wean off the ventilator (see Chapter 42).

6. With the strategy as mentioned, goals are not being met.
    Consider other strategies: (i) pressure controlled ventilation (see chapter 35), (ii) prone position, (iii) tracheal gas insufflation, (iv) high frequency ventilation, and (v) ECMO/ECCO$_2$R.

References

1. Alsous F, Amoateng-Adjepong Y, Manthous CA. Noninvasive ventilation: experience at a community teaching hospital. Intensive Care Med 1999; 25:458-463.
2. Amato MBP, Barbas CSV, Medeiros DM et al. Effect of a protective-ventilation strategy on mortality in the acute respiratory distress syndrome. N Engl J Med 1998; 338:347-354.
3. Anonymous International Consensus Conferences in Intensive Care Medicine: Ventilator-associated lung injury in ARDS. Am J Respir Crit Care Med 1999; 160:2118-2124.
4. Anonymous. Ventilation with lower tidal volumes as compared with traditional tidal volumes for acute lung injury and the acute respiratory distress syndrome. The Acute Respiratory Distress Syndrome Network. N Engl J Med 2000; 342:1301-1308.
5. Antonelli M, Conti G, Rocco M, et al. A comparison of noninvasive positive-pressure ventilation and conventional mechanical ventilation in patients with acute respiratory failure. N Engl J Med 1998; 339; 429-435.
6. Artigas A, Bernard GR, Carlet J, et al The American-European Consensus Conference on ARDS. II. Ventilatory, pharmacologic, supportive therapy, study design strategies, and issues related to recovery and remodelling.

Am J Respir Crit Care Med 1998; 157:1332-1347.

7. Bandouin SV. Ventilator induced lung injury and infection in the critically ill. Thorax 2001; 56(suppl 11): 1150-1157.

8. Briegel J, Forst H, Haller M, Schelling G, Kilger E, Kuprat G, Hemmer B, Hummel T, Lenhart A, Heyduck M, Stoll C, Peter K. Stress doses of hydrocortisone reverse hyperdynamic septic shock: a prospective, randomized, double-blind, single-center study. Crit Care Med 1999; 27:723-732.

9. Brochard L, Roudot-Thoraval F, Roupie E, et al. Tidal volume reduction for prevention of ventilator-induced lung injury in acute respiratory distress syndrome. The Multicenter Trial Group on Tidal Volume reduction in ARDS. Am J Respir Crit Care Med 1998; 158:1831-1838.

10. Brower RG, Shanholtz CB, Fessler HE, et al. Prospective, randomized, controlled clinical trial comparingExamination reveals traditional versus reduced tidal volume ventilation in acute respiratory distress syndrome patients. Crit Care Med 1999; 278:1661-1663.

11. Chatila W, Jacob B, Guaglionone D, Manthous CA. The unassisted respiratory rate-tidal volume ratio accurately predicts weaning outcome. Am J Med 1996; 101:61-67.

12. Cook DJ, De Jonghe B, Brochard L, Brun-Buisson C. Influence of airway management on ventilator-associated pneumonia: evidence from randomized trials. JAMA 1998; 279:781-787.

13. Doyle RL, Szaflarski N, Modin GW, Wiener-Kronish JP, Matthay MA. Identification of patients with acute lung injury. Predictors of mortality. Am J Respir Crit Care Med 1995; 152:1818-1824.

14. Esteban A, Alia I, Gordo F, et al. Extubation outcome after spontaneous breathing trials with T-tube or pressure support ventilation. The Spanish Lung Failure Collaborative Group. Am J Respir Crit Care Med 1997; 156 (2 Pt 1): 459-465.

15. Esteban A, Alia I, Tobin MJ, et al. Effect of spontaneous breathing trial duration on outcome of attempts to discontinue mechanical ventilation. Spanish Lung Failure Collaborative Group. Am J Respir Crit Care Med 1999; 159:512-518.

16. Gadek JE, De Michele SJ, Karlstad MD, et al. Effect of enteral feeding with eicosapentaenoic acid, gamma-linolenic acid, and antioxidants in patients with acute respiratory distress syndrome. Enteral Nutrition in ARDS Study Group. Crit Care Med 1999; 27:1409-1420.

17. Hasibeder WR. Fluid resuscitation during capillary leakage: does the type of fluid make a difference. Intensive Care Med 2002; 28:532-534.

18. Heyland DK, Cook DJ, Griffith L, Keenan SP, Brun-Buisson C. The attributable morbidity and mortality of ventilator-associated pneumonia in the critically ill patient. The Canadian Critical Trials Group. Am J Respir Crit Care Med 1999; 159:1249-1256.

19. Humphrey H, Hall J, Sznajder I, Silverstein M, Wood L. Improved outcome based on fluid management in critically ill patients requiring pulmonary artery catheterization. Am Rev Respir Dis 1990; 145:990-998.

20. Kollef MH, Shapiro SD, Silver P, et al. A randomized, controlled trial of protocol-directed versus physician-directed weaning from mechanical ventilation. Crit Care Med 1997; 25:567-574.

21. Lewandowski K. Small tidal volumes-large benefit? Intensive Care Med 1999; 25:771-774.

22. Marini JJ. A lung-protective approach to ventilating ARDS, Respir Clin North Am 1998; 4:633-663.

23. Martin GS, Mangialardi RJ, Wheeler AP, Bernard GR. Albumin and diuretics in ARDS. Am J Respir Crit Care Med 1999; 159:A376.

24. Meduri GU, Headley AS, Golden E et al. Effect of prolonged methylprednisolone therapy in unresolving acute respiratory distress syndrome: a randomized controlled trial. JAMA 1998; 280:159-165.

25. Meduri GU, Headley AS, Golden E, Carson SJ, Umberger RA, Kelso T, Tolley EA. Effect of prolonged methylprednisolone therapy in unresolving acute respiratory distress syndrome: a randomized controlled trial. JAMA 1998; 280:159-165.

26. Meduri GU, Turner RE, Abou-Shala N, Wunderink R, Tolley E. Non-invasive positive pressure ventilation via face mask: first-line intervention in patients with acute hypercapnic and hypoxemic respiratory failure. Chest 1996; 109:179-193.

27. Quinlan GJ, Margarson MP, Mumby S, Evans TW, Gutteridge JM. Administration of albumin to patients with sepsis syndrome: a possible beneficial role in plasma thiol repletion. Clin Sci (Colch) 1998; 4:459-465.

28. Royall JA. Pulmonary edema and ARDS. In: Fuhrman BP, Zimmerman JJ. (eds). Pediatric Critical Care, 2 ed. St Louis: Mosby: 1998; 457-471.

29. Schuster DP. Predicting outcome after ICU admission. The art and science of assessing risk. Chest 1992; 102:1861-1870.

30. Schuster DP. The case for and against fluid restriction and occlusion pressure reduction in adult respiratory distress syndrome. New Horiz 1993; 1:478-488.

31. Slutsky AS. Mechanical ventilation: American College of Chest Physicians' Consensus Conference. Chest 1993; 104:1833-1859.

32. Stewart TE, Meade MO, Cook DJ, et al. Evaluation of a ventilation strategy to prevent barotrauma in patients at high risk for acute respiratory distress syndrome. Pressure- and Volume-Limited Ventilation Strategy Group. N Engl J Med 1998; 338:355-361.

33. Vallverdu I, Calaf N, Subirana M, Net A, Benito S, Mancebo J. Clinical characteristics, respiratory functional parameters, and outcome of a two-hour T-piece trial in patients weaning from mechanical ventilation. Am J Respir Crit Care Med 1998; 158:1855-1862.

34. Wright PE, Carmichael LC, Bernard GR. Effect of bronchodilators on lung mechanics in the acute respiratory distress syndrome (ARDS). Chest 1994; 106:1517-1523.

Flail Chest and Pulmonary Contusion

60

Introduction

- The term flail chest refers to the paradoxical motion of the chest caused by loss of chest wall stability. Usually, double fractures of three or more contiguous ribs or combined sternal and rib fractures lead to a flail segment. Pulmonary complications such as pulmonary contusion, haemothorax, and pneumothorax can occur in upto 60% of patients with flail chest.

- Flail chest occurs as a result of blunt trauma, although it may also be seen after over aggressive chest compression during cardiopulmonary resuscitation, after total sternectomy, and occasionally, with pathologic fractures such as those due to multiple myeloma. The fourth to ninth ribs are more often fractured because of their protruding positions.

- Flail chest, as a rule, occurs not as an isolated injury but in association with equally severe injuries (e.g. closed head injury, shock, long bone fractures, cervical spine fracture, pelvic fracture, and rupture of liver and spleen). Trauma patients with cervical spine injuries may have "flail like" chest without actual injury to thorax. Quadriplegia may be associated with bilateral paradoxical inward chest wall motion on inspiration due to paralysis of the intercostal muscles and accessory muscles of respiration.

- Pulmonary contusion or 'bruise' to the lung parenchyma is characterized by interstitial and alveolar edema, haemorrhage, and resultant alveolar collapse. Typically, there is a central zone of haemorrhage with a variable sized peripheral ring of edema. Children have very compliant chest walls and typically sustain significant pulmonary contusions without fracture to the bony portions of the thorax. With increasing age, the thoracic wall becomes less compliant, and thus, chest wall damage becomes proportionately greater than parenchymal injury for any given force absorbed.

- When kinetic energy of trauma is transferred to the lung tissue, tears occur in the alveolar- capillary membrane, leading to flooding of damaged alveoli with blood and proteinaceous fluid, and concomitant loss of surfactant. Thus some regions of the injured lung are consolidated while others are collapsed. Areas of micro-haemorrhages scattered around the areas of contusion further increase extent of consolidation. There is an increase in mucous production in the airways in response to the inflammatory reaction, creating segmental mucous plugging, air resorption, and collapse of injured lung segments. The zone of injury is ringed by an area of edema before transition into normal appearing lung parenchyma.

- Adverse effects of flail chest on the respiratory system include: (a) A reduction in functional residual capacity (FRC) and vital capacity (up to 50-60% decrease in both) due to disordered chest wall motion, (b) a reduction in lung compliance due to pulmonary contusion (when present) or microatelectasis, (c) increase in the work of breathing and energy demands of the inspiratory muscles due to alteration of the chest wall mechanics (paradoxical motion of flail segment), (d) hypoxaemia (due to contused lung or to microatelectasis because of splinting from chest wall pain, rapid shallow breathing, weak cough and retained secretions) which further contributes to respiratory muscle dysfunction by reducing energy supply to the muscles, and (e) significant blood loss due to multiple rib fractures. Flail chest in the absence of pulmonary contusion can in itself cause hypoxaemia and result in respiratory failure.

- Hypoxia increases during the first 24-48 hours after injury. As the pulmonary vascular resistance of the injured lung increases, blood is shunted away to the non-injured lung. However, as the inflammatory process progresses, the ability to completely shunt from non-ventilated areas of the lung, is exceeded. In addition, there is increased blood flow (in response to injury) to the periphery of injury to aid in preservation of tissue and healing. The resulting contribution to the pulmonary venous admixture from the contused lung segments with mismatched ventilation perfusion ratios produces an increasing amount of hypoxia. Volume resuscitation of the associated intravascular losses (due to other injuries also) further causes the contused lung segments to "blossom", thereby increasing the extent of hypoxia.

- The initial chest x-ray has been shown to be a poor predictor of outcome in patients with pulmonary contusion. Classically, the radiologic findings of pulmonary contusion lag behind the clinical findings in case of blunt trauma by two to three days, which makes the diagnosis more difficult. The diagnosis should be suspected in patients with known, significant, blunt impact to the chest wall.

- The fundamentals of treatment for patients with chest trauma and pulmonary contusion are standard resuscitative measures, effective analgesia, proper positioning, aggressive pulmonary physiotherapy and optimum oxygenation.

- Oxygen therapy should be administered as required. Nasal cannulas may be used, but an air entrainment mask allows more precise control of inspired oxygen concentration. In a patient who does not achieve optimum oxygenation with mask, who has normal, adequate respiratory drive, is alert, who is able to protect the upper airway, and in whom PaO_2/FiO_2 ratio is more than 150 but under 250, CPAP is probably the best mode of ventilatory support. CPAP reduces venous admixture, improves lung compliance, and increases the efficiency of spontaneous breathing. Mask CPAP is not useful in patients with hypercarbia. When mask CPAP fails, hypercarbia ensues, or when the patient meets the criteria for early intubation and ventilation (even when mask CPAP has not been tried), mechanical ventilation should be instituted.

- The indications for early intubation and ventilation in a patient of flail chest are: (a) Falling PaO_2 (<50 mmHg) on air, (b) PaO_2<60 mmHg with supplemental oxygen (FiO$_2$ ≥ 0.5), (c) rising PaCO$_2$ > 45 mmHg, (d) exhaustion, (e) respiratory rate > 30/min, (f) alveolar –arterial oxygen gradient at FiO$_2$ of 1.0> 450mmHg, (h) maximal inspiratory force ≤ 25 cm H$_2$O, (i) clinical evidence of severe shock, (j) significant associated injuries of the abdomen and head, and (k) waning mental status. Remember, patient should be intubated for respiratory decompensation and NOT for chest wall instability. In case of thoracic trauma patients admitted to the ICU, prolonged mechanical ventilation was primarily determined by presence of bilateral chest injuries, age, and degree of neurotrauma, as concluded in one study. Bilateral thoracic injuries were found to be associated with a 13-fold higher probability of prolonged mechanical ventilation.

- When conventional mechanical ventilatory management has not produced the desired response (adequate gas exchange) and the pattern of injury is unilateral, independent lung ventilation (ILV) may be considered. The prime objective of ILV under these circumstances is differential PEEP. This technique allows application of high level of PEEP to the diseased lung, giving maximum benefit to the injured lung, without adverse effects on the contralateral lung, intrathoracic pressure, cardiac output, and the distribution of ventilation between the two lungs. PEEP applied to the diseased lung can be applied at a higher level than would be tolerated if applied to both lungs (as in conventional ventilation) and can improve oxygenation both by alveolar recruitment in that lung and by diverting blood flow to the normal lung. Low PEEP applied to the normal lung avoids overinflation and reduction in overall cardiac output and allows that lung to receive on increased proportion of cardiac output, compared with the diseased lung.

- Prophylactic antibiotics are not indicated and there is no role of systemic steroids in a patient with flail chest and pulmonary contusion.

- Volume resuscitation of patients with significant pulmonary contusion results in a precarious balance between adequate restoration of lost intravascular volume and iatrogenic pulmonary hypertension followed by excessive pulmonary edema in contused lung segments. Warmed, lactated Ringer's solution should be given in adequate amounts to ensure that the patient is resuscitated to normal haemodynamics and urine output. Avoid overtransfusion. Use furosemide if already overtransfused. But do not use diuretics, or restrict fluids just because patient has pulmonary contusion. Optimizing tissue perfusion is more important. In case of questionable volume status, progressive hypoxia, and reducing urine output, a pulmonary artery catheter may guide therapy and should be introduced sooner rather than later.

- The degree of pneumothorax is usually expressed as a "percent" of pneumothorax. The percent of pneumothorax is often expressed as the distance across which the lung is collapsed from the chest wall as compared to the total lung size. Patients with small pneumothoraces (<10%) and essentially asymptomatic may be left without a tube thoracostomy. A follow-up radiograph should be done at 6 and 24 hours after diagnosis to ensure stability of the pneumothorax. However, tube thoracostomy is clearly indicated for patients requiring general anaesthesia or positive-pressure ventilation, or those with bilateral lung injuries.

- In patients with multible rib fractures or a displaced rib fracture, prophylactic chest tube placement may be indicated when (i) requiring transfer from one facility to another, (ii) requiring positive-pressure ventilation, and (iii) requiring general anaesthesia.
- Haemothorax may compress the lung and interfere with its function. Failure to evacuate the blood may lead to chronic lung entrapment, and massive haemothorax (>1500 mL of blood in the pleural space) may lead to shock and death from haemorrhage. Normaly, 200-300 mL of fluid must collect in the pleural space before it can be detected on a chest x-ray. In case of a small haemothorax (<300 mL) with no associated injuries, it is preferable to observe. However, for a collection of more than 300mL, a chest tube should be placed in the midaxillary line in the 5th to 6th intercostal space, since this area is most devoid of muscles, allowing more rapid and less painful tube placement. Immediate removal of more than 1000 mL of blood from the pleural cavity, or a chest tube output of more than 200 mL /hr for 4 hours, is an indication for thoracotomy.
- Mortality in patients with flail chest injury remains high and depends on associated injuries (especially head injury), the presence of shock on admission, the injury severity score (ISS), concomitant pulmonary contusion, and age. Morbidity is more in patients who are intubated than in those who are not.

GUIDELINES FOR MANAGEMENT OF A PATIENT WITH FLAIL CHEST AND PULMONARY CONTUSION

1. Take care of airway and breathing.
   Check for airway patency; use nasal cannula or air entrainment mask.

2. Restore circulation. Normalize CVP, urine output, and peripheral perfusion.
   Establish an IV access with 16 G cannula; withdraw blood for routine laboratory investigations and blood grouping and crossmatching. Start crystalloids (Ringer lactate or normal saline). Use inotropes, if required.

3. Take a quick history and physical examination, ask for a chest radiograph. Look for associated life-threatening lesions of the thorax. Place a chest tube into the pleural space to evacuate air or blood, if indicated.
   - History may be suggestive of vehicular accident or fall from a height. Patient may complain of chest wall pain. Inspection may reveal rapid, shallow breathing, shortness of breath, dyspnoea, distended neck veins (tension pneumothorax, or cardiac tamponade), haemoptysis, evidence of chest wall trauma (chest wall contusion, subcutaneous emphysema), retraction of chest, or decreased chest wall excursion.
   - Palpation may show tenderness, palpable fractures of ribs, sternum, clavicle or scapula, deviation of trachea (tension pneumothorax, haemothorax).

- On auscultation, the findings may include absent or diminished breath sounds over one or both sides, rhonchi (pulmonary contusion). Hypotension and tachycardia may be because of blood loss, myocardial contusion, or cardiac tamponade.
- A selected group of patients (who meet the criteria) will require early intubation and ventilation.
- Chest radiograph can detect most pneumothoraces, massive haemothorax, or widened mediastinum suggestive of thoracic aortic injury. Other possible findings on radiograph include subcutaneous emphysema, rib fractures, clavicle fractures, sternal fractures, pulmonary contusion, mediastinal widening, or findings suggestive of diaphragmatic rupture.

4. **After initial stabilization, reassess the patient in detail.**
   - (a) **Look for associated injuries.**
   - (b) **Continue monitoring pulse, blood pressure, respiratory rate, skin perfusion, level of consiousness, ECG, oxygen saturation, arterial blood gas analysis, end-tidal CO_2. Review blood investigations.**

   ECG may reveal dysrhythmias, ST-T wave abnormalities, and conduction disturbances.

   ABG may reveal base deficit, hypoxia ($PaO_2 < 70$ mmHg, $PaO_2/FiO_2 < 250$).

5. **Control pain.**

   The goals of pain relief are to facilitate patient ambulation, enhance secretion clearance, and allow coughing and deep breathing. Patients with thoracic injuries receiving adequate pain relief experience significantly fewer pulmonary complications, such as pneumonia.

   - (a) **Parenteral narcotics.**

     Parenteral narcotics and benzodiazepines should be avoided, if possible, in patients with chest wall pain. An oversedated patient cannot sit up, cough effectively, initiate adequate negative inspiratory efforts or participate in respiratory therapy. Further, impaired minute ventilation may result in hypercarbia, resultant pulmonary hypertension and pulmonary edema. If at all these need to be used, these should be utilized in the form of patient-controlled analgesia (PCA).

   - (b) **Epidural analgesia.**

     Studies have confirmed that epidural analgesia can increase FVC, FEV, and FRC over pre-epidural values. Patients with chest wall injuries receiving epidural analgesia can ambulate earlier, cough, deep breathe, and participate in intensive pulmonary physiotherapy. Also, overall ICU stay, hospital stay, morbidity, and mortality are significantly reduced in patients with chest wall injuries treated with epidural analgesia, when compared to patients treated with parenteral narcotics.

   - (c) **Intrapleural analgesia.**

     For patients with severe coagulopathy or spine fractures, who are not candidates for epidural catheter, intrapleural analgesia is an attractive alternative.

   - (d) **Intercostal nerve blocks.**

Intercostal nerve block is simple, effective but somewhat labour-intensive modality for control of chest wall pain. These need to be repeated frequently. These blocks are of great importance for the initial management of chest wall pain in emergency department. An effective technique is to infiltrate the intercostal space just inferior to the rib margin one level above and below the injured rib.

6. **Respiratory care, Humidification, Pulmonary physiotherapy, Suctioning, Early mobilization. Incentive spirometry.**

   Strict bed rest is not recommended for rib fractures, flail chest, and pulmonary contusion. Once pain control has been established, patient should sit up, get into a chair, and ambulate if possible. Bed rest contributes to reduced lung volumes and causes venous stasis. Encourage frequent changes in position. Initiate the patient to cough and deep breathe. If he needs additional motivation, incentive spirometry may be helpful. For patients who are unable to generate sufficient cough, and retain secretions, nasotracheal suctioning may be required. Avoid chest percussion, as it can aggravate pain and result in increased splinting, atelectasis, and hypoxaemia.

7. **Review the oxygenation goal. Add mask CPAP if required. Observe respiratory rate, SpO_2, patient's comfort level.**

   If patient is not being oxygenated optimally with air-entrainment mask, the next step is to add mask CPAP as a means of oxygenation support (provided the patient meets the prerequisites as described before i.e., alert, normocarbia, normal respiratory drive, able to protect airway, and PaO_2/FiO_2 more than 150 but under 250). Start CPAP at 5cm H_2O, at an FiO_2 sufficient to maintain oxygen saturation more than 92%. Increase CPAP in increments of 2 to 3 cm H_2O to maintain the respiratory rate under 25 breaths/min. When mask CPAP is successful, respiratory rate decreases and SpO_2 increases.

   If CPAP reaches 15 cm H_2O without relieving tachypnoea, consider intubation.

8. **Initiate mechanical ventilation.**
   (a) Volume cycled mode.
   (b) PEEP-set to maintain SpO_2 >92% with FiO_2 ≤0.6.
   (c) TV 7-8 mL/kg with modification so as to maintain Pplat < 35 cmH_2O.
   (d) Respiratory rate- to maintain pH >7.25 and a spontaneous respiratory frequency below 25 breaths/min. Add sedation if required.
   (e) Inspiratory time 1-1.5 sec.
   (f) I:E ratio –select so that expiratory flow returns to baseline before delivery of the next mechanical breath (to prevent auto PEEP).
   (g) Decelerating flow waveform.
   (h) Flow triggering.

   Primary goal is to achieve optimum oxygenation with haemodynamic improvment.

   - Although an upper limit of plateau pressure (35 cmH_2O) should not be crossed, in patients with chest trauma with diminished compliance, higher plateau pressures may be required and are considered safe. A better measurement is transpulmonary (alveolar pressure minus pleural pressure) pressure, but it is difficult to measure it clinically.

- If the initial mode selected fails to achieve adequate gas exchange, consider lengthening inspiratory time and utilizing a decelerating flow waveform (if not being used already). Alternatively, use pressure controlled ventilation with long inspiratory time, including inverse ratio ventilation. The prolongation of inspiratory time and decelerating flow waveform improves distribution of ventilation as a result of limitation of maximal regional pressures among lung units with heterogenous time constants (a feature of pulmonary contusion caused by the difference in compliance between the two lungs). However, longer inspiratory times may contribute to reduced cardiac output and patient/ventilator dyssynchrony.

9. Position the patient.
   (a) Semi-Fowler's position.
   (b) Lateral decubitus position.
   (c) Prone position.
   Usually the patient is maintained in a semi-Fowler's position. Several reports have documented improved gas exchange, when patients with unilateral disease (pulmonary contusion, unilateral pneumonia, and atelectasis) are placed in a lateral decubitus position. However, the improvement is not a consistant finding and is not predictable from clinical and laboratory data, ventilatory parameters, or radiographic patterns. Therefore, a trial of the lateral positioning with good lung being down (dependent) should be attempted with careful monitoring of oxygenation, ventilator volumes and pressures, and blood pressure (at the same ventilatory parameters). When negligible difference is noted in oxygenation between the lateral and supine position, lateral position may be discontinued. Prone position may be used in patients who develop ARDS after chest trauma.

10. Independent-lung ventilation (ILV).
    (a) Use the largest size plastic, left sided Robertshaw double-lumen tube.
    (b) Asynchronous ILV is as efficacious as synchronous ILV.
    (c) Sedate and achieve neuromuscular paralysis, if not already.
    (d) Use a ventilator-cycled mode that provides total support.
    (e) Improvement in lung compliance and peak airway pressure in the involved lung is a favourable sign.
       - Criteria for using independent lung ventilation in patients who have unilateral disease (i.e. pulmonary contusion, atelectasis) include, radiographically apparent unilateral or asymmetrical lung disease with one of the following: (i) hypoxaemia refractory to high FiO_2 and generalized PEEP, (ii) PEEP-induced deterioration in oxygenation or shunt fraction, (iii) overinflation of the uninvolved lung with or without collapse of the involved lung, and (iv) significant deterioration in circulatory status in response to PEEP.
       - Since most patients requiring ILV will have been supported with conventional ventilation before initiating ILV, total minute ventilation and

FiO_2, as used for conventional ventilation can serve as starting points for ILV, though the distribution of ventilation and ventilation/perfusion match will undoubtedly change. Start with an initial tidal volume 5-8 mL/kg for each lung (equal tidal volumes to each lung tend to have a better overall response). Frequent adjustments are necessary. Reduction of volume in the involved lung because of excessive pressures frequently necessitates compensatory increases in the contralateral side to maintain desired gas exchange. Determine appropriate PEEP level. Increase PEEP progressively to the diseased lung until the compliance of the two lungs approximates each other. In general, start with 3-5 cmH_2O PEEP to normal lung and 10-15 cmH_2O PEEP to diseased lung. Subsequent changes may be based on clinical, blood gas, and haemodynamic data. ILV is usually required for 2-3 days. After this, the patient either improves and can be switched back to single lumen tube conventional ventilation, or multisystem injury results in ARDS involving both lungs, which also requires transition to a single lumen tube.

11. **Weaning from independent lung ventilation (transition to conventional ventilation with a single lumen tube).**

    While considering a transition to conventional ventilation, give a trial of ventilation with identical settings in the circuits to each lung and assess residual difference in physiology. When majority of the following criteria are met, successful transition to conventional ventilation may be expected: (i) Difference in PEEP in two circuits <5cmH_2O with stable PaO_2, (ii) peak airway difference <5cmH_2O on identical settings in both circuits, (iii) difference in compliance between the two lungs <10mL/cmH_2O, (iv) ratio of end tidal $CO_2 \geq 0.88$, (v) total minute ventilation < 12L/min (sum of the two systems), and (vi) radiographic improvement with decreased asymmetry.

12. **When the patient improves, wean off the ventilatory support.**

    When the patient improves, stabilizes and meets the weaning criteria, patient may be weaned off the ventilatory support.

References

1. Bachman-Mennega B, Biscoping J, Kuhn DFM, et al. Intercostal nerve block, intrapleural analgesia, thoracic epidural block, or systemic opioids application for pain relief after thoracotomy? Eur J Cardiothorac Surg 1993; 7:12-18.
2. Bolliger CT, Van Eeden SF. Treatment of multiple rib fractures: ventilatory management. Chest 1990; 97:943-948.
3. Branson RD. PEEP without endotracheal intubation. Respir Care 1988; 33:598-610.
4. Clark GC, Scheeter WP, Trunkey DD. Variables affecting outcome in blunt chest trauma: flail chest vs, pulmonary contusion. J Trauma 1988; 28:298-304.
5. Dimopoulou I, Anthi A, et al. Prediction of prolonged ventilatory support in blunt thoracic trauma patients. Intensive Care Med. 2003; 29:1101-1105.
6. Duff JH, Goldstein M, McLean AP, et al. Flail chest: a clinical review and physiological study. J Trauma 1986; 8:63-74.

7. Freedland MA, Wilson RF, Bender J. The management of flail chest injury. J Trauma 1990; 30:1460-1468.

8. Fulton RL, Peters ET. The progressive nature of pulmonary contusion. Surgery 1979; 67:499-506.

9. Hurst JM, Dehaven B, Branson RD. Comparison of conventional mechanical ventilation and synchronous independent lung ventilation (SILV) in the treatment of unilateral lung injury. J Trauma 1985; 25:766-770.

10. Hurst JM, Dehaven B, Branson RD. Use of CPAP mask as the sole mode of ventilatory support in trauma patients with mild to moderate respiratory insufficiency. J Trauma 1985; 25:1065-1068.

11. Johnson JA, Cogbill TH, Winga ER. Determinants of outcome after pulmonary contusion. J Trauma 1986; 26:695-697.

12. Mackersie RC, Shackford SR, Hoyt DB, et al. Continuous epidural fentanyl analgesia: ventilatory function improvement with routine use in treatment of blunt chest injury. J Trauma 1987; 27:1207-1212.

13. Nolan J. Fluid resuscitation for the trauma patient. Resuscitation 2001; 48:57-69.

14. Pape HC, Remmers D, Rice J, Ebisch M, Krettek C, Tscherne H. Appraisal of early evaluation of blunt chest trauma: development of a standardized scoring system for initial clinical decision making. J Trauma 2000; 49:496-504.

15. Relihan M, Litwin MS. Morbidity and mortality associated with flail chest injury. J Trauma 1973; 13:663-671.

16. Shackford SR, Virgillo RW, Peters RM. Selective use of ventilatory therapy in flail chest injury. J Thorac Cardiovasc Surg 1981; 81:194-201.

17. Siegel JH, Stoklosa JC, Borg U, et al. Quantification of asymmetric lung pathophysiology as a guide to the use of simultaneous independent lung ventilation in posttraumatic and septic adult respiratory distress syndrome. Ann Surg 1985; 202:425-439.

18. Stow PJ, Grant I. Asynchronous independent lung ventilation. Its use in the treatment of acute unilateral lung disease. Anaesthesia 1985; 40:163-166.

19. Thomas AR, Bryce TL. Ventilation in the patient with unilateral lung disease. Crit Care Clin 1998; 14(4): 743-773.

20. Tuxen D. Independent lung ventilation. In: Tobin MJ (ed). Principles and Practice of Mechanical Ventilation. New York: McGraw-Hill 1994, pp 571-588.

21. Wisner DH. A stepwise logistic regression analysis of factors affecting morbidity and mortality after thoracic trauma: effect of epidural analgesia. J Trauma 1999; 30:799-804.

22. Zandstra DF, Stoutenbeek CP, Bams JL. Monitoring lung mechanics and airway pressure during differential lung ventilation (DLV) with emphasis on weaning from DLV. Intensive Care Med 1989; 15:458-463.

Acute Respiratory Failure due to Chronic Obstructive Pulmonary Disease

61

Introduction

- Chronic obstructive pulmonary disease (COPD) is a chronic, slowly progressive disorder and refers to a triad of distinct disease processes that, as a rule, co-exist. The three disease processes are asthma (airway reaction), emphysema (airway collapse), and bronchitis (airway inflammation).
- Most of the impairment in lung function is fixed, although some reversibility can be produced by bronchodilator (or other) therapy.
- Acute exacerbation of COPD presents as a worsening of the previously stable condition, accompanied by deteriorating lung function.
- In the early stage of ventilatory insufficiency, mild degree of hypoxaemia (PaO_2 <60 mmHg) stimulates the respiratory centre, producing hyperventilation, $PaCO_2$ less than 40 mmHg, and acute respiratory alkalosis (pH> 7.40). As the disease progresses, the work of hyperventilation becomes cost ineffective – that is, more carbon dioxide is produced than is cleared. Despite the body's mechanical hyperventilation, alveolar hypoventilation leads to CO_2 retention and acute respiratory acidosis ($PaCO_2$ 45-60mmHg, pH 7.30-7.35, PaO_2 < 50 mmHg). However, with renal compensation and retention of bicarbonate, the pH returns towards normal. This stage of ventilatory failure is characterized by moderate to severe dyspnoea with use of accessory muscles, paradoxical abdominal motion, and respiratory rate more than 25 breaths per minute. Mental status is usually clear with some degree of anxiety or the beginning of lethargy or disorientation. Finally, with further progression of disease (end-stage disease, with terminal ventilatery failure) patient is usually cyanotic, lethargic, speechless, confused, gasping, and has ineffective respiration (respiratory rate >36 breaths per minute). ABG shows PaO_2 < 50 mmHg, $PaCO_2$ > 60 mm Hg, pH < 7.30, and elevated bicarbonate.
- The management of acute exacerbation includes, treating the reversible elements of bronchospasm, airway inflammation, correcting hypoxaemia, respiratory acidosis, managing secretions, removing or treating precipitating causes/factors, and avoiding iatrogenic complications, like, barotrauma and haemodynamic instability.
- Treatment should start as soon as possible, even before completing the examination of the patient.

- Factors for precipitating an acute exacerbation of COPD include infections (usually viral), pneumonia, pulmonary emboli, myocardial infarction, congestive heart failure, dysrhythmias, pneumothorax, aspiration, neuromuscular weakness, rib or vertebral body fractures, post-surgical thoracoabdominal pain, electrolyte disturbances, pleural effusion, drugs (sedatives, β-blockers), inappropriate use of oxygen, and dysfunction of any other organ (e.g. gastrointestinal haemorrhage).

- Markers of increased mortality include advanced age, need for mechanical ventilation, atrial fibrillation, ventricular dysrhythmia, acute or chronic cardiac disease, associated nonpulmonary organ failure, poor nutritional status and baseline health status, an alveolar-arterial oxygen gradient on room air greater than 40 mmHg or a low PaO_2/FiO_2 ratio.

- Indications for ICU admission of patients with acute exacerbation of COPD include: (a) Severe dyspnoea that responds inadequately to initial emergency therapy, (b) confusion, lethargy, or respiratory muscle fatigue (the last characterized by paradoxical diaphragmatic motion), (c) persistent or worsening hypoxaemia (PaO_2 < 50 mmHg) despite supplemental oxygen or worsening hypercarbia ($PaCO_2$ > 70 mmHg) or respiratory acidosis (pH<7.3), or (d) cardiorespiratory instability that signifies a need or a potential need for ventilator support. Most patients treated with NIPPV for acute respiratory failure should preferably be cared for, in an ICU environment.

- Investigations within 24 hours of admission include complete haemogram, blood counts, urea, sugar, electrolytes, liver function tests, chest radiography, ECG, ABG, ECHO, and cultures for blood and sputum. Monitor the patient's vital signs, SpO_2, end tidal CO_2, and fluid status continuously. Perform ABGs at regular intervals to guide therapy.

- The patient may be considered for discharge if (a) Inhaled bronchodilator therapy is required no more frequently than every 4 hours, (b) patient, if previously ambulatory, is able to walk across the room, (c) patient is able to eat and sleep without frequent awakening by dyspnoea, (d) patient's clinical condition and arterial blood gases have been stable for 12-24 hours, and (e) patient or a responsible relative fully understands the correct use of medication prescribed.

GUIDELINES FOR AN APPROACH TOWARDS A PATIENT WITH ACUTE COPD

1. Assess the severity and initiate the management.
   Immediate airway and ventilatory management depends on clinical findings and oxygen saturation.
   (a) -Increased respiratory effort.
   -No signs of respiratory failure.
   -SpO_2 < 90%.
   -$PaCO_2$ < 40 mmHg.
   -pH> 7.40.
   -Normal mental status.

- Add oxygen by nasal cannula @ 2L/min or by ventimask settings at 24-28% (see Chapter 4).
- Titrate oxygen to achieve an SpO_2 90-92%.
- Add β_2-agonists and anticholinergics (inhalation route).
- Corticosteroids, oral or IV.
- Antibiotics, oral or IV.
- Consider aggravating factors.

(b) -Moderate to severe dyspnoea.
-Respiratory rate >25-30 breaths/min.
-Wheezing.
-Use of accessory muscles.
-Paradoxical abdominal motion.
-Prolonged expiratory time.
-pH 7.30-7.35.
-$PaCO_2$ 45-60 mmHg.
-Mental status clear with some anxiety.

- Add NIPPV (non-invasive positive pressure ventilation). NIPPV is highly effective in avoiding intubation in these patients. NIPPV can be given in the form of CPAP (continuous positive pressure ventilation) or BiPAP (bilevel positive pressure ventilation).
- Oxygen to maintain saturation 90-92%.
- Nebulized β_2–agonists and anticholinergics.
- Corticosteroids IV.
- Antibiotics IV.
- Consider aggravating factors.

(c) -Severe dyspnoea with the use of accessory muscles and paradoxical abdominal motion.
-Respiratory rate >36/min despite NIPPV.
-Worsening tachycardia.
-Patient's subjective sense of exhaustion.
-Life-threatening hypoxaemia (PaO_2 < 40 mmHg or PaO_2/FiO2<200).
-Severe acidosis (pH<7.25-7.30).
-Severe hypercapnia ($PaCO_2$ > 60 mmHg).
-Respiratory arrest.
-Somnolence, impaired mental status.
-Cardiovascular complications (hypotension, shock, heart failure).
-Other complications (metabolic abnormalities, sepsis, pneumonia, pulmonary embolism, massive pleural effusion).
-Patients who fail to improve with NIPPV.

- Address ABC (airway, breathing and circulation).
- Consider preoxygenation/bag ventilation.
- Consider intubation (use wider bore endotracheal tube via orotracheal route preferably).
- Consider ventilation.
- β_2-agonists and anticholinergics with the use of in-line nebulizer .

- Corticosteroids IV.
- Antibiotics IV.
- Aminophylline IV (±).
- Consider aggravating factors.

2. Oxygen therapy.
   (a) Administer oxygen with nasal cannula or venturi mask.
   (b) Increase FiO_2 from 0.24 onwards, gradually, to achieve the goal.
   (c) Monitor $PaCO_2$.
      - $PaCO_2 < 50mmHg$ –continue with lowest FiO_2 to achieve goal.
      - $PaCO_2 > 50mmHg$ and $pH > 7.3$ – maintain oxygen flow.
      - $PaCO_2 > 50mmHg$ and $pH < 7.3$ – consider assisted ventilation.
      - During acute exacerbations, hypoxaemia is mainly caused by worsened ventilation-perfusion mismatch. With increasing obstruction and severity, alveolar hypoventilation (inability of fatigued respiratory muscles to sustain breathing) contributes to hypoxaemia, hypercarbia, and respiratory acidosis. Hypoxaemia and respiratory acidosis, by causing pulmonary vasoconstriction, add load on the right ventricle and can lead to right ventricular failure (necessitating addition of diuretics). Severe hypoxaemia and hypercarbia with respiratory acidosis may also compromise left-ventricular function, precipitate arrhythmias, impair respiratory muscles, and depress mental status. Therefore, correction of hypoxaemia is the immediate priority.
      - Administer oxygen in the lowest concentrations in order to maintain SpO_2 of 90% (PaO_2 of 60mmHg) without CO_2 retention.
      - Take an ABG measurement 15-30 minutes after every change in FiO_2 to monitor worsening hypercapnia (probably due to the Haldane effect and worsening ventilation-perfusion match).
      - A rise in $PaCO_2$ should not stop the administration of oxygen to a hypoxic patient, as patients may progress to respiratory failure despite oxygen therapy but not because of it.
      - High concentrations of inspired oxygen are usually not necessary unless pneumonia, pulmonary edema, or pulmonary embolism is present.

3. Corticosteroids.
   (a) Methylprednisolone: 125 mg IV (one dose) followed by 0.5 – 1mg/kg IV every 6 hours. Switch over to prednisolone after 1-3 days when clear improvement is seen, OR
   (b) Prednisolone 0.5-1mg/kg/24 hr for 10-14 days.
      - Recent data suggest that hospitalized patients treated with systemic corticosteroids have fewer treatment failures, more rapid normalization of spirometric values and shorter duration of hospital stay. Prolonged treatment (more than 2 weeks) does not result in greater efficacy and also increases the risk of side effects. Possible mechanisms of action include decrease in inflammation, microvascular permeability and mucous production and perhaps upregulating β_2-adrenergic receptors in the airway.

4. Antibiotics.
    (a) In ICU: Third generation cephalosporins or β-lactam/β-lactamase inhibitor plus fluoroquinolones, or newer macrolide.
    (b) In outdoor patient: Amoxicillin, co-trimoxazole, or doxycycline.
    (c) For those who fail initial therapy, get guided by sputum cultures.
    - Antibiotics are added in the presence of at least two of these symptoms: increased breathlessness, increased sputum volume, and sputum purulence. An antibiotic is selected which is active against Streptococcus pneumoniae, H.influenzae and Moraxella catarrhalis. In some patients, an additional coverage for Mycoplasma pneumoniae and Chlamydia pneumoniae is required. For hospitalized patients, routine use of antibiotics is justified as they substantially decrease the rate of treatment failures, increase the rate of recovery, and an aetiological role for bacteria in individual cases cannot be excluded (at least one third of exacerbations may be caused by viral infection).
    - β-lactam/β-lactamase inhibitors are: amoxycillin/sulbactum, or ticarcillin/clavulanate, or piperacillin/tazobactum.
    - Fluoroquinolones: levo-, spar-, or gati-floxacin.
    - Macrolides: azithromycin, clarithromycin.

5. β_2–agonists and anticholinergics.
    (a) Salbutamol aerosol 2.5-5 mg every 20-30 minutes or metered dose inhaler (MDI) 0.4 mg (available as 0.1mg/dose) every 20-30 minutes till response is achieved or toxicity appears (e.g. tachycardia, tremulousness, dysrhythmias). Decrease the frequency of administration depending upon the response.
    (b) Ipratropium bromide aerosol 500µg every 4-6 hours, or MDI 40-80 µg (two to four doses) every 4-6 hours.
    - For moderate exacerbations, a β_2- agonist (salbutamol 2.5-5 mg or terbutaline 5-10 mg) or an anticholinergic drug (ipratropium bromide 0.25-0.5 mg) should be given. In case of severe exacerbation or a poor response to either treatment alone, both the drugs may be administered simultaneously. Combination bronchodilator therapy has the potential advantage of convenience and improved patient compliance.
    - Nebulisers may be powered by a wall mounted oxygen supply but in patients with COPD, the nebuliser should be driven by compressed air if the $PaCO_2$ is raised and/or there is respiratory acidosis. Oxygen administration may be continued through nasal prongs at 1-2L/min during nebulisation in order to prevent a fall in oxygen saturation.
    - A response to nebulised bronchodilators in the acute situation does not imply long-term benefit.
    - Consensus statement recommends administration of inhaled β_2-agonists with an MDI rather than a nebulizer unit.
    - Ipratropium, as compared with β_2-agonists, has a delayed onset, equivalent bronchodilator effect, and a greater effect on improvement of oxygenation.

6. Aminophylline.
   (a) In the absence of theophylline therapy in the preceding 24 hours:5 mg/kg ideal body weight over 20-30 minutes.
   (b) Maintenance dose: 0.2 to 0.7mg/kg/hr.
   (c) Monitor serum levels.
   - Role is controversial in acute exacerbation of COPD. The addition of aminophylline to a standard regimen of β_2-agonists, ipratropium and corticosteroids in these patients has not shown benefit in controlled trials.
   - Should not be used routinely and may be added when more standard bronchodilator regimens have failed.

7. Diuretics.
   Indicated in the presence of peripheral edema and increased jugular venous pressure.

8. Mucokinetic medications.
   Maintain oral hydration.
   There is little objective evidence of the effectiveness of nebulized water and saline, and oral expectorants like guaifenesin and saturated iodide. Acetylcysteine may cause reflex bronchoconstriction.

9. Respiratory stimulants.
   Presently, not recommended for routine use.

10. Pulmonary vasodilators.
    There is no evidence that pulmonary vasodilators have any role in patients with COPD and pulmonary hypertension.

11. Treat aggravating factor/precipitating cause.
    (a) Inadequate neuromuscular function.
    (b) Increased resistive load.
    (c) Increased lung elastic load.
    (d) Increased chest wall elastic load.
    - Only a few patients develop ventilatory failure from loss of drive. Far more common are the patients who have adequate drive but have inadequate neuromuscular function, excessive load or both. Important causes contributing to inadequate neuromuscular function include electrolyte disturbances (hypokalaemia, hypophosphataemia, and hypomagnesaemia), myopathy, flattened diaphragm, muscle fatigue (hypoperfusion state, hypoxaemia, and anaemia). Contributors to increased resistive load include bronchospasm, airway edema, secretions, scarring, small sized (<7.5mm ID) endotracheal tube. Contributors to increased lung elastic load (increased lung stiffness) are pulmonary edema (cardiogenic and non-cardiogenic), infection, internal PEEP, and atelectasis. Increased chest wall elastic load could be because of obesity, pleural effusion, pneumothorax, abdominal distension, and rib-fracture.

12. **NIPPV.** Reduces intubation rates, duration of hospitalization, infection rates, and mortality.

    See Chapter 29.

    So strong is the evidence for effectiveness of NIPPV in patients with acute exacerbation of COPD that it has been defined as the gold standard mode of ventilatory support with, endotracheal intubation and mechanical ventilation regarded as second line rescue therapy, when NIPPV fails. The exact time when NIPPV should be started is still a matter of debate, but there are very strong arguments for delivering of NIPPV as soon as the patient develops moderate respiratory acidosis with a pH $\leq$ 7.35 and increased $PaCO_2$. There are three important characteristics of NIPPV in the patients of acute COPD:

    (i)   Improves alveolar ventilation by increasing tidal volume which results in decreased patient effort.

    (ii) It uses facemask in place of an endotracheal tube, thus avoiding all the complications of intubation.

    (iii) It is an intermittent mode of support. NIPPV is usually delivered for only a few hours during a 24-hour period. These patients have a highly stimulated and active respiratory drive and can therefore sustain prolonged periods of spontaneous breathing. Any treatment should provide a reduction in the amount of effort needed and thus, intermittent support seems to be adequate.

13. **Invasive mechanical ventilation.**

    (a) **Set goals of mechanical ventilation.**

    - Ensure rest to the muscles of breathing: Patients in acute respiratory failure are fatigued. One to two days of respiratory muscle rest on mechanical ventilation, therefore, should allow recovery from fatigue. A further period of 1-3 days may be needed to allow bronchospasm to resolve, infection to settle and respiratory mechanics to improve to the point at which resistive work is within tolerable limits for the rested muscles, allowing spontaneous breathing.
    - Avoid auto-PEEP, overdistension, respiratory alkalosis.
    - Avoid patient-ventilator dyssynchrony.
    - Gradually correct the acute hypercapnia back to the baseline PaCO2, if known, or to a level that results in a pH of approximately 7.35 and not to a normal range. Overcorrection of $PaCO_2$ will result in acute alkalosis in the short term and in the long term, a difficulty in weaning because of suppression of respiratory drive related to an alkalaemic pH.

    (b) **Intubate the patient.**
    Prefer ETT size $\geq$ 8mm ID and orotracheal route.
    Orotracheal intubation allows the passage of a widebore endotracheal tube (ETT), which may be of help during weaning by decreasing the airway resistance. Orotracheal intubation also avoids nasal obstruction and nosocomial sinusitis.

    (c) **Gently ventilate manually.**
    Immediately after intubation, use gentle, assisted manual ventilation. Avoid overenthusiastic approach of ventilation to bring back $PaCO_2$ to normal. It

may cause acute respiratory alkalosis, hypokalaemia and arrhythmias. Remember, an acute change in $PaCO_2$ of 10 mmHg causes an acute change in pH of 0.08 and an acute change in pH of 0.1 causes an acute change in serum potassium of 0.5 mEq/L. Therefore, if a $PaCO_2$ of 80mmHg (not uncommon in acute COPD) is brought down suddenly to 40mmHg, it cause a sudden change in pH of 0.32 (4×0.08). This rapid increase in pH (hyperventilation) is associated with a marked intracellular flux of potassium (alkalosis causes potassium to shift into the cells). A change in pH of 0.32 therefore, will decrease serum potassium levels by 1.6 mEq/L. (an initial level of, say, 4mEq/L will drop to 2.4 mEq/L) which might be enough to precipitate arrhythmias.

(d) Pressure ventilation versus volume ventilation.

These patients, when intubated and ventilated, are at increased risk for patient-ventilatory dyssynchrony because of air trapping due to high airway resistance. Pressure ventilation (pressure control or pressure support) may be preferable in these patients, as it appears to prevent dyssynchrony, lowers peak airway pressure and alveolar pressure, and decreases the likelihood of alveolar overdistension. PSV mode can be used not only as a weaning mode but also as a ventilatory mode for some patients with COPD. In many ventilators, however, pressure support is terminated by a 25% reduction in inspiratory flow, or when a definite set flow rate is achieved. In a particular patient, when airway resistance is high, decay of inspiratory flow is too slow for the ventilator to detect the end of inspiration, so flow continues into neuronal exhalation, causing hyperinflation and patient ventilator dyssynchrony. Patients may recruit expiratory muscles to terminate flow, increasing the WOB. If dyssynchrony occurs, the PSV level may need to be reduced.

However, volume ventilation may also be safely used, provided the goals are kept in mind and settings done appropriately.

(e) Mode of ventilation.

- Assist-control.

- SIMV plus PS.

During first 24-48 hours, patient may benefit from controlled ventilation with higher respiratory rates to provide respiratory muscle rest, but avoid auto-PEEP and high plateau airway pressures.

The mode selected should be such that it decreases work of breathing, giving enough rest to the already fatigued muscles. Both modes, assist-control and synchronized intermittent mandatory ventilation (SIMV), are suitable in this situation. In general, respiratory muscles rest more predictably on assist-control mode than SIMV mode. Though SIMV mode (alternate mandatory breaths that provide muscle rest with spontaneous breaths that require patient effort), is intended to provide enough rest to the muscles, studies have demonstrated that significant work is required during both mandatory and spontaneous breaths in this mode even at high assist rate because the respiratory center cannot adapt when assistance varies from breath to breath. Because WOB in SIMV usually exceeds that in assist-control, assist-control mode may be preferred when muscle rest is a priority.

(i) **Peak inspiratory flow rate (PIFR 80-100 L/min).**

In patients with COPD and significant amount of auto-PEEP, high flow rates shorten inspiratory time and increase expiratory time, and thus potentially reduce the degree of auto-PEEP and dynamic hyperinflation. With short inspiratory times, there is an improvement in pulmonary mechanics and gas exchange. The improvement in gas exchange is believed to be due to better ventilation of poorly ventilated alveoli due to prolongation of expiratory time. Similarly, there is increase in static compliance, probably reflecting a decrease in dynamic hyperinflation. Also resistance of the respiratory system as a whole decreases significantly with higher inspiratory flows because of reduced tissue viscosity. Therefore in patients with COPD and significant auto-PEEP, high inspiratory flow rates are recommended, provided plateau airway pressures are not unduly increased.

(ii) **FiO_2 (titrate to maintain SpO_2).**

Titrate the FiO_2 to achieve an SpO_2 of 90% and PaO_2 of 60 mmHg. Studies show that following a period of mechanical ventilation with an FiO_2 sufficient to maintain a normal PaO_2, a further increase in FiO_2 does not result in an increased $PaCO_2$ or a depression of respiratory drive in a group of CO_2-retaining COPD patients. A new ventilation-perfusion relationship is established during ventilation to normoxia and it is not altered by further increase in FiO_2.

(iii) **Tidal volume (7-8 mL/kg body weight).**

Tidal volume of 7-8mL/Kg, prevents excessive air trapping and auto-PEEP, keeps plateau pressure within the desired goal (< 30cm. H_2O) and is usually sufficient to prevent $PaCO_2$ from falling below baseline in patients with COPD. High tidal volumes in these patients may overdistend the lungs, increasing the chances of barotrauma, and may also result in greater depression of cardiac output.

(iv) **Respiratory rate (7-8/min).**

Higher respiratory rates will increase the likelihood of development of auto-PEEP. A reduction in expiratory time, which will occur if the respiratory rate is increased without altering the I:E ratio, increases the possibility of development of auto-PEEP. As such, an increase in resistance (e.g. chronic obstructive pulmonary disease or acute asthma) or compliance (e.g. emphysema) causes increase in time constant and makes the development of auto-PEEP more likely.

(v) **Positive end-expiratory pressure (PEEP) (3-5 cm. H_2O).**

The application of external PEEP, at a level less than or equal to 85% of the auto-PEEP, may decrease auto-PEEP, expiratory resistance and the amount of patient effort to trigger the ventilator without increasing peak alveolar pressures. For example, if the auto-PEEP is 10 cmH$_2$O and trigger sensitivity is set at −1 cmH$_2$O, the patient will need to generate enough muscle pressure to lower airway pressure by 11 cmH$_2$O to trigger a breath. Now, if external PEEP is set at 8 cmH$_2$O, the patient will only need to reduce airway pressure by 3 cmH$_2$O to trigger a breath, thereby reducing WOB. To achieve this effect, PEEP is adjusted to improve patient comfort and decrease auto-

PEEP, but applied PEEP is kept less than or equal to 85% of auto-PEEP or at 10 cm H_2O. Carefully monitor the patient to be sure that applied PEEP does not increase the level of measured auto-PEEP, which would indicate the presence of worsening hyperinflation.

(vi) Waveform (constant or decelerating).

See Chapter 32.

GUIDELINES FOR INITIAL MANAGEMENT OF MECHANICAL VENTILATION

14. Monitor the following parameters and take appropriate measures.
    - Haemodynamic stability.
    - Plateau pressure.
    - Auto-PEEP.
    - ABG.
      - pH 7.30-7.45.
        Auto-PEEP < 3 cm H_2O.
        No haemodynamic instability.
        Plateau pressure < 35 cm H_2O.
        Continue with same settings.
      - pH < 7.30 and auto-PEEP < 3cm H_2O.
        Increase minute ventilation –increase tidal volume if plateau pressure <35cm H_2O, otherwise increase rate.
      - pH < 7.30 and auto-PEEP > 3 cmH_2O.
        Decrease inspiratory time.
        Continue aggressive bronchodilator therapy. Clear secretions.
        Improve ventilator-patient synchrony (i.e. add sedation).
        Increase set PEEP to counterbalance auto-PEEP.
      - pH < 7.20.
        Consider buffer therapy.
      - pH > 7.45 and auto-PEEP >3 cmH_2O.
        Decrease minute ventilation –decrease tidal volume if plateau pressure > 30 cmHO_2, otherwise decrease rate.
        Decrease inspiratory time.
        Continue aggressive bronchodilator therapy.
        Clear secretions.
        Improve ventilator-patient synchrony (i.e. add sedation).
        Increase set PEEP to counterbalance auto-PEEP.
      - Haemodynamic instability.
        Take measures to decrease auto-PEEP.
        Decrease minute ventilation.
        Optimize preload/inotropic support.

15. Adopt general measures.
    General measures include:

- Maintaining fluid balance.
- Meeting daily nutritional needs.
- General ICU care.
- Low molecular weight heparin.
- Use of inotropes as and when indicated.

16. Wean the patient.

See Chapter 42.

Patient should be weaned gradually once weaning criteria are met. NIPPV has also been used to decrease the weaning period in patients with acute COPD, and the results have been encouraging. It shortens weaning time, time in the ICU, decreases the incidence of nosocomial pneumonia, and improves 60-days survival rates.

References

1. Agusti AGN, Noguera A, Sauleda J, et al. Systemic effects of chronic obstructive pulmonary disease. Eur Respir J 2003;21:347-360.
2. Barnes PJ. Chronic obstructive pulmonary disease. N Eng J Med 2000;343:269-280.
3. Campbell S. For COPD a combination of ipratropium bromide and albuterol sulfate is more effective than albuterol base. Arch Intern Med 1999;159;156-160.
4. Canadian Thoracic Society Workshop Group. Guidelines for the assessment and manegement of chronic obstructive pulmonary disease. Can Med Assoc J 1992;147:420-426.
5. Celli BR. Standards for the optimal management of COPD: a summary. Chest 1998;113:283S-287S.
6. Connors AFJ, Dawson NV, Thomas C, et al. Outcomes following acute exacerbation of severe chronic obstructive lung disease. J Respir Crit Care Med 1996;154:959-967.
7. Crossley DJ, McGuire GP, Barrow PM, et al. Influence of inspired oxygen concentration on deadspace, respiratory drive, and $PaCO_2$ in intubated patients with chronic obstructive pulmonary disease. Crit Care Med 1997;25:1522-1526.
8. Dhand R, Duarte AG, Jubran A, et al. Dose-response to bronchodilator delivered by metered-dose inhaler in ventilator-supported patients. Am J Respir Crit Care Med 1996;154:388-393.
9. Dhand R, Tobin MJ. Inhaled bronchodilator therapy in mechanically ventilated patients. Am J Respir Crit Care Med 1997;156:3-10.
10. Eller J, Ede A, Schaberg T, et al. Infective exacerbations of chronic bronchitis: relation between bacteriologic etiology and lung function. Chest 1998;113:1542-1548.
11. Fuso L, Incalzi RA, Pistelli R, et al. Predicting mortality of patients hospitalized for acutely exacerbated chronic obstructive pulmonary disease. Am J Respir Crit Care Med 1995;98:272-277.
12. Gomersall CD, Joynt GM, Freebairn RC. Oxygen therapy for hypercapnia patients with chronic obstructive pulmonary disease and acute respiratory failure: A randomized, controlled pilot study. Crit Care Med 2002;30:113-116.
13. Grossman RF. Guidelines for treatment of acute exacerbations of chronic bronchitis Chest 1997;112:310 S-313 S.
14. Grossman RF. The value of antibiotics and the outcomes of antibiotic therapy in exacerbations of COPD. Chest 1998;113:249 S-255 S.
15. Hamnegard CH, Bake B, Moxham J, et al. Does undernutrition contribute to diaphragm weakness in patients with severe COPD? Clinical Nutrition 2002;21(3):239-243.

16. Hess D, Medoff B. Mechanical ventilation of the patient with chronic obstructive pulmonary disease. Respir Care Clin North Am 1998;4:439-473.

17. Imsand C, Feihl F, Perret C, et al. Regulation of inspiratory neuromuscular output during synchronized intermittent mechanical ventilation. Anesthesiology 1994;80:13-22.

18. Jubran A, Van de Graaff WB, Tobin MJ. Variability of patient-ventilator interaction with pressure support ventilation in patients with chronic obstructive pulmonary diasease. Am J Respir Crit Care Med 1995;152:129-136.

19. Keenan SP, Kernerman PD, Cook DJ, et al. Effect of noninvasive positive pressure ventilation on mortality in patients admitted with acute respiratory failure: a meta-analysis. Crit Care Med 1997;25:1685-1692.

20. Kelles MH. Lung hyperinflation caused by inappropriate ventilation resulting in electromechanical dissociation: A case report. Heart Lung 1992;21:74-77.

21. Lam A, Newhouse MT. Management of asthma and chronic airflow limitation. Are methylxanthines obsolete? Chest 1990;98:44-52.

22. Lapinsky SE, Leung RS. Auto-PEEP and electromechanical dissociation. (letter). N Eng J Med 1996;335:674.

23. MacIntyre NR, Cheng KC, McConnell R. Applied PEEP during pressure support reduces the inspiratory threshold load of intrinsic PEEP. Chest 1997;111:188-193.

24. Madison JM, Irwin RS. Chronic obstructive pulmonary disease. Lancet 1998;352:467-473.

25. Marini JJ. Should PEEP be used in airflow obstruction? (editorial; comment). Am Rev Respir Dis 1989;140:1-3.

26. Marini JJ, Capps JS, Culver BH. The inspiratory work of breathing during assisted mechanical ventilation. Chest 1985;87:612-618.

27. Marini JJ, Smith TC, Lamb VJ. External work output and force generation during synchronized intermittent mechanical ventilation. Effect of machine assistance on breathing effort. Am Rev Respir Dis 1988;138:1169-1179.

28. Moren JL, Green JV, Homan SD, et al. Acute exacerbations of chronic obstructive pulmonary disease and mechanical ventilation: A re-evaluation. Crit Care Med 1998;26:71-78.

29. Murate GH et al. Intravenous and oral corticosteroids for the prevention of relapse after treatment of decompensated COPD. Effects on patients with a history of multiple relapses. Chest 1990;98:845-849.

30. Murphy TF, Sethi S, Niederman MS. The role of bacteria in exacerbations of COPD. A Constructive view. Chest 2000;118:204-209.

31. Pauwels RA. National and international guidelines for COPD: the need for evidence. Chest 2000;117:20 S-22 S.

32. Pearson MG, Alderslade R, Allen SC, et al. BTS guidelines for the management of chronic obstructive pulmonary disease. Thorax 1997;52 (suppl 5): S1-S28.

33. Pauwels RA, Baist AS, Calverley PMA, et al. Global strategy for the diagnosis, management, and prevention of chronic obstructive pulmonary disease. Am J Respir Crit Care Med 2001;163:1256-1276.

34. Rosen RL, Bone RC. Treatment of acute exacerbations in chronic obstructive pulmonary disease. Med Clin North Am 1990;74:691-700.

35. Rossi A, Polese G, Brandi G, et al. Intrinsic positive end-expiratory pressure (PEEPi). Intensive Care Med 1995;21:522-536.

36. Rossi A, Polese G, De Sandre G. Respiratory failure in chronic airflow obstruction: recent advances and therapeutic implications in the critically ill patient. Eur J Med 1992;1:349-357.

37. Saint S, Bent S, Vittinghoff, et al. Antibiotics in chronic obstructive pulmonary disease exacerbations: a meta-analysis. JAMA 1995;273:957-960.

38. Senior RM, Anthonisen NR. Chronic obstructive pulmonary disease (COPD). Am J Respir Crit Care Med 1998;157: S139-S147.

39. Sethi JM, Siegel MD. Mechanical ventilation in chronic obstructive lung disease. Clinics in Chest Medicine. 2000;21(4):799-818.
40. Smith TC, Marini JJ. Impact of PEEP on lung mechanics and work of breathing in severe airflow obstruction. J Appl Physiol 1988;65:1488-1499.
41. Standards for the diagnosis and care of patients with chronic obstructive pulmonary disease. Am J Respir Crit Care Med 1995;152:S77-S120.
42. Tantucci C, Corbeil C, Chasse M, et al. Flow resistance in patients with chronic obstructive pulmonary disease in acute respiratory failure. Effects of flow and volume. Am Rev Respir Dis 1991;144:384-389.

62

Acute Severe Asthma in Adults

Introduction

- Asthma is a chronic inflammatory disorder of the airways in which many cells and cellular elements play a role, in particular, mast cells, eosinophils, T lymphocytes, macrophages, neutrophils, and epithelial cells. In susceptible individuals, this inflammation causes recurrent episodes of wheezing, breathlessness, chest tightness, and coughing, particularly at night or in the early morning. These episodes are usually associated with widespread but variable airflow obstruction that is often reversible either spontaneously or with treatment. The inflammation also causes an associated increase in the existing bronchial hyperresponsiveness to a variety of stimuli.
- Acute severe asthma refers to the presence of one or more of the following: peak expiratory flow (PEF) of 50% or less of the predicted or best, breathlessness that prevents completion of a sentence in one breath, tachypnoea ($\geq$ 25 breaths/min) and tachycardia ($\geq$110 breaths/min).
- Status Asthmaticus refers to severe bronchospasm that does not respond to aggressive therapy within 30-60 minutes.
- Life-threatening asthma is indicated by PEF <33% of the predicted or best, a silent chest, cyanosis, feeble respiratory effort, bradycardia, hypotension, exhaustion, confusion, or coma. Very severe attacks may have oxygen saturation less than 92%.
- Near-fatal asthma (NFA) or severe life-threatening asthma (SLTA) is defined as an attack of asthma associated with a raised $PaCO_2$ (>50 mmHg), respiratory arrest, or a low pH.
- Airway narrowing leads to increased airway resistance, which is reflected in falling PEF and forced expiratory volume in 1 second (FEV_1). The lungs become hyperinflated with marked increase in residual volume (RV) and total lung capacity (TLC). As airway narrowing becomes progressively severe, arterial $PaCO_2$ initially falls as a result of hyperventilation. If airway narrowing increases further, the $PaCO_2$ returns to normal and may then rise steeply, as alveolar ventilation falls. $PaCO_2$ returns from low levels to the normal range when FEV_1 falls to about 25% of predicted normal (or PEF approximately 30% of that predicted). Alveolar hypoventilation can result from progressive airway narrowing, respiratory muscle exhausion, or both. As the asthma becomes more severe, PaO_2 falls progressively due to falling ventilation-perfusion ratio and ultimately, falling ventilation as well. Patients who die from asthma die from hypoxaemia, which is the most serious and dangerous physiological consequence of severe asthma.

- Expiratory airway obstruction in severe asthma leads to hyperinflation, which in turn leads to decrease in respiratory system compliance. It leads to increased inspiratory work of breathing. Hyperinflation also increases dead space fraction (i.e. the proportion of each tidal volume that is wasted, increases with increasing hyperinflation).

- A critically ill asthmatic appears agitated, assumes an upright posture and appears in severe respiratory distress. Tachypnoea, diaphoresis, and the use of accessory muscles of respiration are clearly evident. Breathlessness prevents completion of a sentence in one breath. Pulsus paradoxus is present. Wheezing may be absent indicating severe expiratory obstruction and minimal air movement. Peak expiratory flow test may be difficult for the patient to perform, and when possible, indicates severity of expiratory obstruction. Alteration in consciousness and bradypnoea indicate hypercarbia and impending respiratory arrest.

- Less severe degree of asthma may have less severe signs and symptoms. Generally severity of airflow obstruction cannot be accurately judged when relying on patient's symptoms, signs and laboratory tests. Restlessness and agitation are too non-specific to always indicate hypoxia or hypercapnia. A heart rate more than 120 beats/min is associated with severe obstruction; however, a lesser or normal heart rate does not rule out severe asthma. Respiratory rate also correlates poorly and indicates severe obstruction only if it is greater than 40 breaths/minute. Wheezing correlates poorly with the degree of obstruction, and may be absent when maximal effort produces minimal flow. Use of accessory muscles of respiration, if present, may indicate severe asthma, but if absent, 50% of cases may still have equally severe asthma.

- Measurement of airflow obstruction (FEV_1 or PEF) is very important for the assessment of disease and its response to therapy.

- Obstruction of peripheral airways by inflammation, mucus and bronchoconstriction causes ventilation-perfusion mismatch and hypoxaemia. True shunt in acute asthma averages only 1.5% of the pulmonary blood flow, so correction of hypoxaemia is not a problem. Refractory hypoxaemia is rare and should lead to a search for additional pathology such as pneumothorax, aspiration, lobar atelectasis, and barotrauma.

- Corticosteroids treat airway wall inflammation, potentiate the effects of beta-agonists on smooth muscle relaxation, decrease beta-agonists tachyphylaxis, and decrease mucus production. They are stressed as the first-line of treatment in the management of asthma.

- Ipratropium bromide augments the bronchodilatory effects of beta-agonists in acute asthma.

- Short acting β_2-agonists relax airway smooth muscle, primarily through β_2- adrenergic receptor stimulation, and are the first-line drugs used to treat an acute asthma exacerbation.

- Theophylline, as monotherapy, is inferior to beta-agonists in acute asthma and when added to beta-agonists in the first few hours of treatment, does not confer any additional benefit and may, infact, increase the incidence of tremors, nausea, anxiety, palpitation, and tachycardia. The available data do not allow for strong conclusion regarding the use of theophylline in acute asthma and till definite conclusions could be drawn, it is worth adding theophylline in a patient with poor or incomplete response to treatment with beta-agonists and corticosteroids.

- Subcutaneous epinephrine carries no advantage over inhaled beta-agonists unless patients are unable to cooperate, i.e. those with impaired sensorium or those in cardiopulmonary arrest.
- Magnesium sulfate may be tried in patients who have failed to respond to other drugs. The dose is 30-70 mg/kg (maximum 2-3 g) administered over 20-30 minutes. If the patient has hypomagnesaemia, normalization of serum levels should be achieved.
- Larger and more frequent doses of nebulized drugs are needed in acute asthma because the dose-response curve and duration of activity of these drugs are affected adversely by the degree of bronchoconstriction, airway wall inflammation and edema. The lack of cooperation and breathing pattern of the patient further add on to reduce the delivery of drugs administered by inhalation.
- There is enough evidence to suggest that in non-intubated patients, metered-dose inhalers (MDIs), combined with a spacing device, are just as effective as nebulizers, and they are quicker and cheaper to use.
- In intubated patients, it is difficult to recommend an appropriate route or drug dosages. Nebulized drug is efficacious in the majority of patients, although MDIs are also likely to be effective if used with an appropriate spacing device. Whichever route is used, drug dosages should be titrated either to a beneficial physiological response (as judged by a fall in the airway peak-to-plateau gradient under constant inspiratory flow conditions), or to the development of toxic side effects such as worsening tachyarrhythmias. If there is a significant fall ($\geq$15%) in peak-to-plateau airway pressure gradient after nebulization of 5mg of salbutamol, the dose may be repeated after 1 hour and if the fall is not significant, the same dose may be repeated until a significant decrease in the peak-to-plateau gradient is observed, or toxic side effects occur. However, one should keep in mind the other factors, which can cause high peak pressure (e.g. a kinked or plugged endotracheal tube).
- Plateau pressure has a greater correlation with hyperinflation and the risk for barotrauma since it reflects what really happens at the alveolar level at the end of inspiration. Plateau pressure reflects the volume of lungs since all the airways communicate during inspiration, while auto-PEEP measurement may underestimate the amount of air trapped in the lung owing to complete closure of some airways.
- Using a strategy of ventilating with low tidal volumes and at slower frequencies (in order to limit airway pressures, auto-PEEP, and hyperinflation) may cause hypercapnia. The rise in $PaCO_2$ for each decrement in minute ventilation, however, may be less than expected, since reduction in hyperinflation may reduce dead space. Even when hypercapnia results, it is generally well tolerated as long as $PaCO_2$ does not exceed 90 mmHg and acute increases in $PaCO_2$ are avoided.

- While using small volume nebulizer (SVN), a full volume of 4mL and a flow of 8L/min should be used to power the nebulizer. Many factors affect pulmonary deposition from an SVN during mechanical ventilation: (i) Deposition is less with smaller sized ETT, (ii) more medication is delivered to the ETT if the nebulizer is placed approximately 18 inches from the Y –piece and least amount of aerosol is delivered to the ETT with the nebulizer placed at the Y-piece –the technique that is probably most commonly used in clinical practice, (iii) the inclusion of a humidifier in the ventilator circuit decreases aerosol delivery by 40-50%, and (iv) increasing the inspiratory time and decreasing the respiratory rate augments the aerosol delivery.

- MDI may be placed in a ventilator circuit with the help of a variety of adaptors. Studies have shown that the greatest amount of aerosol is delivered through the ETT with a reservoir device, the least amount with an elbow device, and an intermediate amount with an in-line device. The dose (number of puffs) may need to be adjusted based on the MDI adaptor that is used.

- Use of SVN during mechanical ventilation may be associated with several disadvantages: (i) Contaminated nebulizers can be a source of bacterial aerosols; therefore, it is recommended to clean or disinfect them after each treatment, (ii) the continuous flow from an SVN increases the tidal volume (and associated pressures) delivered when volume ventilators are used, (iii) the continuous flow introduces a bias flow, which makes it more difficult for the patient to generate the trigger pressure required during assited modes of ventilation (e.g. pressure support, assist-control). Use of MDI during mechanical ventilation avoids these problems, and is less time consuming. A MDI is an effective substitute for an SVN in intubated, mechanically ventilated adult patients.

- Antibiotics may not be prescribed routinely, as most of the respiratory tract infections triggering asthma are viral. Antibiotics may be indicated in patients with fever and sputum containing polymorphonuclear leukocytes, with clinical findings of pneumonia, with signs and symptoms of acute sinusitis, and in those patients who have findings suggestive of mycoplasmal or chlamydial infection.

- Strategies to mobilize mucus such as chest physiotherapy or treatment with mucolytics or expectorants, have not proved efficacious in controlled trials.

GUIDELINES FOR THE MANAGEMENT OF AN ADULT WITH ACUTE SEVERE ASTHMA

1. **Assess the severity of the disease.**
   History.
   Physical examination.
   PEF measurement.
   Recognize whether patient has uncontrolled asthma (speech normal, pulse <110 beats/min, respiratory rate <25 breaths/min, PEF >50% of predicted or best), acute severe asthma or has life threatening features (as described before).

2.   Start treatment immediately.
     -Oxygen.
     -Beta-agonists.
     -Steroids.
     -Ask for chest radiograph to exclude pneumothorax.
     - Administer oxygen through air-entrainment mask ($FiO_2 \geq 0.4$). Titrate using pulse oximeter. CO_2 retention is not usually aggravated by oxygen therapy in asthma.
     - Nebulize salbutamol 5 mg (1ml of 5% solution in 2.5 mL normal saline) via oxygen driven nebulizer or 4-6 puffs by MDI with spacer.
     - Give prednisolone tablets 30-60 mg/24 hr, or methyl prednisolone 60-125 mg IV every 6 hourly (or hydrocortisone IV 200 mg 6 hrly), or both if very ill.
     - Avoid sedation of any kind.
     - If patient has any one or more of life-threatening features, add ipratropium 0.5 mg to the nebulizer, or 4-10 puffs by MDI with spacer.
     - Add aminophylline 250 mg over 20 minutes. Do not give bolus aminophylline to patients already taking oral theophyllines, and
     - Measure arterial blood gases.

3.   Reassess the patient after 20-30 minutes.
     -Clinical assessment.
     -Repeat PEF measurement.
     -Oxygen saturation.

     If patient is improving, continue oxygen, prednisolone 30-60 mg daily or hydrocortisone 200 mg IV 6 hourly, nebulized beta-agonist 4 hourly. Stable patient with PEF >75% of predicted may be discharged after a few hours of observation. If patient is not improving, continue oxygen and steroids. Give salbutamol nebulisation every 15-30 minutes for 3 doses, and then every 1-4 hourly, as needed (alternatively use MDI with spacer, 4-6 puffs every 15-30 minutes for 3 doses and then every 1-4 hourly, as needed). Add (if not already started) ipratropium and nebulize 0.5 mg every 30 minutes for 3 doses and then 4-6 hourly, as needed. (Alternatively, use MDI with spacer 4-10 puffs every 20-30 minutes for 3 doses and then 4-6 hourly as needed). Inhalational therapy may be given continuously to severely-obstructed patients until an adequate clinical response is achieved or adverse side effects limit further administration (e.g. excessive tachycardia, arrhythmias, or tremors). Start aminophylline infusion at the rate of 0.4 mg/kg/hr. In an unresponsive patient, use 0.3 mL of 1:1000 subcutaneous adrenaline every 20 minutes for upto 3 doses. Use with caution in patients older than 40 years of age and in patients with coronary artery disease.

4.   Ask for baseline investigations, determine reasons for exacerbations, add antibiotics if indicated.

5.   Continue to monitor clinically and repeat ABG, if indicated.

     Repeat blood gas measurements within 2 hours of starting treatment if (i) initial PaO_2 < 60mmHg, and subsequent SpO_2 < 92%, (ii) $PaCO_2$ normal or raised, or iii) patient deteriorates.

6. **Continue therapy and consider transfer to ICU, if indicated.**
    Consider transfer to ICU if at any stage there is (i) Deteriorating PEF, (ii) worsening or persisting hypoxia or hypercapnia, (iii) exhaustion, (iv) feeble respiration, (v) confusion or drowsiness, and (vi) coma or respiratory arrest.

7. **Consider intubation.**
    A patient having any of the above features should be considered for intubation.

8. **Role of NIPPV.**
    A number of smaller, uncontrolled studies have documented the use of non-invasive positive pressure ventilation as a viable alternative to invasive mechanical ventilation in patients with acute severe asthma. The key factor in the use of non-invasive ventilation is the early initiation of therapy in conjunction with bronchodilators and corticosteroids. Controlled studies using larger number of patients are required before strong recommendations can be made regarding the use of non-invasive ventilation in acute severe asthma.

9. **Invasive mechanical ventilation.**
    (a) **Set goals of mechanical ventilation.**
        - Avoid auto-PEEP and hyperinflation, limit airway pressures.
        - Avoid patient-ventilator dyssynchrony.
        - Ensure optimal gas exchange; accept a higher $PaCO_2$ and low pH, if the situation so demands.
    (b) **Intubate the patient. Prefer orotracheal intubation with a larger sized tube (> 8mm ID).**
        Ask for a chest radiograph to confirm appropriate depth of ETT placement. See Chapter 24.
        Orotracheal intubation allows the passage of a widebore endotracheal tube (ETT), which decreases airway resistance and helps in suctioning tenacious mucus plugs. Orotracheal intubation also avoids nasal obstruction and nosocomial sinusitis.
        A smooth, rapid-sequence induction technique using xylocaine (1.5 mg/kg), induction agents (titrated doses of midazolam and propofol or ketamine) and neuromuscular blocking agent (suxamethonium or rocuronium), is a preferred technique. One must determine whether ETT is in proper position. Breath sounds may not be audible as chest may be silent. Expiratory return of condensate within ETT, SpO_2 of 98-100%, and passing the ETT under vision could be useful clues, but $EtCO_2$ is a confirmatory test. Because of bronchoconstriction, significant resistance may be encountered while ventilating manually. If resistance is not felt, check cuff pressure. If the ETT is properly placed and cuff pressure is adequate, absence of significant resistance to bag ventilation suggests that the original diagnosis of asthma is incorrect and that intubation has bypassed an upper airway obstruction e.g. tumour, foreign body etc.

(c) Immediate post-intubation period.
Hypotension. Desaturation.

It is common to find a patient with silent chest, distended neck veins, decreased blood pressure, difficulty in delivering inspiratory breaths and desaturation in the immediate post-intubation period. The commonest cause of this is a massive auto-PEEP due to enthusiastic manual ventilation, in order to bring back PaO_2 and $PaCO_2$ to normal. The first response to this situation, before fluid challenge, vasopressors, or chest tube is inserted, should be to simply disconnect the ventilator, permitting deflation of the lung, and rapid improvement in blood pressure and saturation. Also these patients are usually hypovolaemic due to decreased oral intake, increased work of breathing, and the use of sedatives and muscle relaxants. Other causes of desaturation in this situation are right mainstem intubation and pneumothorax. Right mainsterm intubation can be excluded by fixing the ETT at the 21 cm mark (in males) on the incisors. Pneumothorax will need chest tube placement, after confirmation.

(d) Connecting a ventilator.
Deep sedation. Paralysis.

When connecting to a ventilator, patient should be deeply sedated, as this is the time when the effect of a short acting muscle relaxant (e.g. suxamethonium) used for intubation, would be wearing off. Otherwise, there is a risk of accidental extubation or the rapid build up of potentially lethal auto-PEEP, as the patient triggers the ventilator at higher frequencies. If sedation is not sufficient to allow a passive patient-ventilator interaction, a brief period of muscle paralysis (i.e. use of vecuronium/atracurium) is indicated. Paralysis augments the beneficial effects of sedation to reduce oxygen consumption, CO_2 production, and lactic acid generation, besides decreasing the risk of barotrauma. After 24-36 hours, paralysis may be discontinued. Generally deep sedation suffices at this time.

See Chapters 7 and 8.

(e) Immediately after connecting the ventilator, monitor the alarms.

High peak pressure alarm might get activated. If high auto-PEEP, kinking or blockage of ETT, or other factors causing mechanical obstruction are not the causes, then high peak airway pressure is probably because of increased airway resistance,and is predictable and acceptable at this stage. The only thing to be done is to reset the peak pressure limit alarm to a higher limit (i.e. may be upto 80-100cmH_2O).

(f) Mode of ventilation.
Pressure ventilation.
Volume ventilation.
Assist-control. SIMV.

- Either pressure or volume modes can be used. With pressure-controlled ventilation, auto-PEEP results in decreased tidal volume and respiratory acidosis. In patients with severe airflow obstruction, it may be difficult to deliver an adequate tidal volume with pressure-controlled ventilation. With volume-controlled ventilation, auto-PEEP results in increased plateau pressure and over-distension. One should use the strategy one is comfortable with, keeping goals in mind.

- To start with, full ventilatory support is usually provided (that is, no spontaneous breathing by the patient). Ventilatory mode is irrelevant in the sedated and paralyzed patient as both, assist-control and SIMV, provide controlled ventilation in this setting. Once patient regains respiratory effort, use SIMV with pressure support. Assist control ventilation may be associated with increased risk of lung hyperinflation. Increasing inspiratory flow rate in this mode increases respiratory rate and thereby may actually decrease exhalation time.

(g) Initial ventilatory settings.

FiO_2 1.0.

TV 6-8 mL/kg.

Peak inspiratory flow rate 80-100L/min.

PEEP 0.

Respiratory rate 8-10/min.

Square waveform.

- The initial ventilatory settings aim at reducing hyperinflation by limiting minute ventilation, using low tidal volumes and respiratory rates and maximizing expiratory time.

  Tidal volume is initially set in the range of 5-8mL/kg and then adjusted to minimize overdistension. Be guided by plateau pressure (avoid > 30cmH_2O). Adopt a strategy of permissive hypercapnia (i.e. allow $PaCO_2$ to rise and tolerate an acidotic pH to prevent overdistension).

- External PEEP has no role in counterbalancing auto-PEEP in a patient who is not attempting to trigger the ventilator. PEEP, as a means to prevent atelectasis or collapse, is not necessary at this stage. In a patient who is triggering the ventilator (after neuromuscular blocking agents have been discontinued), however, external PEEP has been used to counterbalance auto-PEEP. Generally, no more than 10 cmH_2O PEEP is used to counterbalance auto PEEP. But it is difficult to assess the degree of auto-PEEP in a spontaneously breathing patient, and applying external PEEP above the level of auto-PEEP (if it is wrongly assessed) may add to lung hyperinflation. Under these circumstances, using low levels of external PEEP such as 5 cmH_2O (in hyperinflated, actively breathing patient) will decrease inspiratory work of breathing in triggering the ventilator, and are unlikely to increase lung volume. While setting the I: E ratio, the goal is to allow adequate expiratory time to avoid air trapping and minimize auto-PEEP. Use a respiratory rate of 8-10/min with an inspiratory time of around 1 second, high peak inspiratory flow rate and a square waveform, to prolong expiratory time.

- Once the patient is settled, FiO_2 should be titrated to maintain saturation above 90%.

10. Guidelines for initial management of mechanical ventilation.
    Monitor the following parameters:

ABG.
Auto-PEEP.
Haemodynamic stability.
Plateau airway pressure.
Peak airway pressure.

A decrease in gradient $P_{peak} - P_{plat}$ at a constant airflow reflects an improvement in airway resistance and can be used to monitor the degree of airflow limitation.

- pH > 7.20, P_{plat} < 30 cm H_2O, haemodynamic stability — continue with same settings.
- pH < 7.20, P_{plat} < 30 cmH_2O — increase minute ventilation until P_{plat} nears 30cmH_2O.
  If pH improves — continue with the same settings.
  If pH still < 7.20, Pplat near 30 cm H_2O — consider slow bicarbonate infusion.
- P_{plat} > 30 cm H_2O – decrease minute ventilation until P_{plat} nears 30 cm H_2O, improve patient-ventilator synchrony (i.e. add sedation), and continue aggressive bronchodilator therapy.
- Haemodynamic instability (e.g. hypotension) – decrease minute ventilation, optimize preload/inotropic support, take measures to decrease auto-PEEP.

11. Consider weaning.

Once bronchospasm improves, airway resistance begins to fall and $PaCO_2$ normalizes, withdraw sedative agents and neuromuscular blocking agents, start decreasing the respiratory rate on SIMV and gradually reduce pressure support to 5-8 cm H_2O. When patient tolerates a trial of spontaneous breathing, consider an early extubation.

References

1. ACCP Mechanical Ventilation Consensus Group: mechanical ventilation. Chest 1993; 104:1833-1859.
2. Corbridge TC, Hall JB. The assessment and management of adults with status asthmaticus. Am J Respir Crit Care Med 1995; 151:1296-1316.
3. Corne S, Gillespie D, Roberts D, et al. Effect of inspiratory flow rate on respiratory rate in intubated patients. Am J Resp Crit Care Med 1996; 153:A375.
4. Dhand R, Tobin MJ. Inhaled bronchodilator therapy in mechanically ventilated patients. Am J Respir Crit Care Med 1997; 156:3-10.
5. Darioli R, Perret C. Mechanical controlled hypoventilation in status asthmaticus. Am Rev Respir Dis 1984; 129:385-387.
6. Expert Panel Report 2: Guidelines for the diagnosis and management of Asthma. National Asthma Education Program, National Heart, Lung, and Blood Institute, National Institutes of Health, Bethesda, Maryland: Publication No 97-4051, April 1957.
7. Feihl F, Perret C. Permissive hypercapnia: How permissive should we be? Am J Respir Crit Care Med 1994; 150:1722-1737.
8. Heickling KC, Henderson SJ, Jackson R. Low mortality associated with low volume pressure limited ventilation and permissive hypercapnia in severe adult respiratory distress syndrome. Intensive Care Med 1990; 16:372-377.

9. Hess Dr. Aerosol therapy. Respir Care Clin N Am 1995; 1:239

10. Jain S, Nicola A, et al. Ventilation of patients with asthma and obstructive lung disease Crit Care Clinics 1998; 14(4): 685-705.

11. Leathermann J. Life-threatening asthma. Clin Chest Med 1994; 15:453-479.

12. Manthous CA, Hall JB. Update on using therapeutic aerosols in mechanically ventilated patients. J Crit Illness 1996; 11:457.

13. Marini JJ, Caps JS, Culver BH. The inspiratory work of breathing during assisted mechanical ventilation. Chest 1989; 87:612-618.

14. Marini JJ. Should PEEP be used in airflow obstruction? Am Rev Respir Dis 1989; 140:1-3.

15. Meduir GU, et al. Noninvasive positive pressure ventilation in status asthmaticus Chest 1996; 110:767-774.

16. Metha S and Hill NS. Non-invasive ventilation. Am J Respir Crit Care Med. 2001; 163:540-577.

17. Ranieri VM, Grasso S, Fiore T, et al. Auto-positive end-expiratory pressure and dynamic hyperinflation. Clin Chest Med 1996; 17:379-394.

18. Rodrignez-Roison R, Ballestar E, Roca J, et al. Mechanisms of hypoxemia in patients with status asthmaticus requiring mechanical ventilation. Am Rev Respir Dis 1989; 139:732-739.

19. The British Guidelines on asthma management-position statement. Thorax 1997; 52(Suppl.1): S1-S21.

20. Tuxen DV, Williams TJ, Sheinkestel CD, et al. Use of a measurement of pulmonary hyperinflation to control the level of mechanical ventilation in patients with acute severe asthma. Am Rev Resp Dis 1992; 146:1136-1142.

21. Tuxen DV. Determental effects of PEEP during controlled mechanical ventilation of patients with severe airflow obstruction. Am Rev Respir Dis 1989; 140:5-9.

63

Diabetic Ketoacidosis

Introduction

- Diabetic ketoacidosis (DKA) is a state of severe, uncontrolled diabetes due to insulin deficiency and an excess of counterregulatory hormones (epinephrine, glucagon, cortisol, and somatostatin) and is characterized by high blood glucose, ketone body formation and acidosis.
- The signs and symptoms of DKA result from hyperglycaemia (dehydration, hyperosmolality, osmotic diuresis, electrolyte depletion) or ketoacidosis (acidosis, osmotic diuresis).
- Diagnostic features of DKA are glucose: (> 300mg/dL), pH (< 7.3), bicarbonate (< 18 mEq/L), serum osmolality $\leq$ 320 mOsm /kg, dehydration, and presence of ketone bodies in blood (positive at 1:2 dilution) and in the urine.
- Mild DKA is characterized by arterial pH between 7.25-7.30, serum bicarbonate 15-18 mEq/L, anion gap more than 10 and a mentally alert patient. A patient with moderate DKA has an arterial pH between 7.00-7.24, serum bicarbonate 10-15 mEq/L, anion gap more than 12, and he may be alert or drowsy. A stuporose or comatosed patient with an arterial pH less than 7.00, serum bicarbonate less than 10 mEq/L and an anion gap of more than 12, is typical of severe DKA.
- Typical total body deficits in DKA include water (100 mL/kg), sodium (7-10mEq/kg), chloride (3-5 mEq/kg), potassium (3-5 mEq/kg), phosphate (5-7mmol/kg), calcium (1-2 mEq/kg), and magnesium (1-2 mEq/kg).
- There is a shift of potassium, magnesium, and phosphate from the intracellular to extracellular space due to acidosis and hyperosmolarity. The initial serum levels of potassium, magnesium and phosphate in DKA may be normal, even with profound total deficits, because of dehydration with profound haemoconcentration.
- Glucose in the renal tubules draws water, sodium, potassium, magnesium, calcium, phosphate and other ions from the circulation into the urine. This osmotic diuresis, with poor intake and vomiting, produces the profound dehydration and electrolyte imbalance associated with DKA.
- The common precipitating causes of DKA are infection, treatment errors, and newly presenting type 1 diabetes. In about 25-40% of cases, no obvious cause is found.
- The goals of treatment in the management of DKA are: (a) To improve circulatory volume and tissue perfusion, (b) to correct electrolyte abnormalities, (c) to decrease blood glucose, and (d) to clear the serum and urine of ketoacids at a steady state. Remember, the primary goal is not to restore blood glucose but

to reverse the ketoacidotic state. Anion gap must be calculated at regular intervals to judge the success of therapy (success means narrowing and eventually normalization of anion gap).

- The endpoint of therapy in DKA is a blood glucose level of 150-250 mg/dL and correction of acidosis. Despite aggressive management, complications are common and include shock, hypoglycaemia, hypokalaemia, hypophosphataemia, hypomagnesaemia, cerebral edema, pulmonary edema, cardiac arrhythmias, myocardial infarction and arterial thrombosis.

- Emergency surgery for patients with DKA should be delayed until initiation of treatment with fluids, electrolytes and insulin, and not till correction of ketoacidosis. Infact, correction of surgical illness is necessary to manage DKA.

- The hyperosmolarity produced by hyperglycaemia and dehydration is the most important determinant of the patient's mental status. Calculated effective osmolality of more than 340 mOsm/kg is likely to be associated with altered level of consciousness. Infact, the occurence of stupor or coma in diabetic patients in the absence of a definite elevation of effective osmolality ($\geq$ 320mOsm/kg), should be investigated for other causes of altered mental status. Effective osmolality may be calculated by the following formula: 2[measured Na {mEq/L}] + glucose {mg/dL}/18.

- Studies have shown that patients at risk for cerebral edema are those who receive fluid resuscitation at a rate greater than $4L/m^2$ per day, or those who usually present with low sodium values and during treatment have a decrease in serum sodium concentration or fail to show a rise in serum sodium level as blood glucose falls. In the management of cerebral oedema, mannitol has been shown to be helpful, while hyperventilation and dexamethasone have not been proved to be effectiv.

- The anion gap is calculated by subtracting the sum of chloride and bicarbonate anions from the sodium concentration: [Na-(Cl+HCO_3)]. The normal anion gap is 12±2 mEq/L and represents the normal quantity of unmeasurable anions. Because bicarbonate anions are replaced by acetoacetate and β-hydroxybutyrate in DKA, and because these ketone bodies are not measured as anions in electrolyte penals, the sum of bicarbonate and chloride is reduced, increasing the anion gap.

- Delta anion gap refers to "calculated anion gap-16". Delta HCO_3 is equal to "25-measured arterial HCO_3". One can use the delta anion gap/delta HCO_3 ratio, which represents the fraction of the plasma bicarbonate deficit that is accounted for by the retention of anions, to define the type of acid-base disorder in DKA. A ratio of equal to or higher than 0.8 represents increased anion gap acidosis and DKA, a ratio of 0.4-0.8 represents a mixed acidosis, and a ratio of less than 0.4 indicates hyperchloraemic acidosis.

GUIDELINES FOR THE MANAGEMENT OF DIABETIC KETOACIDOSIS

1. Take the history and examine the patient.
   - The relevant points include, a recent history of increased thirst, polyuria,

polyphagia, visual blurring, weakness, weight loss, nausea, vomiting, and abdominal pain, the latter especially common in children.

- The ketonaemia may be responsible for the abdominal pain and nausea but hypokalemia can also worsen gastroparesis and cause an ileus. Remember, effective treatment of DKA should decrease the intensity of or cure the abdominal pain within 6-12 hours. If it does not respond or worsens further, a surgical condition is more likely.
- Physical examination findings in a patient with DKA include drowsiness (±), tachypnoea with Kussmaul's respiration, tachycardia, small volume pulse, cool peripheries, postural or supine hypotension, peripheral cyanosis, and the odour of acetone in the breath.

2. **Confirm the diagnosis by laboratory tests.**
    - Relevant initial laboratory investigations include full blood count, blood sugar, urinary ketones, serum electrolytes, arterial blood gases, blood urea, serum creatinine, osmolality (measured or calculated), anion gap, ECG, X-ray chest and cultures (blood, urine, sputum).
    - Elevated haematocrit may be suggestive of dehydration.
    - WBC count is often raised to 15-20,000/mm^3 with a neutrophil leucocytosis. It does not signify infection in the absence of obvious clinical signs.
    - Blood urea is usually raised as a feature of prerenal impairement secondary to dehydration.
    - ECG is important (a) to exclude underlying silent myocardial infarction, especially in those over 40 years of age or with long duration of diabetes and (b) to diagnose potassium disturbances.
    - The serum sodium value is often misleading in DKA. Sodium is often low in the presence of significant dehydration because it is strongly affected by hyperglycaemia, hypertriglyceridaemia, salt-poor fluid intake, and increased gastrointenstinal, renal, and insensible losses. Hyperglycaemia causes shift of water from cells into the vessels, resulting in dilutional hyponataremia. Lipids also dilute the blood, thereby further lowering the value for sodium.
    - In the absence of marked lipaemia, the true value of sodium may be approximated by adding 1.3–1.6 mEq/L to the sodium value of the laboratory report, for every 100 ml/dL glucose over the normal value. For example, if serum sodium is reported as 130 mEq/L with a blood sugar of 1200 mg/dL, the true serum sodium value is 148 mEq/L, indicating a free water deficit and intracellular dehydration.
    - Serum potassium may be corrected, for the influence of acidosis, by subtracting 0.6 mEq/L from the laboratory potassium level for every 0.1 decrease in pH on ABG analysis. For Example, if serum potassium level is 5 mEq/L and pH is 6.9, the corrected potassium value would be only 2.6 mEq/L, representing severe hypokalaemia. Further, with ongoing insulin therapy, the patient will need considerable potassium replacement.

3. Replace fluids:
    First fluid - N-saline 500 mL over 10 minutes.
    Second fluid - N-saline 1000 mL plus KCl 20-40 mEq/L over 1-2 hours.

Third fluid - same as for second fluid.
Fourth fluid - same amount and composition over 2-4 hours.
Fifth fluid - same as for fourth fluid.
Sixth fluid - same as for fifth fluid.

- Normal saline or half normal saline is the recommended fluid. Administration of Ringer lactate is controversial because lactate is converted to glucose.
- The composition of fluid (NS or half NS) should be based on serum sodium and serum osmolality measurements (if possible). If serum sodium exceeds 150mEq/L, and vital signs are stable, use half-normal saline.
- Fluid infusion beyond 4 hours should be guided by intake, urinary output, CVP, and clinical assessment of volume status (postural blood pressure changes, tachycardia, poor skin turgor, lack of sweating, and dry mucous membrane), to replace 50% of estimated deficit by 8 hours.
- Corrected sodium concentration higher than 140 mEq/L, or calculated effective plasma osmolality more than 340 mOsm/kg, are associated with the larger fluid deficit.
- While replacing fluids, the induced change in serum osmolality should not exceed 3 mOsm/kg H_2O/hr. This may be of importance, especially in patients with cardiac compromise.
- When the blood glucose becomes less than 250-300 mg/dL, a dextrose solution (5% or 10%) should be started to avoid hypoglycaemia during insulin therapy.
- In patients who are anuric (acute tubular necrosis or end-stage renal disease), fluids may be restricted. Insulin administration and electrolyte management form the basis of therapy. Patients having oliguria, secondary to severe dehydration and hypotension, are likely to respond to fluid administration and urine output can be taken as an index of rehydration.
- If a patient has polyuria at the onset, a decrease in urine volume indicates a decrease in plasma glucose concentration and a decrease in the severity of glucosuria.
- In patients with severe hypotension (on admission), an infusion of a plasma expander (e.g. 500 mL haemaccel) may be necessary before starting saline infusion.

4. Start insulin therapy.
   (a) 0.1 U/kg regular insulin as IV bolus, followed by 0.1 U/kg/hr as a continuous infusion (half life of insulin is 3-10min).
   - Decrease IV insulin infusion to 0.05 U/kg/hr, when blood glucose is 250-300mg/dL and the HCO_3^- is more than or equal to 18 mEq/L.
   (b) Adjust insulin infusion every 2 hours based on blood glucose concentration (Table 63.1).

   When blood glucose is < 200 mg/dL, $HCO_3^- \geq$ 18mEq/L, pH>7.3, and serum ketones are negative at 1:2 dilution, and the patient is taking orally, change to subcutaneous insulin.

Table 63.1: Adjustment of insulin infusion based on glucose concentration

Blood glocose (mg/dL)	Dose of insulin
<100	Decrease by 1 U/hr and give 25 mL 50% dextrose
100-160	Decrease by 1 U/hr
161-220	No change
221-280	Increase by 1 U/hr
> 280	Give 8 U IV bolus and increase by 1 U/hr

- In the past, higher doses of insulin were used, but they were associated with a greater incidence of iatrogenic hypoglycaemia and hypokalaemia and are not more effective than low-dose therapy.

- Insulin adheres to the walls of glass and polyvinyl bottles, and tubings, thereby altering the exact amount of insulin being administered. Running approximately 10 units of the insulin infusion (e.g. 100 mL of a solution having 50 units of regular insulin in 500 mL N-saline) through the tubing accomplishes adherence and reduces alterations in the delivered concentration of the remainder of the infusate.

- With this dose and route, the blood glucose concentration decreases at a rate of 75-100 mg/dL/hr. The presence of infection may reduce the rate of decline to approximately 50mg/dL/hr. If the patient fails to respond in an expected manner, as stated above, within 2-3 hours, double the infusion rate every hour, until the blood glucose level starts to fall.

- The decrease that occurs in blood glucose concentration while treating DKA is not mainly due to increased glucose utilization by peripheral tissues but is due to dilution of glucose in the body by infused fluids, enhanced glucose excretion in the urine, and inhibition of hepatic glucose production.

- Rapid lowering of plasma osmolarity, i.e. by rapid reduction in blood sugar levels (>100 ml/dL/hr), can lead to the development of cerebral edema, and is more likely in children than in adults.

- If blood glucose is not very high but there is moderate to severe metabolic acidosis (i.e. pH<7.2), simply reducing glucose will delay recovery of the acidosis. In this situation, maintain insulin infusion rate, say, at 5 units/hr to suppress lipolysis and prevent hypoglycaemia by infusing sufficient glucose as a 5% or 10% solution (250-500 mL/hr), until the arterial pH has risen to more than 7.2.

- Correction of acidaemia is usually delayed because of the slower metabolism of ketone bodies. It is estimated to take twice the time to restore bicarbonate and pH to controlled levels than it takes to reduce blood glucose to 200 mg/dL. In general, the time required for normalizing bicarbonate or blood pH, is same as that required for clearing the sensorium in obtunded or comatosed patients.

5. **Replace potassium.**
Maintain serum K^+ between 4-5 mEq/L. Potassium supplementation should be guided by the serum potassium levels (Table 63.2).

Table 63.2: Potassium supplementation

Serum K^+ (m Eq/L)	Supplementation in replacement fluid
> 5	No supplementation required
4-5	Add 20 mEq/L
3-4	Add 30-40 mEq/L
< 3	Add 40-60 mEq/L

- Assure urinary output before potassium supplementation.
- Hyperkalaemia is expected in patients with DKA despite a large deficit because of severe acidosis. Approximately 2% of patients with DKA may have initial serum potassium levels more than 6 mEq/L because of severe dehydration and prerenal impairement.
- The presence of normokalaemia or hypokalaemia at presentation suggests that the potassium deficit is greater than 3-5 mEq/kg and may be of the magnitude of 5-10 mEq/kg.
- Severe hypokalemia is most frequently due to concomitant use of diuretics, nasogastric suction, or persistent vomiting.
- Potassium is not added to the initial 500-1000 mL of 0.9% saline because initially, serum potassium levels are commonly normal or elevated and initial fluids are given at a faster rate. Most of the decline in serum potassium is due to insulin-mediated reentry of potassium into the intracellular compartment. Once insulin therapy has started, potassium supplementation should begin, as insulin therapy without aggressive potassium replacement can lead to profound hypokalaemia.
- Oral potassium supplements (2-4 g/24 hr) should be given for 5-7 days after an episode of severe DKA to fully replenish the total body potassium.

6. **Assess the need for bicarbonate therapy. Target of therapy: raise bicarbonate level to 10-12 mEq/L. Do not correct pH above 7.0**
   - With insulin therapy, ketoacids are metabolized to bicarbonate and pH gets corrected on its own.
   - Bicarbonate replacement is not routinely recommended in the treatment of DKA.
   - Bicarbonate replacement is indicated if bicarbonate concentration is less than 8-10 mEq/L, $PaCO_2$ is 10-12 mmHg, pH is less than 7.0, or cardiorespiratory collapse seems imminent.
   - If severe acidosis (pH < 7.0) persists inspite of fluid replacement and insulin therapy for 1-2 hours, infuse sodium bicarbonate at following rate:

- pH<6.9 - infuse 100 mEq sodium bicarbonate added to 400mL sterile water, at a rate of 200 mL/hr.
- pH between 6.9 and 7.0 - add 50 mEq sodium bicarbonate to 200 mL sterile water and infuse at a rate of 200 mL/hr.
- It is recommended that 15 mEq KCL be given for every 50 mEq of bicarbonate, to avoid hypokalaemia.

- Hypertonic (8.4%) sodium bicarbonate should not be used as it causes thrombosis of the peripheral veins, and excessive sodium load may precipiate pulmonary edema in vulnerable patients.

7. **Replace magnesium.**

If serum magnesium level is less than 1.8 mEq/L, or tetany is present, give magnesium sulphate 5 g in 500 mL of 0.45% saline over 5 hours.

8. **Replace calcium.**

For symptomatic hypocalcaemia, give 10-20 mL of 10% calcium gluconate (100-200 mg elemental calcium), as indicated.

9. **Phosphate replacement.**

Not routinely recommended.

10. **Adopt general measures.**

- Protection of airway in the unconscious patient.
- Nasogastric aspiration should be considered in patients who are drowsy and have been vomiting. Acute gastric dilatation is common in DKA, with the associated risk of aspiration of gastric contents.
- Urinary catheterization is not a must, but should be considered in the elderly, in those with impaired renal function, or in those with prolonged hypotension unresponsive to fluid challenge.
- Central venous pressure (CVP) monitoring may be helpful for monitoring fluid therapy, especially in those with cardiac failure, renal failure or septic shock, or in those who remain hypotensive, despite adequate fluid replacement as a result of severe acidosis.
- Find out and treat the underlying precipitating factors, if any. Use antibiotics, when there is clear-cut evidence of infection.
- Low dose heparin: Because DKA is often associated with low grade disseminated intravascular coagulation, low dose heparin should be considered in those with higher risk of venous thromboembolic disease, and in those with severe dehydration or immobility.

11. **Monitor the patient at regular intervals.**

- Monitor blood glucose at 1 hourly intervals for the first four hours, at 2 hourly intervals for the next 4-8 hours, and then 8 hourly till 24 hours.
- Measure arterial or venous blood gases (and bicarbonate) at zero hours and then at 4, 8 and 24 hours after baseline.
- Following the initial arterial blood gas measurement, venous blood may be used to follow the pH, as it is easy to obtain and is less painful. Venous pH is about 0.03 lower than the arterial pH.

- Urine ketones at 0 hours, 4 hours, 8 hours and then at 8 hourly intervals till 24 hours.
- Calcium, magnesium, and phosphate at baseline and then 8 hourly during the first 24 hours.
- Clinical, assessment 2 hourly during the initial 4 hours, and then at 4-8 hour interval for 24 hours.

References

1. Adrogue HJ, Wilson H, Boyd AE, Suki WN, Eknoyan G. Plasma acid-base patterns in diabetic ketoacidosis. N Engl J Med 1982;307:1603-1610.
2. Alberti KGMM. Low dose insulin in the treatment of diabetic ketoacidosis. Arch Intern Med 1977;137:1367-76.
3. Beigelman PM: Severe diabetic ketoacidosis (diabetic coma): 482 episodes in 257 patients: experience of three years. Diabetes 1971;20:490-500.
4. Caroll P, Matz R. Uncontrolled diabetes mellitus in adults: experience in treating diabetic ketoacidosis and hyperosmolar coma with low-dose insulin and uniform treatment regimen. Diabetes Care 1983;6:579-585.
5. DeFronzo RA, Matsudu M, Barrett E. Diabetic Ketoacidosis: a combined metabolic-nephrologic approach to therapy. Diabetes Rev 1994;2:209-238.
6. Ennis ED, Stahl EJVB, Kreisberg RA. The hyperosmolar hyperglycemic syndrome, Diabetes Rev 1994;2:115-12.
7. Fisher JN, Kitabchi AE. A Randomized study of phosphate therapy in the treatment of diabetic ketoacidosis. J Clin Endocrinol Metab 1983;57:177-180.
8. Fisher JN, Shahshahani MN, Kitabchi AE. Diabetic ketoacidosis: low dose insulin therapy by various routes. N Engl J Med 1977;297:238-247.
9. Foster DW, McGarry JD. The metabolic derangements and treatment of diabetic ketoacidosis. N Engl J Med 1983;309:159.
10. Hillman K. Fluid resuscitation in diabetic emergencies: a reappraisal. Intensive Care Med 1987;13:4-8.
11. Kitabchi AE, Sacks HS, Young RT, Morris L. Diabetic ketoacidosis: reappraisal of therapeutic approach. Ann Rev Med 1979;30:330-357.
12. Kitabchi AE, Wall BM. Diabetic ketoacidosis. Med Clin North Am 1995;79:9-37.
13. Kreisberg RA. Diabetic ketoacidosis: new concepts and trends in pathogenesis and treatment. Ann Int Med 1978;88:681-695.
14. Morris LR, Murphy MB, Kitabchi AE. Bicarbonate therapy in severe diabetic ketoacidosis. Ann Int Med 1986;105:836-840.
15. Van der Meulen JA, Klip A, Grinstein S. Possible mechanism for cerebral oedema in diabetic ketoacidosis. Lancet 1987;2:306.
16. Viallon A, Zeni F, Lafond P, Venet C, Tardy B, Page Y, Bertrand JC. Does bicarbonate therapy improve the management of severe diabetic ketoacidosis? Crit Care Medicine 27, December 1999
17. Wetterhall SF, Olson DR, DeStefano F, et al. Trends in diabetes and diabetic complications, 1980-1987. Diabetes Care 1992;15:960.

Guillain–Barré Syndrome 64

Introduction

- Guillain–Barré syndrome (GBS) is an acute, inflammatory, demyelinating polyneuropathy, affecting the peripheral nervous system. It is immune mediated, and is preceded by an infectious episode in 60% of cases. Infection with the bacterium Campylobacter jejuni is responsible for up to 40% of GBS cases, and is often associated with a more severe form of disease with prolonged disability.
- Two features must be found before a diagnosis of Guillain–Barré syndrome can be made : progressive motor weakness in both arms and both legs, and areflexia. Other features strongly supporting the diagnosis are: (a) Progression of symptoms over days to weeks, (b) relative symmetry of symptoms, (c) mild sensory symptoms or signs, (d) cranial nerve involvement, especially bilateral weakness of facial muscles, (e) recovery beginning 2 to 4 weeks after progression ceases, (f) autonomic dysfunction, (g) absence of fever at the onset, (h) elevated protein concentration in CSF with fewer than 10 cells/mm^3, and (i) typical electrodiagnostic features.
- Factors associated with poor prognosis are age, greater than 60 years, rapid progression to severe weakness (less than 1 week), need for ventilatory support, and mean compound muscle action potential amplitudes from distal stimulation less than 20% of normal.
- Clinical indications for admission to intensive care unit (ICU) include:
  (a) Rapid progression of motor weakness.
  (b) Severe respiratory and autonomic dysfunction.
  (c) Autonomic instability: hypertension, hypotension, tachyarrhythmias, bradycardia, and conduction block.
  (d) Bulbar weakness.
  (e) Ventilatory failure.
  (f) Presence of complications: aspiration, pulmonary embolism, infection and myocardial infarction.
- Acute Guillain–Barré syndrome can compromise respiratory system in many ways: (a) Abnormal central respiratory drive, either because of chronic neuromuscular fatigue with central adaptation, or due to sensory deafferentaition of respiratory muscles with reflex modulation of central ventilatory drive, (b) inadequate protection of the upper airway - inability to swallow, and weak or ineffective cough, (c) respiratory muscle weakness, leading to decreased ability to generate large volumes, ineffective cough, progressive microatelectasis, decreased pulmonary compliance, increased intrapulmonary

shunt, increased work of breathing, hypoxia, hypercarbia, and ventilatory failure, and (d) pulmonary complications – pneumonia, atelectasis with or without lobar collapse, and pulmonary embolism.

- Frequent monitoring of two bedside parameters – vital capacity (VC) and maximum inspiratory pressure (MIP), is the single, most important technique for assessing the progress of GBS.

- Patients with marginally compensated ventilatory status may decompensate in the night time, even without any worsening of their underlying neuropathy. This is due to a decrease in the contribution of the rib cage excursion to breathing and inability of the diaphragm (affected and weak) to effectively compensate for this, added burden on diaphragm by supine position, an increased dead space because of rapid, shallow, irregular respiration during REM sleep, and reduced secretion clearance during sleep.

- Indications for intubation and ventilatory support include, vital capacity less than 15-18 mL/kg or less than 1 L, inability to handle oral secretions, impending ventilatory failure (difficulty in swallowing, coughing, speaking, chest signs of aspiration), MIP $\leq$ 30 cm H_2O, hypoxaemia (PaO_2 < 70 mmHg on room air, or alveolar–arterial PO_2 difference more than 300 mm Hg with FiO_2 of 1.0) and hypercapnia. Respiratory rates in excess of 30/min, coupled with TV less than 5 mL/kg, are associated with increased WOB, ventilatory muscle fatigue, and the development of ventilatory failure. A rapid shallow breathing index (f/TV) of >105 breaths/ min/L is associated with a difficulty in maintaining effective spontaneous ventilation. Arterial blood gases should not be relied upon for deciding whether patient needs respiratory support. Blood gases FOLLOW the clinical condition rather than precede it. Hypoxaemia develops first, as a result of atelectasis; hypercapnia occurs late in the course of acute ventilatory failure. The average $PaCO_2$ at the time of intubation, when FVC is less than 12 mL/kg, was 43 mmHg in two large series of GBS patients.

- Sharshar et al followed up 772 patients and identified six predictors of the need for mechanical ventilation:

(i)   Time from GBS onset to admission < 7 days.

(ii) Inability to cough.

(iii) Inability to stand.

(iv) Inability to lift the elbows.

(v)   Inability to lift the head.

(vi) Raised liver enzymes.

They concluded that patients with at least one predictor should be admitted to the ICU. Most patients (> 85%) with 4 predictors will require mechanical ventilation. The authors agreed with the findings in another study, that bulbar dysfunction and a decrease in vital capacity, are also early warning signs of the need for mechanical ventilation. According to a recent retrospective study, VC < 20 mL/kg, maximal inspiratory pressure < 30 cm H_2O, and a maximal expiratory pressure < 40 cm H_2O, or a reduction of > 30% in VC, maximal inspiratory pressure and maximal expiratory pressure were associated with progression to respiratory failure.

- Autonomic dysfunction is commonly associated with acute GBS. Its manifestations include, fixed tachycardia and other arrhythmias, transient hypertension, transient or orthostatic hypotension, reduced sweating, and parasympathetic discharges with flushing, chest tightness, and profuse bronchorrhea. β-blockers may be helpful for tachycardia and hypertension. Life-threatening bradycardia usually responds to atropine, but may sometimes require a temporary pacemaker.
- General management of GBS includes prevention of ventilatory failure, malnutrition, bedsores and thromboembolism, and treatment of autonomic neuropathy, pain and psychological stress. Specific immunotherapeutic intervention includes plasma exchange or intravenous immunoglobulins. Steroids have not been demonstrated to be efficacious, and are not recommended.
- NIPPV is not of much value in these patients, as they usually have difficulty in swallowing and clearing secretions, making invasive positive pressure ventilation as the preferred means of ventilatory support.

GUIDELINES FOR ASSESSING A PATIENT OF ACUTE GBS

1. **History of illness.**

   Take history, with special reference to the duration and the rate of progression of illness.

2. **Clinical examination: Pulse rate and rhythm, blood pressure, respiratory rate and pattern of respiration, retraction of muscles, efficiency of cough, mobility of soft palate, gag reflex, quality of voice.**
   - Asses the patient every 4-6 hours.
   - Patient may have sweating, mild tachycardia, and the need to take a breath in the middle of a brief sentence because of increased WOB. Various arrythmias with fluctuating blood pressure could be because of autonomic disturbances. Patients may not complain of dyspnoea. Breathing is usually shallow and rapid inspite of hypoventilation. Retraction of intercostals and scalene muscles may not be marked and obvious because these muscles usually are weakend earlier than diaphragm. Once diaphragmatic weakness is present, breathing becomes paradoxical with abdominal inversion during inspiration. Abdominal muscle weakness is manifested as a diminution in the strength of the cough. Nasal voice, poorly pronounced speech (dysarthria), poor mobility of the soft palate when saying "ah", and a decreased or abolished gag reflex, indicate bulbar dysfunction.

3. **Assess tidal volume and vital capacity in both erect and supine positions.**
   - Ask the patient to count as fast as possible, using a single exhalation. The patient's ability to count from 1 to 25 rapidly in one breath reflects a vital capacity of more than 20 mL/kg. With VC falling below 25 mL/kg, accumulation of secretions (with risk of infection and airway obstruction) increases and intubation is often required.

- A vital capacity of 15-18 mL/kg is a sign of imminent respiratory failure, and of less than 10-12 mL/kg signals overt respiratory failure.
- When diaphragmatic weakness is a major component of ventilatory failure, imminent decompensation is reflected more accurately in the fall in VC, when adopting a supine posture. VC drops by 19% in normal subjects, and by as much as 55% in patients with diaphragmatic paralysis.

4. **Water drinking test.**

   Patient's ability to swallow (and protect his airway) can be judged by asking him to drink a glass of water. Observe whether the water comes out of the nose, or whether it make the patient cough.

5. **Maximal static pressures: PI max, PE max.**

   Measurement of respiratory muscle strength is useful, and there exists a good correlation between PI max and atelectasis, and PE max and cough efficacy. In general, healthy males and females generate a PI max of about 120 cm H_2O and 90 cm H_2O respectively, and a PE max of about 180 cm H_2O and 140 cm H_2O respectively. A PI max of more than 30 cm H_2O is thought to correlate with adequate strength for unassisted breathing, whereas a normal $PaCO_2$ cannot be maintained if the PI max is less than 20 cm H_2O. Similarly, an effective cough is generally not possible when maximal expiratory pressure is less than 40 cm H_2O. These tests (VC, PI max, and PE max), if performed too frequently, can lead to fatigue of the patient and altered results.

6. **Chest examinations.**

   Patient may have decreased breath sounds, areas of consolidation, rattling of secretions, all pointing to impending decompensation. Cyanosis, wheezes and severe breathlessness are late signs, and patients with weakness of neuromuscular apparatus often decompensate dramatically, leading to respiratory arrest.

7. **Arterial blood gas (ABG) analysis.**
8. **Examine other systems of body, including the nervous system.**

GUIDELINES FOR VENTILATORY MANAGEMENT

1. **Consider chest physical therapy, incentive spirometry, adequate humidification, and aerosolized bronchodilators, if required.**

   In the early stages, initiate therapy when patient shows signs of ineffective cough, atelectasis or retained secretions. Be careful, however, as chest percussion and airway suctioning may result in dangerous arrhythmias, hypotension and even cardiovascular collapse in the presence of autonomic dysfunction.

2. **Endotracheal intubation.**

   Ideally intubation should be done several hours before ventilatory decompensation.

(a) Reassess the patient.
- Patient may be dehydrated: These patients have difficulty in swallowing and sweat too much. Ask history of intake. If required, give the patient 500-1000 mL of IV fluid.
- Patients often have autonomic dysfunction. There is an exaggerated hypotensive response to drugs used for anaesthesia to intubate the trachea. Also, there is a constant potential for sudden vagal dominance and severe bradycardia.

(b) Monitor the patient.
Make sure that the heart rate, ECG, oxygen saturation and blood pressure monitoring is available during laryngoscopy and intubation.

(c) Atropine and other drugs.
Give IV atropine before tracheal intubation, or have it ready to administer at the first sign of bradycardia. Vasoconstrictors (epinephrine) and antiarrhythmic drugs (xylocaine) should be kept ready.

(d) Avoid succinylcholine.
There is a potential for lethal hyperkalaemia after succinylcholine administration, due to extrajunctional chemosensitivity of denervated muscles to succinylcholine.

(e) Perform intubation.
- When sufficient time is available: Topical anesthesia of the airway and intubation with the help of the fiberoptic bronchoscope and short acting sedatives is a preferable alternative.
- In case of emergency, perform intubation using rapid sequence technique, including pre-oxygenation, cricoid pressure, atropine, xylocaine, and low dose of thiopental / propofol. Short acting, non-depolarizing muscle relaxant can be added, if required.

3. Mechanical ventilation.
(a) Goals.
- Provide adequate lung inflation.
- Aggressive airway management
- Maintain eucapnia.

(b) Mode of ventilation: Assist control, SIMV+PS or PSV.
There is no evidence to favour any particular mode. Depending upon the patient's ability to generate a breath, total or partial ventilatory support may be used.

(c) Tidal volume: 12-15 mL/kg.
These patients typically have normal lungs and are at low risk for barotrauma. Start with 6-8 mL/kg tidal volume, readjust, to meet the patient's demands and to relieve the feeling of dyspnoea, as long as pressures are low (lung protective).

(d) Inspiratory flow rates $\geq$ 60 L/min
Such patients are more comfortable with high inspiratory flow rates. Adjust to satisfy patient's inspiratory needs.

(e) **Flow waveform.**
   Constant or descending ramp.
(f) **PEEP: 5-10 cm H_2O.**
   To relieve dyspnoea and maintain normal FRC.
(g) **FiO_2.**
   Titrate to maintain PaO_2 and SpO_2. It should not be a problem to maintain oxygenation unless parenchymal injury is present e.g. pneumonia or aspiration.

4. **Tracheostomy. Consider in 2nd week.**
   With the use of intravenous immunoglobulins or plasmapheresis, recovery is good in around two-thirds of the patients, and it is worthwhile waiting until the end of the 2nd week, to be able to predict more accurately, the future course of the disease.

5. **Weaning.**
   See Chapter 42.

References

1. Asburry AK, Cornblath DR. Assessment of current diagnostic criteria for Guillain –Barre syndrome Ann Neurol 1990; 27(suppl):S21-S24.
2. Chakrabarty A, Chatterjee SK. Management strategies in acute Guillain –Barre syndrome: Do's, Don'ts and Don't knows. Advanc N Clin Neurosc 1992; 2:165-174.
3. Hughes RAC. Intravenous IgG in Guillain–Barre syndrome. Br Med J 1996;313:376-377.
4. Kankam CG, Sallis R. Guillain –Barre syndrome. Postgrad Med 1997; 101:279-290.
5. Lawn ND, Fletcher DD, Henderson RD, et al. Anticipating mechanical ventilation in Guillain-barre' syndrome. Arch Neurol 2001; 58 : 893-898
6. Pentland B, Donald SM. Pain in the Guillain–Barre syndrome: a clinical review. Pain 1994; 59:159-164.
7. Ropper AH. The Guillain–Barre syndrome–Current Concepts. N Eng J Med 1992; 326(17):1130-1136.
8. Sharshar T, Chevret S, Bourdain, F. et al. Early predictors of mechanical ventilation in Guillain-Barre' syndrome. Crit Care Med 2003; 31(1): 278-283.
9. Slutsky AS. Mechanical ventilation. American College of Chest Physicians Consensus Conference. Chest 1993;104:1833-1859.
10. Teitelbaum JS, Borel CO. Respiratory dysfunction in Guillain–Barre syndrome. Clin Chest Med 1994; 15(4): 705-713
11. Unterborn JN, Hill NS. Options for mechanical ventilation in neuromuscular diseases. Clin Chest Med 1994; 15(4):765-779.
12. Van der Meche FGA, Van Doorn PA. Guillain–Barre syndrome and chronic inflammatory demyelinating polyneuropathy: immune mechanisms and update on current therapies. Ann Neurol 1995; 37(51):S14-S31.

Head Injury 65

Introduction

- Injury to the brain can be classified as immediate (primary) or delayed (secondary). Once an injury occurs, little can be done to modify the course of primary damage but secondary brain damage is potentially preventable. Minimizing secondary brain injury is the key to the optimal management of the head-injured patient.
- Various factors contribute to secondary brain damage, including extracranial and intracranial factors.
  - (a) *Extracranial factors*: (i) Hypoxaemia (hypoventilation, thoracic injury, aspiration pneumonia, anaemia), (ii) hypotension (hypovolaemia, cardiac failure, sepsis, spinal cord injury), (iii) hypercapnia (respiratory depression), (iv) hypocapnia (hyperventilation-spontaneous or induced), (v) hyperthermia (hypermetabolism, stress response, infection), (vi) hyperglycaemia (hypothermia, IV infusion of dextrose, stress response), and (vii) hyponatraemia (hypotonic fluids, excessive sodium loss).
  - (b) *Intracranial factors:* (i) Raised intracranial pressure and/or brain shift (mass lesion, vascular engorgement, edema (increased brain water content)), (ii) vasospasm (traumatic sub-arachnoid haemorrhage), (iii) seizures (cortical brain injury), and (iv) infection (skull base fracture, compound depressed skull fracture).
- As many as 40% of the patients with head injury may have subarachnoid haemorrhage in the initial CT scan and neurological recovery is significantly worse in these patients. Vasospasm is caused by the release of breakdown products of haemoglobin into the CSF. The mainstay of management includes maintenance of adequate blood pressure, avoiding hypovolaemia, and use of calcium channel blocker, nimodipine.
- The aim of treatment of brain injury is to restore oxygen supply to the injured neurons (which are exquisitively sensitive to the effect of cerebral ischemia or hypoxemia) by controlling intracranial pressure (ICP), maintaining cerebral blood flow (CBF) and cerebral oxygen delivery, and minimizing the increased metabolic requirement of oxygen, seen in the injured brain.
- Normal autoregulation is lost in head injury. CBF, and hence cerebral oxygen delivery, is then critically dependent on cerebral perfusion pressure (CPP), which is dependent on ICP and mean arterial blood pressure (MAP). Normal ICP is 5-10 mmHg and MAP is 80-90 mmHg. Straining or coughing can cause transient elevations of ICP above 15 mmHg. Sustained ICP greater than 20

mmHg is considered abnormal. The values between 20 and 40 mmHg indicate moderate intracranial hypertension (ICH). An ICP greater than 40 mmHg represents severe, life-threatening intracranial hypertension.

- Although there is controversy over whether the therapeutic strategy should be ICP targeted or CPP targeted, two recent studies have concluded that treatment protocols should concentrate upon reduction in raised ICP before preservation of a high CPP, since "a CPP greater than 60 mmHg appears to have little influence on the outcome." Thus, there are indications that a change in treatment policy should occur towards ICP-targeted therapy, where prevention and treatment of intracranial hypertension is the first priority.

- There are no reliable non-invasive indicators of intracranial hypertension (ICH) in patients with severe head injury. Indications for ICP monitoring include a GCS score of 8 or less after resuscitation, combined with any one of the following: abnormal CT finding, a systolic blood pressure of 90mmHg, motor posturing, or age above 40 years. ICP monitoring may be considered for patients with GCS score above 8 if they require treatment that prevents serial neurological examinations, e.g. prolonged anaesthesia for operative treatment of multiple injuries or prolonged pharmacologic paralysis for ventilatory management, or those requiring PEEP therapy.

- Pyrexia is extremely frequent in the acute phase after head injury. The incidence is higher in severe cases and it is an independent predictor of a longer ICU stay. Avoidance of pyrexia should be a major aim in the management of severe head injury. However, very often, this is difficult to achieve.

- Mannitol reduces the intracranial volume by inducing an osmotic pressure gradient in regions where the blood/brain barrier is intact, drawing fluid out of the extracellular space into the vessels. Serum osmolarity must be kept lower than 320 mOsm/L. In higher doses, mannitol can cause acute renal failure, especially when used alongwith nephrotoxic drugs (antibiotics, vasoconstrictors), or in the presence of sepsis. Combination with other diuretics such as furosemide does not seem to be useful, as there is added risk of hypovolaemia. There are other suggested beneficial, systemic and cerebral haemodynamic effects of mannitol.

- Operative treatment: A surgically significant epidural haematoma, or acute subdural haematoma should be evacuated immediately. A conservative approach is generally adopted for small haemorrhagic contusions or other small intracerebral lesions. Specific indications for operation include: (i) Clinical deterioration, (ii) A thick extracerebral clot more than 1 cm in size, (iii) Intracerebral haematoma of more than 25-30 mL, (iv) midline shift > 5 mm, (v) enlargement of contralateral ventricle (temporal horn), (vi) obliteration of basal cisterns/third ventricle, and (vii) raised or increasing ICP.

GUIDELINES FOR THE MANAGEMENT OF HEAD INJURY

Initial Resuscitation

1. Maintain an airway:oral suction, chin lift or jaw thrust, insertion of an oral airway, intubation, and cricothyroidotomy.

   Initial ABC approach is the same as for all critically ill patients. The underlying logic is simple. Airway problems will kill before breathing problems, which will kill before circulatory problems, which will kill before neurological problems!

   - In general, all patients who are not verbalizing and cannot follow commands, should be promptly intubated. Virtually all patients with a GCS score of 8 or less meet these criteria. Other indications include, loss of protective laryngeal reflexes, ventilatory insufficiency (PaO_2 < 60 mmHg, $PaCO_2$ > 45 mmHg), and spontaneous hyperventilation ($PaCO_2$ < 25 mmHg).
   - Intubation is best facilitated using rapid-sequence induction, with thiopental sodium (2-3 mg/kg IV) or propofol (1-2 mg/kg IV) or if the patient is hypotensive, with ketamine (1mg/kg) plus midazolam (0.05-0.1mg/kg). Inj. succinylcholine (1-1.5 mg/kg) should be preceeded by xylocaine 1.5 mg/kg.
   - Nasotracheal intubation is best avoided until fracture of the base of the skull has been excluded because it is associated with higher complication rate.
   - A nasogastric tube should be positioned through the mouth, on account of the risk of fractures of the skull base and ethmoid bone.
   - In patients with major facial or upper airway trauma, a cricothyroidotomy may be necessary to provide an airway.
   - In general, the decision to intubate a head-injured patient should include a decision to ventilate as well (in order to control the rise in ICP).
   - Sedation/analgesia should be continued, using short acting drugs (see Chapter 7) so that neurological assessment can be made at regular intervals.

2. Breathing.

   Breathing may need to be assisted in cases of associated chest injury, presence of instability of the chest wall, pneumothorax or haemothorax. While ventilating these patients, the aim should be to achieve SpO_2 > 95%, PaO_2 > 90 mmHg and a $PaCO_2$ of approximately 35 mmHg.

3. Circulation.

   - Establish venous access with wide-bore cannulae (two lines are preferable). Take samples for grouping/crossmatching and baseline investigations, including coagulation profile. Infusion of saline (0.9% NaCl, osmolality 308 mOsm/kg) is preferred to Ringer's lactate (osmolality 273 mOsm/kg). Monitor fluid balance using clinical parameters i.e. pulse rate, blood pressure, temperature, capillary refill, SpO_2, and urine output. Maintain euvolaemia. After initial 1-2 liters of crystalloid infusion, colloids and/or blood, may be added, if necessary.

- Start mannitol (before stabilization) only if signs of herniation (unequal or dilated pupils) are present.
- Avoid hypotonic solutions such as 5% glucose.

4.   **Disability/neurological assessment.**

Make a rapid assessment. Assess whether the patient is alert, responds to verbal commands or pain, or is unresponsive. Examine the pupils for size, equality and reaction to light.

5.   **Once the patient is stable, make a detailed assessment.**

(a)   **History.**

Gather information from those accompanying the patient, regarding the mode and time of trauma, any loss of consciousness, or occurrence of convulsions even for a short time, immediately after the trauma. Any other history regarding use of drugs, alcohol, allergies or other diseases is also useful.

(b)   **Assess consciousness level.**

Use Glasgow coma scale (GCS). A GCS of 8 or less for a period of at least 6 hours is labelled as severe head injury.

(c)   **Examine pupils.**

A dilating pupil that reacts more and more sluggishly to light, may indicate the presence of an intracranial mass lesion on the same side. While examining pupils, light in the room should not be too bright.

(d)   **Examine limb response.**

Assess symmetry of the limb responses to standard stimuli.

(e)   **Examine for presence of extracranial injuries.**

Rule out cervical spinal cord, abdominal, chest, (pneumothorax, pericardial tamponade), and pelvic trauma. These injuries could contribute to hypotension and/or hypoxia.

6.   **Ask for X-ray skull, CT scan of the head, X-rays of the chest, cervical spine, pelvis, or other regions as indicated by clinical examination and the mechanism of injury.**

- Radiological work-up should be delayed until the patient is fully stable and on mechanical ventilation, if required.
- Skull fracture and depressed level of consciousness strongly indicate the presence of an intracranial haematoma. A CT scan may reveal haematomas, brain contusion and focal or generalized swelling of the brain. Indications of a CT scan in a patient of head injury include: (a) fracture skull associated with confusion or impairment of consciousness, focal neurological signs, seizures or any other neurological symptoms or signs, (b) confusion or other neurological disturbances persisting after resuscitation, even in the absence of a fracture, (c) deteriorating level of consciousness or developing focal neurological signs, (d) neurologically well patient with CSF leak or other penetrating injury, and (e) worsening headache or vomiting, especially in a child.
- If on admission, CT scan was negative, it may be repeated within 24 hours or within 12 hours if the patient was hypotensive at the time of admission or has coagulation disorders.
- If the admission CT scan was not negative, it may be repeated within 24

hours, if it was first done later than 6 hours after the trauma, and the patient presents no risk factors. Or within 12 hours, if it was done within the first 3-6 hours following the trauma.

- Negative findings in the first CT scan must not induce a sense of false security.

Care in the ICU

Care in the ICU is mostly supportive, with little specific therapy, other than surgical evacuation of mass lesions and management of traumatic SAH. Current guidelines followed by most centers are, to maintain ICP less than 20 mmHg, to target a CPP $\geq$ 70 mmHg, and to maintain normovolaemia and normal blood chemistry.

1. **Elevate the head end of the bed to 30°.**

  This position can lower the ICP without reducing either cerebral perfusion pressure or cerebral blood flow (CBF), by improving the jugular venous outflow. Calibrate the ICP transducer and the arterial blood pressure transducer at the same level, ideally at the level of external auditory meatus. In case the patient needs to be transported out of the ICU for any reason, it is better to lower the head end to the flat position 15-30 minutes before transport, so that any alteration in ICP or other physiological parameters can be corrected in the ICU rather than during transport.

2. **Consider sedation and analgesia.**

  Sedatives and analgesics blunt the adverse effects on ICP that result from movements, coughing and bucking on the ventilator and from routine nursing care, such as turning and bathing the patient. Consider morphine/fentanyl and diazepam/lorazepam combination, after correcting the hypovolaemia. Propofol (a good sedative) may also be considered, as it lowers the cerebral metabolic rate. Because it is rapidly eliminated, it may allow a reliable examination till 15-20 minutes after discontinuation. The disadvantages include cost, risk of hypotension with the loading dose, or increased rate of infusion and possibility of hyperlipidaemia.

3. **Administer mannitol.**

  Mannitol should be started as soon as hypovolaemia is corrected and blood pressure is more than 100 mmHg. Mannitol is given as an IV bolus infusion of 0.25–1.0 g/kg. Evidence suggests that the efficacy of mannitol does not differ significantly over the dose range between 0.25 g and 1.0 g/kg. Thus, smaller doses may be used, whenever possible.

4. **Consider neuromuscular blocking agents.**

  When patient-ventilator dyssynchrony persists inspite of adequate sedation and analgesia, neuromuscular blockade may be considered. This dyssynchrony increases the intrathoracic pressure, interfering with cerebral venous outflow, which in turn increases the intracranial pressure. Muscle relaxants should preferably be administered by continuous intravenous infusion to have a stable control on intracranial dynamics (See Chapter 8). Use of these agents should always be associated with adequate sedation and analgesia.

5. **Control blood pressure.**

   - Occurrence of hypotension (mean arterial blood pressure, MAP, < 90 mmHg), any time in the course of head injury, is associated with nearly a two-fold increase in mortality, as it can lead to cerebral ischaemia. Initially, the preload is optimised with crystalloids, colloids/blood as is appropriate. Later on, inotropes and pressor agents (dopamine, noradrenaline) are added to achieve the goal of MAP > 90mmHg. Any extracranial cause of hypotension should be excluded. It has been suggested that the routine administration of 250 mL of hypertonic saline as the first resuscitation fluid may further improve recovery.

   - A systolic blood pressure greater than 160 mmHg after head injury may result from sympathetic hyperactivity. Do not treat this if associated with an untreated intracranial mass lesion because a higher blood pressure is required to maintain cerebral perfusion. However, hypotension should be treated in the post operative period as it can increase CBF and ICP, exacerbate cerebral edema, and increase the risk of recurrent haemorrhage. It often resolves with sedation; but if it doesn't, sympathetic blocking agents like propranolol, esmolol, and labetalol or centrally acting α-agonists like methyldopa are added. Vasodilators e.g. hydralazine, nifedepine, and sodium nitroprusside should be avoided as they can increase the ICP.

6. **Consider anticonvulsants.**

   There is no evidence that early prophylactic treatment with anticonvulsants decreases the incidence of late post-traumatic seizures. However, there is evidence that early prophylactic treatment with anticonvulsants does prevent early onset of seizures. It is recommended that phenytoin be given to all patients who have subdural haematomas or parenchymal brain injury, and that it be withdrawn after 7-10 days if the patient does not have seizures. Prophylactic treatment for delayed seizures, is therefore, not recommended. Frank seizures are treated with diazepam/lorazepam and a longer acting anticonvulsant, e.g. phenytoin 15-20 mg/kg is given as a loading dose followed by maintainance therapy. (See Chapter 66).

7. **Control body temperature.**

   Fever is a potent cerebral vasodilator and thus raises the ICP. ICP increases by 3-4 mmHg for every 1°C rise in temperature. Fever also increases cerebral metabolic requirements (10-13% per °C rise). Furthermore, brain temperature, can be as much as 0.5°C to 2.0°C higher than the body temperature. Therefore fever should be treated aggressively with antipyretics, cooling blankets and antibiotics when the core body temperature exceeds 38°C. It is best to avoid management of escalating ICP in febrile patients until the body temperature has been controlled.

8. **Correct anaemia.**

   Normally cerebral blood flow increases to compensate for a decrease in arterial oxygen content (CaO_2). After head injury however, the cerebral vasculature may not be able to dilate in response to a decrease in CaO_2 (loss of metabolic autoregulation). Even if metabolic autoregulation is present, the increase in

CBF, that results from anaemia, can increase the ICP. For these reasons, it is recommended to maintain haemoglobin level of 10 g% or higher in all patients with severe head injury.

9. **Monitor the patient.**
    Minimal recommended monitoring includes ECG, SpO_2, end-tidal CO_2, CVP, temperature, invasive blood pressure, and ICP monitoring in all severe head injury patients. Clinical recording should include 1-2 hourly charting of blood pressure, body temperature, level of sedation, ventilatory settings, Glasgow coma scale, pupil size and reaction. During the initial 2-3 days, sedation should be stopped to assess the patient at least every 12 hours. Hourly urine output measurement is also important as, in case of brain damage, an oliguric or polyuric response may suggest hyper- or hypo-secretion of antidiuretic hormone (ADH). Serum biochemistry should also be kept within normal limits.

10. **Corticosteroids.**
    Not recommended for treatment of ICH (intracranial hypertension).

11. **Management of ICP.**
    Medical treatment of ICH can be divided into two broad categories: general measures to limit factors that may exacerbate or cause ICH and specific measures. The causes of ICH include: (a) Obstruction of venous outflow (positioning of the head and neck, poor adaptation to mechanical ventilation, pneumothorax), (b) cerebral vasodilatation (fever, hypercapnia, hypotension, seizures), (c) arterial hypertension (pain, visceral stimuli, inadequate sedation], (d) shivering, (e) low serum sodium, and (f) instrument malfunction.
    - When a sustained ICP of greater than 20 mmHg is refractory to general measures, specific therapies are added in a stepwise fashion until ICH is controlled. These include, CSF drainage, hyperventilation, barbiturate coma, and hypothermia.

12. **Care of nutrition.**
    Replace 140% of resting metabolism expenditure in non-paralysed patients and 100% of resting metabolism expenditure in paralysed patients using enteral or parenteral formulas containing at least 15% of calories as protein by the seventh day after injury. When using enteral nutrition, the preferable option is the use of jejunal feeding by gastrojejunostomy due to ease of administration and avoidance of gastric intolerance.

13. **Other therapeutic aspects.**
    Other therapeutic measures include stress ulcer prophylaxis, respiratory care management, maintenance of fluid-electrolyte balance, control of infection, and physiotherapy.

Initiation of Mechanical Ventilation
1. Calculate predicted body weight.
2. Initial ventilatory settings:
    (a) Mode – volume ventilation in control mode or assist-control mode.

Volume controlled ventilation is preferred since it delivers constant volume of gases in the presence of changing lung mechanics, does not carry any significant detrimental effects when applied to the normal lung, and helps to prevent atelectasis and hypoxemia. Pressure controlled ventilatory modes are contraindicated because the minute volume, and therefore $PaCO_2$ can vary. PSV, combined with SIMV, can be used as a weaning mode for these patients.

(b) Tidal volume: 10-12mL/kg.

(c) Respiratory rate: 10-12 breaths/min.

(d) Flow pattern: decelerating.

(e) PEEP: ≤ 5 cmH$_2$O

(f) FiO$_2$: 1.0

(g) PIFR: 60-70 L/min

Adjust respiratory rate to keep $PaCO_2$ at desired level.

3. Set goals.

(a) FiO$_2$

FiO$_2$ should be as low as possible to maintain PaO_2 >90 mmHg and SpO_2 > 95%. These goals have been recommended to cover the devastating effects of hypoxia.

(b) PaCO$_2$

In the first 24 hours after injury, maintain the $PaCO_2$ at approximately 35 mmHg. After 24 hours, maintain $PaCO_2$ between 30-35 mmHg. Hyperventilation probably has its most deleterious effects during the first 24 hours after a severe head injury, when the CBF is typically at its lowest. Adjust minute ventilation (RR and TV) to keep the $PaCO_2$ at the desired level and to keep mean airway pressure at its lowest level. Settings that act to increase mean airway pressure may exacerbate ICP by impeding venous return to the chest. Switch over to SIMV mode as soon as the patient's condition improves, keeping the number of mechanical breaths to a minimum and allowing the patient to breathe spontaneously. Excessive hyperventilation to a $PaCO_2$ level of less than 30 mmHg should be considered for a short period (about 30 minutes) as a separate and more extreme measure, should be attempted only in the presence of clinical signs of transtentorial herniation (pupillary dilatation, hypertension, bradycardia) or when all other means of ICP control have failed. It should generally be accompanied by a concomitant monitoring of cerebral blood flow whenever facilities are available.

(c) PEEP

- Whenever pulmonary edema is present, addition of PEEP may be required to allow the FiO$_2$ to be lowered to less toxic levels. PEEP can adversely affect ICP and BP (increases ICP and decreases BP). The severity of the effect on ICP depends both on intracranial and pulmonary compliance. Usually, when PEEP is needed, lungs are poorly compliant, and the use of PEEP does not cause significant effect on the venous pressures or on the ICP. Furthermore, positioning the patient with the head elevated at 30-45º, reduces the effect of PEEP on ICP. Only the minimum required PEEP should be used.

- Termination of PEEP is performed in a stepwise fashion, with careful monitoring of haemodynamic parameters and the ABG, over one to two days. Abrupt discontinuation of PEEP can lead to a reflexive hypertension, with subsequent elevation of ICP through engorgement of cerebral tissues (with defective autoregulation).

4. Adjusting/titrating $PaCO_2$.

Adjustments in $PaCO_2$ in a patient undergoing controlled ventilation can be made by using a simple formula:

$$\text{Required minute ventilation} = \frac{\text{measured } PaCO_2 \times \text{patient's minute ventilation}}{\text{desired } PaCO_2}$$

References

1. Bartlett J, Kett-White R, Mendelow AD, et al. Guidelines for the initial management of head injuries. Recommendations from the society of British Neurological surgeons. Br J Neurosurg 1998;12(4): 349-359.
2. Bayir H, Clark RSB, Kochanek PM. Promising strategies to minimize secondary brain injury after head trauma. Crit Care Med 2003; 31(Suppl): S112-S117.
3. Chestnut RM. Avoidance of hypotension: Condition sine qua non of successful severe head-injury management. J Trauma 1997, 42(Suppl): S4-S14.
4. Finfer SR, Cohen J. Severe traumatic brain injury. Resuscitation 2001;48:77-90.
5. Gopinath SP, Robertson CS. Intensive Care Unit management. In: Marion DW (ed). Traumatic Brain Injury. New York: Thieme Medical Publishers, 1999, pp 101-118.
6. Grande PO, Naredi S. Clinical studies in severe traumatic brain injury: a controversial issue. Intensive Care Med 2002;28:529-531.
7. Guerra WK, Gaab M, Dietz H, et al. Surgical decompression for traumatic brain swelling: indications and results. J Neurosurg 1999;90:187-196.
8. Gutman MB, Moulton RJ, Sullivan, et al. Risk factors predicting operable intracranial haematomas in head injury. J Neurosurg 1992; 77(1):9-14.
9. Haydel MJ, Pheston CA, Mills TJ, et al. Indications for computed tomography in patients with minor head injury. N Engl. J Med 2000; 343:100-105.
10. Hsiang J, Chestnut RM, Crisp CB, et al. Early routine paralysis for ICP control in severe head injury: is it necessary? Crit Care Med 1994; 22:1471-1476.
11. Jennet B, Bond M. Assessment of outcome after severe brain damage. A practical scale. Lancet 1975;I:480-484.
12. Jones PA, Andrews PJ, Midgley S, et al. Measuring the burden of secondary insults in head-injured patients during intensive care. J Neurosurg Anesthesiol 1994;6(1):4-14.
13. Kelly DF. Emergency department management. In: Marion DW (ed). Traumatic Brain Injury, New York: Thieme Medical Publishers, 1999, pp 67-79.
14. Maas AIR, Dearden M, Teasdale GM, et al. EBIC-guidelines for management of severe head injury in adults. Acta Neurochir (wien) 1997; 139:286-294.
15. Myburgh JA. Respiratory and cardiovascular support. In: Reilly P, Bullock R (eds). Head Injury. London: Chapman & Hall Medical, 1997, pp 333-361.
16. Oakley PA, Coleman NA, Morrison PJ. Intensive Care of the trauma patient. Resuscitation 2001;48:37-46.
17. Patel HC, Menon DK, Tebbs S, et al. Specialist neurocritical care and outcome from head injury. Intensive Care Med 2002; 28:547-553.

18. Polderman KH, Joe RTT, Peerdeman SM, et al. Effects of therapeutic hypothermia on intracranial pressure and outcome in patients with severe head injury. Intensive Care Med 2002; 28:1563-1573.

19. Procaccio E, Stocchetti N, Citerio G, et al. Guidelines for the treatment of adults with severe head trauma J Neurosurg Sci 2000;44: (Part I)1-10 and (Part-II) 11-18.

20. Stocchetti N, Rossi S, Zamier ER, et al. Pyrexia in head-injured patients admitted to intensive care. Intensive Care Med 2002;28:1555-1562.

21. Valadka AB, Pepe PE. Prehospital management. In: Marion DW(ed). Traumatic Brain Injury. New York: Thieme Medical Publishers, 1999, pp 55-65.

22. Wilkens I, Menon DK, Matta B. Management of comatosed head injured patients. Are we getting any better? Anaesthesia 2001; 56:350-369.

23. Zinc BJ. Traumatic brain injury. Emerg Med Clin North Am 1996; 14(1): 115-150.

24. Zornow MH, Prough DS. Fluid management in patients with traumatic brain injury. New Horizons 1995; 3(3):488-498.

Introduction

- A seizure is an episode of abnormal neurologic function caused by an abnormal electrical discharge of brain neurons. Seizure represents the clinical attack experienced by the patient; however, some patients with epileptic EEG discharges may not experience any clinical symptoms.

- Status epilepticus (SE) is defined as either continuous seizure activity for 30 minutes or more, or occurrence of two or more seizures without full recovery of consciousness between the attacks. Even a marked increase in seizure frequency (i.e. three seizures in 60 minutes, even with recovery) or duration (i.e. a seizure lasting more than 5 minutes), may constitute an emergency that should be treated as SE.

- Tonic-clonic status epilepticus generally follows a predictable sequence of events. These events are classified as early (phase I) and late (phase II) SE. The transition from phase I to phase II usually occurs after 30 to 60 minutes. The events refer to autonomic, systemic, cerebral, and metabolic changes.

- During phase I *(phase of compensation)*, cerebral metabolism is greatly increased because of seizure activity, but compensatory mechanisms are sufficient to meet the metabolic demands, and cerebral tissue is protected from hypoxia or metabolic damage. The changes include: (a) *Autonomic and cardiovascular changes*: (i) initial hypertension, (ii) increased cardiac output and central venous pressure, (iii) massive catecholamine release, tachycardia, cardiac dysrhythmias, (iv) increased temperature, and (v) salivation, vomiting, and incontinence; (b) *systemic and metabolic changes*: (i) hyperglycaemia and (ii) lactic acidosis; (c) *cerebral changes*: (i) increased cerebral blood flow (may be upto 900% increase), (ii) increased cerebral oxygen consumption (may be up to 300% increase), (iii) compensated cerebral energy state, and (iv) increased lactate and glucose concentrations.

- During phase II *(phase of decompensation)*, the greatly increased cerebral metabolic demands cannot be met fully, resulting in hypoxia and altered cerebral and systemic metabolic patterns. Similarly, autonomic and cardiorespiratory functions may progressively fail to maintain homeostasis. The changes include: (a) *Autonomic and cardiovascular changes*: (i) systemic hypoxia, (ii) falling cardiac output and blood pressure, (iii) respiratory and cardiac impairment (pulmonary edema, pulmonary embolism, respiratory collapse, cardiac failure, dysrhythmia), and (iv) hyperpyrexia; (b) *systemic and metabolic changes*: (i) hypoglycaemia, hyponatraemia, hypokalaemia/hyperkalaemia, (ii) metabolic and respiratory acidosis, (iii) rhabdomyolysis, myoglobulinuria, renal failure, (iv) disseminated intravascular coagulopathy, multiorgan failure, and (v) leucocytosis; (c) *cerebral changes*: (i) failure of cerebral autoregulation (cerebral blood flow now becomes dependent on systemic blood pressure). (ii) hypoxia, hypoglycaemia, falling lactate concentrations, (iii) falling cerebral energy state, and (iv) rise in intracranial pressure and cerebral edema.

- Avoiding or controlling these changes is important for limiting the morbidity and mortality. It is not clear how long a seizure must occur before permanent neurologic sequalae ensue, but it does appear that the longer the seizures are allowed to progress, the more would be the chances for the permanent CNS injury to occur. Also, the longer the seizure is allowed to continue, the more difficult it is to control.
- Frequent causes of tonic-clonic SE include: (a) withdrawal from antiepileptic drugs, (b) withdrawal from alcoholic or sedative drug, (c) metabolic disorder (hypocalcaemia, hyponatraemia, hypoglycaemia, hepatic or renal failure), (d) sleep deprivation, (e) acute new brain insult (meningitis, encephalitis, cerebrovascular accident, trauma, or anoxic-ischaemic injury), (f) drug intoxication (e.g. cocaine, amphetamines, tricyclics, or isoniazid), (g) eclampsia, and (h) idiopathic, where no cause is found.
- SE due to anoxia, stroke, drug toxicity, CNS infection, and multiple medical illnesses predicts a worse outcome. The mortality due to SE in the adult and elderly population, is 14% and 38% respectively, with an overall rate of 22%. Death may result from the basic disease process causing SE, medical complications, or overmedication.
- In a convulsing patient, initial supportive, therapeutic, and diagnostic measures, should be taken up simultaneously. The main priority, as far as supportive measures are concerned, is to preserve the vital functions, that is, protect the airway, maintain breathing, support the circulation, and correct any metabolic abnormality.
- During an acute episode, the therapeutic end point, while administering anticonvulsants, is to stop clinical and more importantly, electrical seizure activity by giving the appropriate drugs in adequate doses. After the acute episode has been controlled, achieving optimum drug concentration becomes the more important consideration for preventing recurrence of the seizure.

GUIDELINES FOR MANAGING A PATIENT WITH STATUS EPILEPTICUS

1. Confirm the diagnosis.

   Diagnose status epilepticus by observing continued seizure activity or one additional seizure.

2. Establish/maintain airway, assist breathing, if required.
   - Position the head and jaw of the patient to promote drainage of secretions.
   - If required, clear the airway by suctioning and ensure its patency.
   - If possible without undue force, insert an oral airway.
   - Administer oxygen either by nasal cannula or mask.

- Maintain a low threshold for intubation and initiation of ventilatory support, as respiratory compromise can result either from continued seizure activity, pulmonary edema, the drugs used, or from aspiration.
- Assume these patients to be having a full stomach. Use rapid sequence technique with preoxygenation with 100% oxygen and apply cricoid pressure for intubation. Use short acting neuromuscular blocking agent (e.g. vecuronium), whenever required. Perform oro-tracheal intubation.
- Administering an antiepileptic drug is top priority, because managing the airway and assisting respiration are much easier after the convulsion has stopped.

3. **Establish an IV line, draw venous samples, and initiate monitoring. Assess oxygenation with a pulse oximeter.**

   Draw venous samples for blood sugar, serum electrolytes, urea, creatinine, liver function tests, calcium, magnesium, complete blood count and antiepileptic drug levels (if facility exists). Use IV fluid without glucose, as glucose is not compatible with phenytoin. Consider other investigations, as soon as the patient is stable. These include ECG, ABG, X-ray chest, X-ray cervical spine and head (if indicated), coagulation profile and blood cultures. CT scan of the head and CSF examination should be considered, whenever indicated.

4. **Administer 50 mL of 50% glucose. In children, use 10% glucose in a dose of 5 mL/ kg.**

   There is some evidence that glucose, given to a normoglycaemic person, will worsen or intensify the status. Therefore, sugar should only be given if there is a reason for suspecting hypoglycaemia.

5. **Consider thiamine 100 mg IV and magnesium 1-2 g IV.**

   In a patient with history of alcoholism or of poor nutrition (or who is malnourished), thiamine and magnesium should be administered. This is especially important if intravenous glucose is to be given, as glucose infusions can precipitate Wernicke's encephalopathy in susceptible individuals.

6. **Administer lorazepam IV up to 0.1 mg/kg at the rate of 2 mg/min (maximum dose 8 mg), in children 0.1 mg/kg.**
   OR
   Diazepam IV 5 mg every 5 minutes up to 20 mg (IV infusion 3 mg/kg/24 hr).
   In children: 0.25-0.50 mg/kg at less than 2-5 mg/min (IV infusion: 200-300 mg/ kg/24 hr).

   Lorazepam is the drug of choice in the early stages of the status. A single intravenous injection is highly effective, has an onset of action in 3 minutes (2 minutes with diazepam), with a longer duration of action of 12-24 hours (15-30 minutes with diazepam), a smaller risk of cardiorespiratory depression than diazepam, and little risk of drug accumulation. Lorazepam is a stable compound which is not likely to precipitate in solution, and is relatively unaffected by hepatic or renal disease. Lorazepam is also more effective than phenytoin or phenobarbital as the initial drug. The main disadvantage of lorazepam is a stronger tendency for tolerance to develop, the drug being usually effective for about 12-24 hours only.

7. Administer phenytoin IV 15-18 mg/kg diluted in normal saline at a rate less than 50 mg/min. In children: 18-20 mg/kg is administered at a rate less than 25 mg/min. Monitor ECG and blood pressure.
   - Phenytoin should not be mixed with any glucose-containing IV fluid and should not be given IM due to erratic absorption. Due to myocardial depression and the effects of the diluent, ethylene glycol, phenytoin should be infused at a rate not greater than 50 mg/min in adults and a rate of 25 mg/min is safer in elderly and in children. It has been suggested to infuse phenytoin slowly (less than 50 mg/min) if lorazepam is successful in stopping the seizures, and infuse phenytoin rapidly (less than 150 mg/min), if lorazepam is unsuccessful in stopping the seizures.
   - Renal or hepatic diseases do not affect the loading dose. Phenytoin is contraindicated in the presence of second-or third degree AV block, in myocardial infarction and congestive heart failure.

8. If status persists, give an additional dose of 5-10 mg/kg phenotoin IV
9. If still not controlled, give phenobarbital IV 10-20 mg/kg at 50-75 mg/min. The maintenance dose is 1-4 mg/kg/24 hr.
   In children: 15-20 mg/kg is given at a rate less than 100 mg/min, maintenance dose being 3-4 mg/kg/24 hr. Monitor end-tidal CO_2, SpO_2, and ECG.
   When phenobarbital is given after a benzodiazepine, the risk of apnea or hypopnea is high, and assisted ventilation may be required.

10. Give additional dose of phenobarbital 5-10 mg/kg IV, if required.
11. If status persists, add thiopentone 100-250 mg IV bolus over 20 seconds with further 50 mg boluses every 2-3 minutes until seizures are controlled, followed by a continuous IV infusion to maintain a burst suppression pattern on the EEG (usually 3-5 mg/kg/hr). SLOWLY withdraw, 12 hours after the last seizure.
   OR
   Midazolam 0.2 mg/kg slow IV, at a rate not exceeding 4 mg/min, can be repeated once after every 15 minutes, and then 0.05-0.4 mg/kg/hr is given as an infusion.
   OR
   Propofol 1-2 mg/kg IV bolus, repeated if necessary, and then followed by continuous infusion of 5-10 mg/kg/hr initially, later reducing to 1-3 mg/kg/hr. When seizures have been controlled for 12 hours, slowly taper the infusion over the next 12 hours.
   - In most patients, if seizures continue for more than 60 minutes inspite of the therapy outlined above, full anaesthesia is required. In some emergency situations (e.g. postoperative states, severe or complicated convulsive status, patients already in ICU), patient should be anaesthetized early.
   - Depth of anesthesia should be such that all clinical and EEG epileptic activity is abolished (often requiring sedation to the point of burst suppression on the EEG). Monitor cerebral activity either with EEG or a cerebral function monitor (if facility is available).
   - Admit the patient in ICU, if not already done so. Place CVP and arterial catheters. Ventilate the patient. Monitor blood pressure, heart rate and

ECG. Use IV fluids and dopamine to treat hypotension (if it occurs).

- Thiopentone has been used for long in the treatment of SE. Its disadvantages, however, include profound hypotension (requiring inotropes) and a tendency to accumulate. Recovery may be delayed after a prolonged therapy.

12. Monitor the patient continuously.
    - Pulse, blood pressure, CVP.
    - Temperature
    - ECG, SpO_2.
    - Input-output record.
    - Arterial blood gases.
    - EEG/cerebral function monitor (whenever facility is available).
        - During the first 30-45 minutes, status epilepticus is usually associated with hypertension. Later on, the compensatory physiological mechanisms begin to fail if seizure activity continues. Hypotension develops because of seizure related autonomic and cardiopulmonary changes and due to drug therapy. In the terminal stages, the fall in blood pressure may be severe. At this time cerebral autoregulation breaks down progressively, and thus cerebral blood flow becomes increasingly dependent on the systemic blood pressure. At the same time, the metabolic demands of the epileptic cerebral tissue are high, and if not met, can result in ischaemic damage. Therefore, systolic blood pressure should be maintained at normal or high-normal levels during prolonged status by using vasopressors, if necessary.
        - Cardiac dysrhythmias are common in prolonged status, and are associated with a high mortality. ECG monitoring should be continued for at least 12-24 hours after the status epilepticus has been controlled.
        - Hyperthermia, which results primarily from an increased motor activity, should be treated promptly with passive cooling and antipyretics, as it may contribute to brain damage.
        - Overhydration should be avoided, as it can exacerbate cerebral edema, a complication seen in the later stages of status epilepticus. If there is no evidence of shock or hypotension in the acute phase, infuse isotonic fluids at the rate of 2-3mL/kg/hr. Use CVP and input-output record as guides.
        - All patients in status epilepticus develop acidosis, which usually resolves promptly when SE terminates. In severe acidosis, however, bicarbonate infusion should be given.
        - Rhabdomyolysis from prolonged seizures can give rise to myoglobinuria, which may cause acute tubular necrosis and renal failure. Optimum hydration, forced diuresis and urinary alkalinization with bicarbonate, can prevent renal failure. Neuromuscular blockade arrests the rhabdomyolysis in cases of refractory SE.
        - Steroids and osmotic agents (e.g. mannitol) **may be** used to treat the cerebral edema that results from prolonged SE, especially in children, but their efficacy has not been established.

13. Identify and treat the precipitating factor, if any.

History taking, physical examination and investigations are helpful in finding the possible cause of SE. Antibiotics should be used whenever indicated.

References

1. Aminoff MJ, Simon RP. Status epilepticus: causes, clinical features and consequences in 98 patients. Am J Med 1980; 69:657-666.
2. Bleck TP. Convulsive disorders: Status epilepticus. Clin Neuropharmacol 1991;14(3):191.
3. Browne TR, Mikati MA. Status epilepticus. In: Roper AH, ed. Neurological and neurosurgical intensive care, 3rd ed. New York: Raven Press, 1993:383-410.
4. Igartua J, Silver P, Maytal J, Sagy M. Midazolam coma for refractory status epilepticus in children. Crit Care Med 1999; 27:1982-1985.
5. Lothman E: The biochemical basis and pathophysiology of status epilepticus. Neurology 1990; 40 (suppl 2): 13.
6. Lowenstein DH, Alldredge BK. Status epilepticus. N Engl J Med 1998; 338:970-976.
7. Treatment of convulsive status epilepticus: recommendations of the Epilepsy Foundation of America's Working Group on Status Epilepticus. JAMA 1993; 270:854 859.
8. Treiman DM, Meyers PD, Walton NY, et al. A comparison of four treatments for generalized status epilepticus. N Engl J Med 1998; 339:792-798.

Appendices I–XIII

I: ACUTE RESPIRATORY FAILURE (ARF)

Classification

A. Post-operative Respiratory Failure
Causes:
1. Reduced lung volume due to:
   - Elevated diaphragm.
   - Abdominal distension
     (Intestinal paralysis, ileus).
   - Atelectasis.
   - Retention of secretions.
   - Pulmonary edema.
   - Pleural effusion.
   - Pneumothorax.
2. Reduced movement of the diaphragm and chest wall due to:
   - Pain.
   - Central suppression.
   - Abdominal distension.
3. Impediment to coughing:
   - Pain.
   - Central suppression (e.g. sedation).
   - Abdominal distension.
   - Tenacious bronchial secretions.

B. Hypoperfusion States Causing Respiratory Failure
1. Cardiogenic (e.g. myocardial infarction).
2. Hypovolaemic (e.g. haemorrhage, dehydration).
3. Septic (e.g. endotoxaemia, bacteraemia).
   Ventilatory therapy may be indicated in these patients to stabilize gas exchange and to minimize the steal of limited cardiac output by the working respiratory muscles until the hypoperfusion state is corrected.

C. Acute Hypoxaemic Respiratory Failure
- Diseases usually involving the pulmonary component.
- Diseases affecting gas exchange between the alveolus and the pulmonary capillary blood.
- Associated metabolic (lactic) acidosis.

- $PaO_2 < 60mmHg$ or $SpO_2 <90\%$ on $FiO_2 > 0.5$.
- Hypoxaemia predominates ± hypercarbia.

Causes:

1. Shunt (e.g. atelectasis, pulmonary edema, pneumonia, pulmonary embolism).
2. Ventilation/perfusion mismatch or venous admixture;$\dot{V}/\dot{Q}$ ratio above zero but less than 1 (e.g. asthma, COPD).
3. Hypoventilation and high $PaCO_2$ (respiratory arrest).
4. Low FiO_2, low barometric pressure, and toxins (e.g. fire, altitude, CO poisoning).
5. Inadequate diffusion equilibrium (e.g. anaemia, high cardiac output; typically a contributing factor rather than the primary cause).

D. Acute Hypercapnic Respiratory Failure

- Diseases usually involving the extra-pulmonary component.
- Impaired alveolar ventilation.
- Associated respiratory acidosis.
- $PaCO_2 > 55mmHg$ with acidosis or a sudden rise in $PaCO_2$ from baseline with acidosis.
- Hypercapnia predominates ± hypoxaemia.

Causes:

1. Work capacity overwhelmed by increased workload from:
   (a) Low compliance (e.g. ARDS, chest burns, pleural effusion, obesity, pneumonia).
   (b) High resistance (e.g. asthma, COPD, airway tumour or obstruction).
2. Increased CO_2 production in the presence of limited capacity for work (e.g. diet, COPD).
3. Increased dead space ($\dot{V}/\dot{Q}$ ratio > 1) requiring increased minute ventilation in the presence of limited capacity for work (e.g. emphysema).
4. Work capacity decreased.
   (a) Decreased central drive (e.g. drug overdose, central hypoventilation syndrome).
   (b) Neuromuscular disease (e.g. myasthenia gravis, Guillain-Barre syndrome).
   (c) Mechanical disadvantage (e.g. hyperinflation, auto PEEP).
   (d) Atrophy (e.g. malnutrition, long-term paralysis, and corticosteroids).
   (e) Metabolic disturbances (e.g. acidosis, decreased oxygen delivery).
   (f) Exhaustion.

Indications for Initiating Mechanical Ventilation in ARF

1. Rapidly worsening physiologic variables: hypotension, tachycardia, tachypnoea, hypoxaemia, hypercarbia and acidosis.

2. Impending fatigue of the respiratory muscles.
   (a) Presence of severe dyspnoea & diaphoresis.
   (b) Prominent use of accessory muscles.
   (c) Paradoxic movement of the abdomen.
   (d) Upward trends in respiratory rate.
   (e) Upward trends in arterial carbon-dioxide tension.
3. Inability to protect airway and/or expectorate secretions.
4. Evidence of compromised cardiac function.
5. Increasing confusion, restlessness, and/or exhausion.

Objectives of Mechanical Ventilation in ARF

1. To improve pulmonary gas exchange.
   (a) Reverse hypoxaemia.
   (b) Relieve acute respiratory acidosis.
2. To correct incomplete lung inflation.
   (a) Increase lung volume.
       (i) Prevent and reverse atelectasis.
       (ii) Improve lung compliance.
   (b) Prevent further lung injury.
3. To permit lung and airway healing.
4. To improve cardiac function:
   By reducing myocardial oxygen demand.
5. To relieve respiratory distress.
       (a) Decrease oxygen cost of breathing.
       (b) Reverse respiratory muscle fatigue.

While the patient is on mechanical ventilation, it is important to avoid iatrogenic injury caused by:
   (a) Complications of endotracheal tube.
   (b) Complications of positive pressure ventilation.
       (i) Barotrauma.
       (ii) Volutrauma.
       (iii) Reduced cardiac output.
       (iv) Oxygen toxicity.
       (v) Ventilator-associated pneumonia.

References

1. Davidson AC, Treacher DF. Respiratory failure: new horizons, new challenges. In: Davidson C, Treacher D (eds). Respiratory Critical Care. London: Arnold, 2002, pp 278-293.
2. Ponte J. Assisted ventilation: 2 Indications for mechanical ventilation. Thorax 1990; 45:885-890.
3. Slutsky AS. Mechanical ventilation. American College of Chest-Physicians' Consensus Conference. Chest 1993; 104:1833-1859.
4. Tobin MJ. Mechanical ventilation. N Engl J Med 1994;300:1056-1061

II: CONVERSION FACTORS FOR IMPORTANT MINERALS

1 mEq Na = 1 mmol Na = 23 mg Na
1 g Na = 43 mEq Na = 43 mmol Na
1 mEq K = 1 mmol K = 39 mg K
1 g K = 26mEq K = 26 mmol K
1 mEq Cl = 1 mmol Cl = 35 mg Cl
1 g Cl = 29 mEq Cl = 29 mmol Cl
1 mEq Mg = 0.5 mmol Mg = 12 mg Mg
1g Mg = 82 mEq Mg = 41 mmol Mg
1 mEq Ca = 0.5 mmol Ca = 20 mg Ca
1 g Ca = 50 mEq Ca = 25 mmol Ca
1 mmol P = 2 mEq HPO_3 = 31 mg P

III: MINERAL CONTENT IN VARIOUS COMPOUNDS AND SOLUTIONS

1 g NaCl = 393 mg Na = 17 mEq Na
1 g $NaHCO_3$ = 273 mg Na = 12 mEq Na
1 g $MgSO_4$. $7H_2O$ = 99 mg Mg = 8.1 mEq Mg
1 g calcium gluconate = 93 mg Ca = 4.6 mEq Ca
1 g KCl = 524 mg K = 13 mEqK
50 mL of 7.5% $NaHCO_3$ = 1 g Na = 44 mEq Na
1000 mL saline solution = 9 g NaCl = 3.5 g Na = 154 mEq Na
1000 mL lactated Ringer's solution = 3 g Na = 130 mEq Na

IV: INTRAVENOUS ELECTROLYTE SOLUTIONS (mmol/L)

	Na^+	K^+	$HCO3^-$	Cl^-	Ca^{++}	Dextrose mg/ml
Normal saline	150	–	–	150	–	–
Dextrose saline (0.18% saline +4% dextrose)	30			30	–	40
5% Dextrose.	–	–	–	–	–	50
Ringer's lactate solution	131	5	29 (as lactate)	111	2	–

V: SUGGESTED GUIDELINES FOR ADMINISTRATION OF ELECTROLYTE SOLUTIONS

Electrolyte

(a) Sodium (chloride)
(b) Calcium (chloride, gluconate)

Administration guidelines

(a) Sodium. Hypertonic saline (3%) may be given for severe hyponatraemia (<120 mEq/L) when the patient is symptomatic. The amount of hypertonic saline solution needed can be calculated by the following formula: mEq Na=(0.60) (body weight in kg) (125 – Na). Discontinue infusion when serum Na reaches 120-125 mEq/L and begin water restriction.
3% hypertonic saline has a sodium concentration of 513 mEq/L.

(b) Calcium. Administer slowly (no faster than 50 mg/min for $CaCl_2$; 100 mg/min for Ca gluconate) into a central line (in an emergent situation, may be given into a peripheral line if no central access is available).
May be administered by continuous infusion via peripheral intravenous line. Maximum concentration should not exceed 20 mg/ml.
Administer boluses in a dextrose or saline solution with no additives. Calcium is incompatible with many medications. Boluses are not administered with parenteral nutrition solutions.

Monitoring

(a) Sodium. Monitor serum sodium frequently. Administer through large vein. The serum sodium concentration should be raised by no more than 10 mEq/L in the first 24 hours, and by no more than 18 mEq/L in the first 48 hours (i.e. at a rate of approximately 0.5 mEq/L per hour).
Maximum rate: 1 mEq/kg/hr.

(b) Calcium. Monitor intravenous site closely. Necrosis and sloughing will occur with extravasation.
Monitor patients receiving digoxin and calcium supplements closely because elevated calcium levels precipitate digoxin-related arrhythmias.
(Monitor for bradycardia, hypotension, and cardiac arrhythmias.)

VI: ELECTROLYTE CONTENT OF GASTROINTESTINAL SECRETIONS

Type of secretion	Volume/24hr (mL)	Na (m Eq/L)	Cl (m Eq/L)	K (m Eq/L)	HCO$_3$ (m Eq/L)	Mg (m Eq/L)
Salivary	1500	60	15	20	50	0.6
Stomach	2500	60	90	10	0	0.1-3.4
Pancreatic fistula	>1000	140 (135-155)	75 (60-100)	5 (4-6)	80 (70-90)	0.2-0.7
Bile	600	145 (135-155)	100 (80-110)	5 (4-6)	45 (35-50)	0.2-3.0
Mid-jejunum	3000	105 (70-125)	100 (70-125)	5 (3.5-6.5)	45	—
Ileostomy	—	120 (90-140)	105 (60-125)	5 (4-10)	20 (15-50)	—
Diarrhoea	—	25-50	20-40	35-60	35–45	0.9-13.9

References

1. Cerra F. Manual of Critical Care. St. Louis: Mosby-Year Book; 1987.
2. Thoren L. The magnesium content of fluids lost from the gastrointestinal tract. Acta Chir Scand 1963; 306(suppl):13-16.

VII: NORMAL RANGES FOR BLOOD GAS ANALYSIS

Measure	Normal range
pH	7.36-7.44
PaO$_2$	Over 90 mmHg on room air
PaCO$_2$	35-45 mmHg
Actual HCO$_3$	21-28 mmol/L
Standard HCO$_3$	21-27 mmol/L
Base excess	± 2 mmol/L

Formula to adjust PaO$_2$ for age:

$$PO_2 = 100.1 - 0.325 \, (age)$$

Reference

Knudson RJ. How age affects the normal lung. J Respir Dis 1981;2:74-84.

VIII: GLASGOW COMA SCALE

			Score
Best eye opening response	Open	- Spontaneously - To verbal command - To pain	4 3 2
	Closed	- No response	1
Best motor response	To verbal command	- Obeys	6
	To painful stimulus	- Localizes - Flexion – withdrawal - Abnormal flexion (decorticate) - Extension - No response	5 4 3 2 1
Best verbal response		- Oriented and converses - Disoriented and converses - Inappropriate words - Incomprehensible sounds - No response	5 4 3 2 1

- Localizes means localizing to painful stimuli. It is best tested by a painful stimulus on the supraorbital ridge producing flexion/abduction of upper limbs.
- Abnormal flexion means flexion at elbow and wrist, pronation of forearm and adduction of thumb into palm of hand.
- Extension means extension at elbow, pronation of forearm and flexion of wrist. Occasionally supination of the forearm is present.
- Severe head injury (GCS $\leq$ 8) has a mortality of approximately 40%.
- Moderate head injury (GCS 9-12) has a mortality of approximately 4%.
- Minor head injury (GCS 13-15) has a mortality of approximately 0.4%.
- The prognostic value of the GCS is greatest in the immediate post injury phase. Obtain an initial GCS score within 1 to 2 hrs after injury. Avoid scoring until hypotension or hypoxia have been stabilized. Use an ocular score of 1 for patients with severe periorbital swelling.

References

- Lyle DM, Pierce JP, Freeman EA, et al. Clinical course and outcome of severe head injury in Australia. J. Neurosury. 1986; 65:15-18.
- Teasdale G and Jennet B. Assessment of coma and impaired conciousness, a practical scale. Lancet 1974;ii: 81-83.

IX: LUNG INJURY SCORE

Component	Value
• Chest roentgenogram score	
- No alveolar consolidation	0
- Alveolar consolidation confined to 1 quadrant	1
- Alveolar consolidation confined to 2 quadrants	2
- Alveolar consolidation confined to 3 quadrants	3
- Alveolar consolidation in all 4 quadrants	4
• Hypoxaemia score	
- PaO_2/FiO_2 >300	0
225-299	1
175-224	2
100-174	3
< 100	4
• PEEP score (during mechanical ventilation)	
- PEEP $\leq$ 5cm H_2O	0
6-8cm H_2O	1
9-11cm H_2O	2
12-14cm H_2O	3
$\geq$ 15 cm H_2O	4

The final value is obtained by dividing the aggregate sum by the number of components that were used.

	Score
No lung injury	0
Mild to moderate lung injury 0.1-2.5	
Severe lung injury (ARDS)	> 2.5

X: CHECKLIST OF THE CRITERIA FOR DIAGNOSIS OF BRAIN-STEM DEATH

We, the following members of the Board of medical experts after careful personal examination hereby certify that Mr/Mrs/Ms ....
aged about ....
son of / wife of / daughter of ....
resident of ....
is dead on account of permanent and irreversible cessation of all functions of the brain-stem. The tests carried out by us and the findings therein are recorded in the brain-stem death Certificate annexed hereto.

Dated:_______________________   Signature...

1. R.M.P., Incharge of the Hospital in which brain-stem death has occurred.

2. R.M.P., nominated from the panel of names approved by the Appropriate Authority.

3. Neurologist/Neuro-Surgeon nominated from the panel of names approved by the Appropriate Authority.

4. R.M.P. treating the aforesaid deceased person

Brain-Stem Death Certificate

(A) PATIENT DETAILS:

   1. Name of the patient   Mr/Mrs/Ms

         ________________________   ________________________

        S.O./W.O./D.O.   Mr

         ____

         Sex________________Age ________________

   2. Home address

   3. Hospital number

   4. Name and address of next of kin or person responsible for the patient (if none exists, this must be specified)

5. Has the patient or next of kin agreed to any transplant?

____

____

____

6. Is this a Police Case?

                           Yes________________No________________

(B) PRE-CONDITIONS:

1. Diagnosis: Did the patient suffer from any illness or accident that led to irreversible brain damage? Specify details_______________________________

____

    Date and time of accident/onset of illness _______________________

    Date and onset of non-responsive coma _______________________

2. Findings of Board of Medical Experts:

   (1) The following reversible causes of coma have been excluded:

      ntoxication (Alcohol)

      Depressant Drugs

      Relaxants (Neuromuscular blocking agents)

	First Medical Examination		Second Medical Examination	
	1st	2nd	1st	2nd
Primary hypothermia				
Hypovolaemic shock				
Metabolic or endocrine disorders				
Tests for absence of brain-stem functions				

   (2) Coma

   (3) Cessation of spontaneous breathing

   (4) Pupillary size

   (5) Pupillary light reflexes

   (6) Doll's head eye movements

   (7) Corneal reflexes (Both sizes)

   (8) Motor respons in any cranial nerve distribution; any responses to stimulation of face, limb or trunk.

   (9) Gag reflex

 (10) Cough (Tracheal)

 (11) Eye movements on caloric testing bilaterally.

 (12) Apnoea tests as specified.

 (13) Were any respiratory movement seen?

____

Date and time of first testing: _______________________

Date and time of second testing: _______________________

This is to certify that the patient has been carefully examined twice after an interval of about six hours and on the basis of findings recorded above.

Mr/Mrs/Ms ________________________ is declared brain-stem dead

1. Medical Administration Incharge of the hospital   2. Authorised specialist

3. Neuroligst/Neuro-Surgeon   4. Medical Officer treating the patient

NB   I. The minimum time interval between the first testing and second testing will be six hours.
II.No.2 and No.3 will be co-opted by the Administrator Incharge of the hospital from the Panel of experts approved by the appropriate authority.

References

1. Pande GK, Patraik PK, Gupta S, Sahni P. Brain Death and organ transplantation in India. Proceedings of a workshop. Nail Med J India 1990: 59-61.
2. The Gazethe of India: Extraordinary. Part II - Sec. 3(U). Ministry of Health and Family Welfare. 20th Oct, 1995.

XI: VENTILATION MONITORING CHART

Name :   **Date:**
MRD No. :   **DOD:**

Ventilatory parameters											
Time											
Mode of ventilation											
FiO_2 (%)											
Tidal volume (ml)											
Frequency (/min)											
I:E ratio											
Minute volume (L)											
P.I.F.R. (L/min)											
Insp. Pause (sec)											
P.S.V. (cm H_2O)											
PEEP/CPAP (cm H_2O)											
Trigger sens											
Flow (L/min)											
Pressure (cmH$_2$O)											
Pr. Alarm limit											
High (cm H_2O)											
Low (cm H_2O)											
Patient Parameters											
Pt. Vent. Syn.											
Tidal vol. *Spont. (ml)*											
Control (ml)											
Frequency *Spont. (/min)*											
Control (/min)											
Airway Pr.											
Peak (cm H_2O)											
Plateau (cm H_2O)											
Mean (cmH$_2$O)											
Compliance											
Auto PEEP											
CHECK											
ETT size											
ETT cuff pressure											
Vent. tubing water											
Humidifier temp (°C)											
Chest tube											

XII: INVESTIGATIONS CHART

Name :   **Age:**   **MRD No. :**

Date							
Haemoglobin							
TLC							
DLC							
Platelet Count							
Blood Sugar							
Blood Urea							
Serum creatinine							
Sodium							
Potassium							
Calcium							
Magnesium							
Phosphorous							
Chloride							
Serum Bilirubin							
Serum Protein *Total*							
Albumin							
Globulin							
SGOT							
SGPT							
Alkaline phosphatase							
Urine *Glucose*							
Albumin							
Microscopy							
E.C.G.							
X-ray chest							
Coagulation profile							
CT/ Ultrasound							
CSF *Cytology*							
Biochemistry							
Others							

Name : **Age :** **MRD No. :**

Culture Report

Date							
TRACHEA							
Sensitivity							
Resistance							
BLOOD							
Sensitivity							
Resistance							
URINE							
Sensitivity							
Resistance							
WOUND / PUS							
Sensitivity							
Resistance							

Change of ETT / Catheters

Date						
I/V site						
ETT						
Tracheostomy						
CVP line						
Foleys catheter						
Ryles tube						
Epidural Catheter						

XIII: DAILY PROGRESS CHART

Name: Age :   M/F :   Date :   Day of ICU stay :   Diagnosis :   Faculty :

Wt. :   MRD No.:   Unit/Wd.:   Bed :   N Staff : M   E   N   Resident : M :
    N :

TIME									INTAKE (ML)		OUTPUT (ML)			TREATMENT
LEVEL OF CONSC.										8am-8pm	8pm-8am		8am-8pm	8pm-8am
Pupils									IV		Urine			
Pulse (/min)									NG		NG			
BP: S/D (mmHg)									Oral		Drain			
RR (/min)									12hrs		12hrs			
SpO$_2$ (%)									24hrs Total		24hrs Total			
ETCO$_2$ (mmHg)									Time			Vol.		
CVP (cm H$_2$O)														
PCWP (mm Hg)														
Chest wall mov.														
Air entry														
Secretions *Colour*														
Character														
Suction Freq.														
MIF (cm H$_2$O)														
Vital capacity (L)														
Inotropes (µg/kg/mt) *Dopamine*														
Dobutamine														
Noradrenaline														
Abdomen *BS*														
Distension														
Wound														
MOTOR POWER *RUL*														
LUL														
RLL														
LLL														
Bed sores														
Temperature (°C)														
Intake (ml)														
Urine Output (ml)														
RTA (ml)														
Stool														

PLAN

BS - Bowel sounds   RLL - Right lower limb
RUL - Right upper limb   LLL - Left lower limb
LUL - Left upper limb   RTA - Ryle's tube aspirate

Index